Communication Disability in Aging:

From Prevention to Intervention

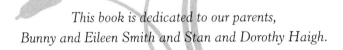

This book is dedicated to our parents,
Bunny and Eileen Smith and Stan and Dorothy Haigh.

Communication Disability in Aging:
From Prevention to Intervention

Linda E. Worrall, BSpThy, PhD
Associate Professor
Communication Disability in Ageing Research Unit and the
Australasian Center on Ageing
The University of Queensland
Australia

Louise M. Hickson, BSpThy (Hons), MAud, PhD
Associate Professor
Communication Disability in Ageing Research Unit
The University of Queensland
Australia

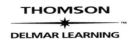
THOMSON
™
DELMAR LEARNING

Australia Canada Mexico Singapore Spain United Kingdom United States

THOMSON

DELMAR LEARNING

Communication Disability in Aging: From Prevention to Intervention
by Linda E. Worrall and Louise M. Hickson

Executive Director **Health Care Business Unit:** William Brottmiller	**Developmental Editor:** Juliet Byington	**Editorial Assistant:** Chris Manion
	Executive Marketing Manager: Dawn F. Gerrain	**Production Editor:** James Zayicek
Executive Editor: Cathy L. Esperti	**Channel Manager:** Jennifer McAvey	

For permission to use material from this text or product, contact us by
Tel   (800) 730-2214
Fax   (800) 730-2215
www.thomsonrights.com

Library of Congress Cataloging-in-Publication Data

Worrall, Linda.
   Communication disability in aging/Linda E. Worrall, Louise M. Hickson.
     p. cm.
   Includes index.
   ISBN 0-7693-0015-4
   1. Communicative disorders in old age. I. Hickson, Louise M. II. Title.

RC429.W67 2003
618.97'6855--dc21

                                                    2002031512

NOTICE TO THE READER

Contents

PREFACE

$\mathcal{M}$ost speech-language pathologists and audiologists are aware that their nation's population is aging. In preparation for this, many educational institutions are incorporating gerontology into their curriculum. This text is designed to fill the need for a comprehensive communication disability in aging text for students of audiology and speech-language pathology. Practicing clinicians will also find new information in this text. Although other worthwhile books have been written on this topic, they fail to ignite the interest of readers in the field of gerontology—arguably not the most glamorous area of our professions. For this reason, we have taken a positive view of aging because we consider that the traditional deficit approach reinforces the stereotype of frail and dependent older people. Positive experiences of older people have been found to be the most significant determinants to health professionals' desire to work with the older population. Certainly, if the professions of speech-language pathology and audiology are going to respond to the challenge of global population aging, there is an urgent need to both educate and enthuse future generations of clinicians about the unique field of gerontological speech-language pathology and audiology.

In addition to taking a positive view of aging, we have also placed much emphasis on functional approaches to gerontology. Functional approaches focus on the effects of an impairment on the everyday lives of older people. In the past, functional communication approaches had been largely restricted to intervention for chronic disabilities such as aphasia, whereas now it has application to the broader domain of gerontological audiology and speech-language pathology. A continuum of care approach has also been taken so that preventive issues as well as intervention issues are addressed. With an increasing interest in healthy aging by many older people and policy makers around the world, speech-language pathology and audiology must market the notion of healthy communication in older people.

Modern day gerontological audiology and speech-language pathology is based on a number of premises that are reflected in this text. They include the following:

1. Health and disease form a continuum.
2. A broad holistic approach is required so that the person, the environment, and the community are as important as the communication impairment.
3. Both deficit-oriented and anti-agist models of communication must be included in speech-language pathology and audiology practice.
4. Prevention is better than cure.
5. Gerontological audiology and speech-language pathology is practiced differently in different settings, that is, in the hospital/rehabilitation unit, the community, and the residential care facility for the aged.
6. Policy issues are as important as theory and practice issues in gerontological speech-language pathology and audiology.

By taking a holistic approach to gerontological speech-language pathology and audiology, we have encountered areas that have not been well researched or explored in the literature. This particularly holds true for the activity, participation, and quality of life dimensions of communication disability in aging. We have, therefore, used much of our own research and clinical material to support these areas. We recognize the limitations to using this material, but consider that there are many benefits to sharing this knowledge with novice and experienced clinicians alike.

ORGANIZATION OF THE TEXT

The text is divided into four sections. Section I is an introduction to some of the fundamental issues in communication disability in aging. Chapter 1 reviews the changing demographics that have made gerontology a topic of interest for many health professionals. It also emphasizes the high prevalence of communication changes in older people and the importance of communication to the aging process and quality of life in older adults. Chapter 2 introduces the theoretical underpinnings of communication disability in aging, including the World Health Organization's (WHO) International Classification of Functioning, Disability and Health (2001) that forms the foundation of the scope of practice for gerontological audiology and speech-language pathology described in the text. Chapter 3 presents three models of practice for working with older people and argues the case for an integrated model of best practice.

Section II of the text uses the WHO model to describe the communication changes that occur with increasing age. This section also focuses on assessment, with many assessments being reprinted. Chapter 4 reviews the impairments that affect communication. Chapter 5 defines the effect of such impairments by describing the everyday communicative activities of older people with and without specific communication disorders. Chapter 6 describes the effect of communication changes on participation and quality of life in older people.

Section III outlines approaches to practice in three different gerontological settings. Chapter 7 focuses on the community setting and promotes a preventive or health promotion role for audiologists and speech-language pathologists. Chapter 8 discusses the hospital setting and the management of older people with specific communication disabilities. A socioenvironmental approach is also advocated in which speech-language pathologists and audiologists take responsibility for improving the access of older people to communication in the hospital. This approach will contribute to making hospitals more age-friendly. In Chapter 9, the effect of the restricted communication environment in residential care facilities for the aged is discussed in some detail. Again, audiologists and speech-language pathologists are increasingly aware of the benefits of interventions aimed at the environment and again, an integrated approach is advocated that incorporates the dimensions of the WHO model.

Chapter 10 summarizes the information in each of the three sections and discusses the theoretical, practice, and policy issues emerging from these. The speech-language pathology and audiology clinicians of the future must overcome many obstacles to provide a relevant, efficient, and effective service to older people. This concluding chapter stresses the importance of creating an enthusiastic, knowledgeable, and skilled workforce to meet the needs of an aging population.

Each chapter begins with an abstract. Most chapters contain case studies that illustrate the concepts discussed. At the end of each chapter, there is a key point summary, a list of class activities to assist learning, a recommended reading list, and references. Appendixes for Chapters 5, 6, and 7 contain representative and illustrative forms and tools to demonstrate the types of resources available for use once speech-language pathologists and audiologists begin working with older individuals with communication disabilites.

HOW TO USE THIS TEXT

It is recognized that various audiology and speech-language pathology curricula have differing amounts of time dedicated to gerontological issues. For this reason, if time is limited, all three chapters in Section I can be used separately to overview the issues in the area, facilitate understanding of the major theories that underlie the practice, and appreciate the different models of service delivery that operate in this area. Alternatively, the whole text can be used as the basis of a comprehensive course in gerontological speech-language pathology and audiology.

ABOUT THE AUTHORS

Both authors are experienced clinicians who have been teaching and researching communication disability in aging for over a decade. Together they formed the Communication Disability in Ageing Research Unit (www.shrs.uq.edu.au/cdaru) within the Department of Speech Pathology and Audiology at The University of Queensland, Brisbane, Australia. This research unit combines the speech-language pathology expertise of Dr. Linda Worrall and the audiology expertise of Dr. Louise Hickson. Numerous publications have evolved from this collaboration, and these publications have earned the authors an international reputation. Both authors have practiced their professions in the United Kingdom as well as in Australia, and Dr. Hickson has also practiced throughout Southeast Asia. Dr. Worrall has also co-edited a book with Dr. Carol Frattali called *Neurogenic Communication Disorders: A Functional Approach.*

ACKNOWLEDGMENTS

Like most books, this text was written with a great deal of support from many people. Tangible support was provided by Madeline Cruice and Jillian Sellars who tracked down authors and publishers around the world to get their permission to use published materials. They also perfected the art of referencing and formatting the text. Invaluable moral support was provided by our friend and "book coach," Suzanne Marshall. We also thank our postgraduate students and research staff in the Communication Disability in Ageing Research Unit (Louise Cahill, Madeline Cruice, Bronwyn Davidson, Jenny Egan, Brigette Larkins, Chris Lind, Robyn McCooey, Dorothea Schmidt, and Edwin Yiu) who have let us use some of their ideas and results so generously. Thank you also to Juliet Byington from Delmar Learning who coaxed us through the last few chapters.

Our deepest gratitude must also go to our families who have continued to support our need to write this text. To Simon, Elizabeth, Jennifer, Victoria, Sheila, and Geoffrey Worrall and Peter, William, Alexander, and Robert Hickson, thank you all for your patience, and we promise not to do it again—for a while.

FEEDBACK

Please send your questions, suggestions, and comments to us at cdaru@uq.edu.au.

Dr. Linda Worrall and Dr. Louise Hickson

Overview

This section begins with a chapter summarizing the relevance of the study of communication disability in aging for speech-language pathologists and audiologists. The topic is important for clinicians because the proportion of older people in society is increasing, communication disability is highly prevalent in the older population, and age-related communication changes can have a significant negative effect on the quality of older people's lives. Chapter 2 contains a detailed discussion of the theories underpinning practice in this area: the World Health Organization's International Classification of Functioning, Disability, and Health (WHO, 2001) framework for considering the effects of aging and health conditions; the health-disease continuum; healthy aging constructs; and Communication Accommodation Theory. In the final chapter in this section (Chapter 3), models of practice for speech-language pathology and audiology with older people are discussed, and best practice in different settings is described.

Chapter 1

Introduction to Aging and Communication

Why learn about communication in aging? It is important for audiologists and speech-language pathologists to study this topic because (a) there is a growing proportion of older people in the population, (b) communication problems are highly prevalent in older people, and (c) communication problems can have serious implications for the quality of life of the older person. This chapter introduces these three major issues in aging and highlights the potentially important role of the speech-language pathologist and audiologist in maintaining quality of life for older people.

Working with older people has not been viewed by audiology and speech-language pathology students as a particularly glamorous or desirable area of practice. Negative views about aging are common in society, and students also hold such views. Students typically list words such as *wrinkled*, *forgetful*, *disabled*, *deaf*, *gray*, and *nursing home* when asked to do a free association with the word *aging*. These stereotypes are agist, meaning there is discrimination or prejudice on the basis of age alone. It is important that speech-language pathologists and audiologists reflect on their perceptions of aging and work to eliminate discrimination in clinical practice.

Because of changing demographic trends, current students of audiology and speech-language pathology will face very different caseloads than previous generations faced. If adequate funding for services is available, older people are likely to make up the majority of caseloads (Shadden & Toner, 1997). Therefore, it is important that gerontological speech-language pathology and audiology be viewed as a specialty area of the professions and be given priority in curricula and professional education programs. This text was written for that purpose: to provide specialty training in gerontology so that the professions of audiology and speech-language pathology can meet the need for services in the coming decades. This chapter introduces the reasons why the study of communication in aging is so critical: the realities of worldwide population aging, the high prevalence of communication problems that occur with age, and the negative effects of those communication problems on the everyday lives of older people.

The Aging Population

Population aging refers to the demographic trend of an increasing proportion of older people within a population. A more everyday term for this phenomenon is to describe a country as *graying*. Population aging is an often-encountered concept, frequently referred to in media reports with negative words such as *crisis*, *burden*, and *problem*. Negative perceptions of population aging arise because of public concern about the potential economic cost of health care and other social services for growing numbers of older people. Moody (2000) also points out that part of the reason for the fear of population aging is that "many of us are locked into images of decline that are based on prejudiced or on outdated impressions of what individual aging entails" (Prologue, p. xxx). The World Health Organization (WHO) (1998) points out that population aging is, in fact, a triumph of social development and public health and that it should be viewed as a challenge rather than a crisis. Global population aging is occurring because of a decrease in fertility rates and an increase in life expectancy. Fewer children are being born, and adults are living longer.

Audiologists and speech-language pathologists who work with older people need to be knowledgeable about population aging. The main reason for them to study demographic trends is to monitor the effect population aging may have on their professions. Questions such as "What effect will population aging have on speech-language pathology and audiology services?" and ultimately "Are we prepared for this change?" are being asked by professionals. The following sections summarize the major issues in population aging.

When Are People Old?

We are all aging, but when does a person become old? Being old is a relative concept. For example, a 10-year-old child's perception of old might be different from a 50-year-old person's perception. Should being old be determined by chronological age (i.e., number of years lived) or biological age (i.e., how the body has aged)? Chronological age and biological age are not the same concept. There is a great deal of variability in the functional abilities of people who are the same chronological age. For this reason, researchers argue that it is more appropriate to consider aging in terms of biological changes rather than years of life. Nevertheless, chronological age is almost always used as a marker for being old, as it is convenient and more straightforward to quantify and apply (Chodzko-Zajko, Ringle, & Vaca, 1995). The age at which someone is classified as being old varies worldwide, but is typically 60 or 65 years in developed countries, with the latter most commonly used. In some developing countries where life expectancy is lower, the definition of old age is also lower (Sen, 1994).

An approach increasingly being applied in gerontological research is to classify older people into subgroups of young-old and old-old, with the cutoff for these groups being 75 or 80 years. Just as it is inappropriate to compare a 30-year-old with a 60-year-old, it is most inappropriate to cluster 60-year-olds and 90-year-olds in the same category (Tinker, 1996). Classification schemes of older adults based on age vary, but a commonly used system classifies the young-old as aged between 65 and 75, the old-old as between 75 and 85, and the very old as 85 years and older (e.g., McCallum & Geiselhart, 1996; Moody, 2000). In terms of the life cycle, the young-old are considered to be in the third age of life, and the old-old are in the fourth age. The first age is childhood when there is a period of dependence, immaturity, and education. The second age is associated with independence, maturity, employment, and responsibility. The third age is associated with retirement from the workforce and personal fulfillment; and the fourth age is an era of final dependence (Tinker, 1996).

What Is the Demographic Trend?

Projecting the growth of populations is crystal ball gazing; however, many scientists have refined techniques for predicting population trends. Information about population statistics change over time, and the reader is directed to Internet sources such as the International Federation on Aging (www.ifa-fiv.org) and WHO (www.who.int) for the most recent statistics. Information about particular countries usually can be obtained from national organizations. Examples in the United States are the Administration on Aging (www.aoa.dhhs.gov), the Census Bureau (www.census.gov), the Federal Interagency Forum on Age-Related Statistics (www.agingstats.gov), and the National Institute on Aging (www.nih.gov/nia); in the United Kingdom, the Center for Policy on Aging (www.cpa.org.uk); and in Australia, the Australian Bureau of Statistics (www.abs.gov.au). Addresses for some specific Web documents are contained in the reference list at the end of the chapter. Figure 1–1 summarizes important statistics used by many of the lead agencies and publications in the study of aging worldwide. Figure 1–2 illustrates how the proportion of older people in the population is growing. The

By 2020, the number of people over 60 years of age will exceed 1,000 million, of whom 700 million will live in developing countries (WHO, 1999).
Average life expectancy of the world's population was 41 years in the 1950s, 62 years in 1990, and is projected to be 70 years in 2020 (WHO, 1998).
Population aging is most rapid in developing countries. The United Nations predicted in 1985 that the total population of the developing world will increase by 45% in 2020, while the older population will increase by 80% (Sen, 1994).
In 1996, the countries with the oldest populations were Italy, Greece, Sweden, Belgium, and Spain. The United Kingdom was 9th–oldest, and the United States was 25th-oldest (International Federation on Aging, 1996).
By 2020, the countries with the oldest populations will be Japan followed by Italy, Greece, and Switzerland (WHO, 1998).
By 2050, 20% of all Americans will be 65 or older (United States Census Bureau, 2000).
In the United States, the number of centenarians nearly doubled in the 1990s, and it is predicted that the centenarian population may reach 834,000 by the middle of the 21st century (United States Census Bureau, 1999).
In the United States, the number of people over 85 years, who are most in need of help, will reach at least 7 million in 2020 and double again when the baby boomers reach 85 years of age in 2040 (National Institute on Aging, 1997).
By 2030, more than 70% of 8-year-olds in the United States will have a living great-grandparent (National Institute on Aging, 1997).

FIGURE 1–1. Statistics on population aging throughout the world.

rates of change are different from country to country; however, the trend is global, with both developed and developing countries showing rapid increases in the next few decades.

There are three important aspects of the demographic trend that have implications for health care service providers. First, because of increases in life expectancy and decreases in disability rates, the most significant proportional increases are occurring for the oldest old-age groups. For example, the proportion of the older population over 85 years in the United States in 1997 was 10%, and this is projected to increase to 20% by 2050 (Administration on Aging, 1998). Second, because women live longer than men, there are more older women than men, particularly in the old-old group (McCallum & Geiselhart, 1996). In 2000 in the United States, almost half of all older women (45%) were widows

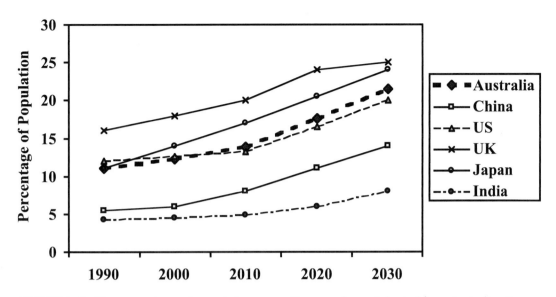

FIGURE 1–2. The percentage of populations over 65 years of age. Adapted from Australian Bureau of Statistics (1996), Tinker (1996), United Nations (1992), and United States Census Bureau (2000).

(Administration on Aging, 2001). Thus, there will be an increasing number of older people requiring audiology and speech-language pathology services, and the majority of clients will be women living alone. It may be necessary, therefore, to give greater consideration in intervention programs to social support and to enhancing opportunities for communication than has been necessary in the past.

Finally, in developed countries, the most rapid growth in the aging population is occurring for minority groups. In Australia, the increase in the percentage of older people who are non-English-speaking immigrants is far greater than the increase in the Australian-born population (McCallum & Gieselhart, 1996). The situation is similar in the United States. Between 1999 and 2030, the white older population in the United States will grow by 81% compared with 131% for the African-American population and 328% for the Hispanic population (Administration on Aging, 2001). This changing mix in the older population will mean that clinicians need to be aware of the cultural and linguistic diversity of their clients.

Health Conditions and Aging

In a discussion of health and aging, it is necessary to differentiate between diseases that occur with age and chronic disability in aging. Aging is not a disease or a disability, but growing older is associated with an increased likelihood of disease, disability, or both. The most common diseases of old age accounting for 75% of deaths in people over 65 years of age in the

United States are heart disease, stroke, and cancer (National Center for Health Statistics, 1995). Other common causes of death in the United States are chronic obstructive pulmonary disease, pneumonia and influenza, diabetes mellitus, accidents, nephritis, Alzheimer's disease, and septicemia. Age-related diseases are particularly relevant to speech-language pathologists and audiologists because some (e.g., stroke, Alzheimer's disease, Parkinson's disease) are associated with communication and swallowing impairments (see Chapter 4).

A chronic disability does not necessarily cause death, but is a health problem that persists for an extended period of time. The three most prevalent chronic conditions of old age are arthritis, hypertension, and hearing impairment (Weinstein, 2000). Vision impairment is also common, a fact that has implications for the management of older people with communication disability. Co-morbidity, or the co-occurrence of one or more chronic disabilities, is a feature of aging. For example, in a study of communication impairments in residents of care facilities for the aged, Worrall, Hickson, and Dodd (1993) reported that 70% of residents had more than one communication impairment (see Chapter 9).

In the future, WHO expects that the increase in life expectancy will result in an epidemic of chronic disabilities (WHO, 1999). Developing countries that are adopting unhealthy Western lifestyle habits such as smoking, sedentary living, and diets high in fat and sugar are likely to be particularly affected. Frequently, the emphasis of health promotion programs is on the prevention of diseases; however, it could also be argued that a focus on the prevention of chronic disabilities of aging is appropriate. Many older people may lose their independence and quality of life because of unrecognized and untreated chronic disabilities such as visual impairment, hearing impairment, cognitive impairment, and physical immobility.

Prevalence of Communication Changes With Age

The importance of population aging for clinicians is that communication changes with age. This occurs for two reasons: (a) the aging process alone can affect communication, and (b) with aging, there is an increased prevalence of diseases and disabilities that can affect communication. In this book, the term *healthy aging* is used in relation to the normal changes that occur with aging, and the term *pathological aging* refers to changes that occur because of a particular age-related disease or disability.

Many studies have documented changes to communicative abilities in healthy older people who do not have an identifiable disease such as stroke, Parkinson's disease, or Alzheimer's disease. A summary of the impairments in hearing, language, conversational discourse, speech, and voice is shown in Table 1–1, and these impairments are described in considerable detail in Chapter 4. The communication changes that occur with age range

TABLE 1–1

SUMMARY OF COMMUNICATION IMPAIRMENTS ASSOCIATED WITH HEALTHY AGING.

Communication System	Description of Impairment
Hearing	Decreased sensitivity to pure tones Decreased ability to discriminate speech in adverse listening conditions
Language	Decreased speed and ability to retrieve words Decreased ability to comprehend with increased complexity of the message
Conversational discourse	Difficulty understanding complex and lengthy discourse Decreased efficiency and increased ambiguity in expression Increased degree of topic maintenance, decreased cohesion, decreased rate, increased number of words per clause, and overall increase in number of words.
Speech	Decreased respiratory support for speech output Imprecise articulation Slower rate of speech
Voice	Increase in pitch for males Decrease in pitch for females Decreased vocal quality

Note: From Caruso and Max (1997), Cherney (1996), Ripich (1991), Shadden (1988), and Shadden and Toner (1997)

from highly prevalent conditions such as hearing impairment to subtle changes to articulation as a result of dentures, or vocal changes due to the ageing of the vocal folds. The changes that older people report most difficulty with are hearing and word retrieval. Hearing impairment is highly prevalent in older people, with approximately 60–70% (see Hickson & Worrall, 1997, for a review) of older people experiencing hearing impairment. There are no known prevalence statistics for word-retrieval impairment despite it being a common complaint of older people. In summary, healthy older people may have a range of communication-related impairments that generally go undetected and unrecognized in the community.

Many older people are fortunate to live without a serious disease in their later years. However, others experience diseases such as dementia, stroke, heart disease, arthritis, cancer, osteoporosis, or diabetes. These age-related diseases or pathologies are part of the process of pathological aging. Many of these diseases have a significant, and perhaps a sudden, effect on the already declining communication abilities of older persons. Conditions that have a direct effect on communication are dementia, stroke, cancer of the head and neck, traumatic brain injury, and progressive neurological disorders such as Parkinson's disease or amyotrophic lateral sclerosis. The most prevalent disease in older people that has an effect on communication is dementia of the Alzheimer's type (DAT). One in 10 people over 65 years of age in the United States have DAT, and this figure increases to 50% of those over 85 years of age (Hopper & Bayles, 2001). Bryan and Maxim (2002) have emphasized the evidence for communication intervention that maintains communication in people with DAT and has called for speech-language pathologists to be more involved in intervention programs for DAT. Audiologists likewise have a vital role in diagnosis with the DAT population, as it is sometimes difficult to determine the differential effects of DAT from the effects of a hearing impairment.

Speech-language pathologists are often called upon to provide assessment and intervention for older people who have aphasia, dysarthria, apraxia, dysphagia, or aphonia as a result of neurogenic age-related diseases. Neurogenic diseases such as stroke and Parkinson's disease are highly prevalent in the aging population, and communication-related impairments are frequently a sequela of these chronic health conditions. A description of the communication and swallowing impairments associated with all the health conditions that affect communication is contained in Chapter 4.

The nature of acquired neurogenic communication disorders is adequately covered in other texts; however, when such disorders occur in older people there are other factors, specific to aging, that must be considered. To illustrate this scenario, a case study of Mr. Byrne is presented.

Providing a service within a gerontological framework is broader than retaining a discipline-specific perspective. Aged care is always multifaceted and considers not only pre-existing disorders associated with increased age, but also the effect of the multiple disabilities in older people within the context of their own adaptation to the later years of their life. It is, therefore, important for speech-language pathologists and audiologists to understand the theoretical foundations of gerontology. These theories are described in Chapter 2.

Effects of Age-Related Communication Changes

Communication is fundamental to older peoples' quality of life for many reasons (see Figure 1–3). Older people need communication to adapt to change, to maintain friendships, to participate in life, and to learn new things. It is assumed that quality of life depends on communication because it is implicit in many of the core components of quality of life such as participation in relationships, expression of self, and autonomy. Communication dis-

Case Study: Mr. Byrne

Mr. Byrne, a 76-year-old who was diagnosed with Parkinson's disease 2 years ago, has mild naming difficulties and mild dysarthria. When managing this case, two main age-related factors emerge: the multiplicity of his disabilities and his psychological response to aging. Apart from the symptoms of Parkinson's disease (i.e., tremor, fatigue, depression, muscle rigidity), Mr. Byrne also has a mild-to-moderate hearing loss, a loss of mobility, and low vision, despite a cataract being removed. These other conditions are affecting his communication. He, therefore, has a multiplicity of disabilities that not only individually affect his communication, but also interact in a synergistic manner. In addition, Mr. Byrne's psychological reaction to aging has been to adopt an old person persona in which he attributes all decline to the unstoppable effects of old age. When conventional interventions were first offered (i.e., hearing aid fitting and dysarthria treatment), Mr. Byrne refused both forms of intervention. He considered that he was too old to learn new tricks. However, upon Mrs. Byrne's insistence, he attended a session to learn how to speak more clearly. The pacing strategies helped a little, but his hearing impairment made therapy difficult. During the session, he began asking questions about Parkinson's disease. He and his wife decided to attend the local Parkinson's disease support group following a recommendation from the speech-language pathologist. At the meetings, they met another older person who had been successfully fitted with an in-the-ear hearing aid. Mr. Byrne finally overcame his belief that nothing could be done for "old codgers like me" and was successfully fitted with a hearing aid. His improved hearing ability brought him back to speech-language pathology for more dysarthria therapy. He continues to attend the support group meetings and occasionally returns for refresher courses to maintain intelligibility. This case illustrates how the multiplicity of disorders and effects of aging interrelate in the management of older people with communication disabilities.

abilities, therefore, have the potential to adversely affect older people's lives in a number of ways. Social withdrawal, and feelings of isolation, dependence, and depression have all been reported (e.g., Bess, Lichtenstein, Logan, Burger, & Nelson, 1989; Le Dorze & Brassard, 1995). In a study of communication and quality of life in healthy older people and people with aphasia, Cruice (2002) found that older people generally appreciated the importance of communication, but that communication was most highly valued by people who had experienced a loss of communication skills. Healthy older people were more likely to take their communication abilities for granted. Older people with aphasia were acutely aware of the far-reaching effects of communication difficulties on quality of life.

In this text, the effects of communication changes with age are described using the WHO model (2001) or the *International Classification of Functioning, Disability, and Health* (see Chapter 2, Figure 2–1). In this model, the effects of a health condition are described in terms of the effects on body structure and function, activities, and participation. Impairments refer to changes

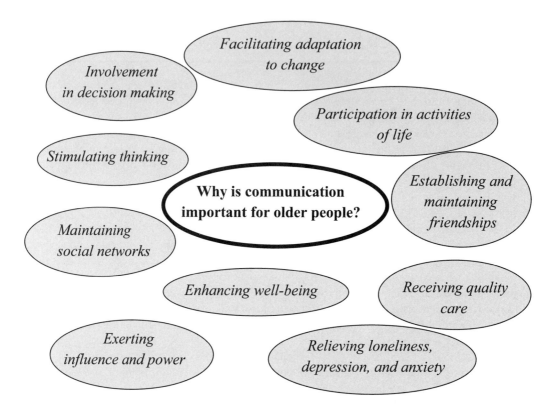

FIGURE 1–3. Reasons why effective communication is important for older people. Adapted from Lubinski (1995, 1997).

at the body level (e.g., reduced sound acuity); activity limitations are changes at the level of the person (e.g., inability to hear conversation); and participation restrictions are the effects of these on broader aspects of life (e.g., withdrawing from social situations). Environmental factors (e.g., residential situation) and personal factors (e.g., personality) are also taken into account. This model has been adopted to describe the scope of practice for speech-language pathology (American Speech-Language-Hearing Association [ASHA], 2001) and has particular relevance to gerontological practice in both audiology and speech-language pathology (Hickson & Worrall, 2001). Chapter 2 describes the WHO model in more detail, and Chapter 3 presents some options for the application of the model in practice settings.

Chapter 4 contains a description of the communication and swallowing impairments associated with both healthy and pathological aging and how they can be assessed. Chapter 5 describes the activity limitations and appropriate methods of assessment. Chapter 6 discusses participation restrictions, quality of life issues, and assessments of participation and quality of life. Although quality of life is not explicitly part of the WHO model, it is often considered to be a similar concept to participation.

Many communication clinicians would agree that the ultimate goal of intervention is to improve the quality of life of clients, and ASHA has stated "the provision of speech, language, and hearing services to older people is critical to the maintenance of quality of life" (ASHA, 1988, p. 84). To achieve better quality of life for older clients, it is argued in this text that clinicians should provide assessment and intervention at all levels of the WHO model. Chapters 7, 8, and 9 provide examples of intervention programs for community, hospital, and residential care settings for the aged, respectively.

In summary, the increasing number of older people with communication difficulties has major implications for the role of speech-language pathologists and audiologists. It is currently estimated in the United States that 19% of the overall speech-language pathology caseload and 33% of the overall audiology caseload are older people. By 2050, these caseloads are expected to increase to 39% and 59%, respectively (Shadden & Toner, 1997). It is, therefore, timely for clinicians to carefully consider their roles with older people and to be proactive about how to meet the challenge of population aging. Future clinicians will need skills in being responsive to change and, indeed, in initiating change. Audiologists and speech-language pathologists must not be afraid to debate issues and become involved. To this end, a list of possible debate topics for the classroom or small groups is presented in the Class Activities section at the end of this chapter. Done well, these debates can stimulate interest in this significant area of audiology and speech-language pathology.

Key Points

- Global population aging is having and will continue to have a significant effect on speech-language pathology and audiology caseloads.

- Typically, old age begins at 65 years, with people younger than 75 years or 80 years being termed the young-old, and people over 75 or 80 years being termed the old-old.

- The proportion of people in the old-old age group is the fastest growing, with most of these being women.

- In developed countries, there is a rapid growth in the proportion of older people from minority groups.

- The major causes of death in older people are heart disease, cancer, and stroke.

- The most common chronic disabilities of aging are arthritis, hypertension, and hearing impairment.
- Co-morbidity or the co-occurrence of disabilities is common in older people.
- There are many age-related changes to communication in healthy older people, with the most common being hearing impairment and word-retrieval problems.
- In the older population, there is an increased prevalence of diseases and disabilities that can affect communication.
- Dementia of the Alzheimer's type is the most prevalent disease in older people that affects communication.
- Gerontology brings a broader perspective to case management than discipline-specific management.
- Communication is important to quality of life in older people.
- The effects of communication changes with age can be framed using the WHO model.

CLASS ACTIVITIES

- Do a free association with the word *aging*. Were the responses predominantly negative?
- Search the Internet for sources of information about aging in your country.
- Talk with an older person. Does he or she have impairments in hearing, vision, speech, and so forth? How easy is it to communicate with the older person?
- Organized debates are a good method for stimulating thought and discussion. The debates need not be formal. Some preparation by students, however, is important. Two groups of students (three in each group) are allocated to either the *for* or *against* sides of the argument. A chairperson is also chosen. The role of the chairperson is to set the rules of the debate as well as chair the debate on the day. Winners of the debate can be determined through a voting system, an independent panel, or simply by the volume of applause for each team.

  Potential debate topics include

  1. Are speech-language pathologists and audiologists agist?
  2. Involvement in policy is not the role of an audiologist or speech-language pathologist.
  3. Communicative decline is an inevitable part of aging.
  4. Courses in adult communication disability and aural rehabilitation prepare us for working with the older population generally.

RECOMMENDED READING

Ripich, D. (Ed.). (1991). *Geriatric communication disorders*. Austin, TX: Pro-Ed.

Sen, K. (1994). *Aging: Debates on demographic transition and social policy*. London: Zed Books Ltd.

Shadden, B. B. (Ed.). (1988). *Communication behavior and aging: A sourcebook for clinicians*. Baltimore: Williams & Wilkins.

Shadden, B. B., & Toner, M. A. (1997). Introduction: The continuum of life functions. In B. A. Shadden & M. A. Toner (Eds.), *Aging and communication* (pp. 3–17). Austin, TX: Pro-Ed.

Tinker, A. (1996). *Older people in modern society*. London: Longman Ltd.

Weinstein, B. E. (2000). *Geriatric audiology*. New York: Thieme.

REFERENCES

Administration on Aging. (1998). *A profile of older Americans*. http://www.aoa.dhhs.gov

Administration on Aging. (2001). *A profile of older Americans*. http://www.aoa.dhhs.gov

American Speech-Language-Hearing Association. (1988, March). Position statement: The roles of speech-language pathologists and audiologists in working with older people. *ASHA*, pp. 80–84.

American Speech-Language-Hearing Association. (2001). *Scope of practice in speech-language pathology*. Rockville, MD: Author.

Australian Bureau of Statistics. (1996). *Projections of the population of Australia, States and Territories 1995-2051*. Canberra: Australian Government Publishing Service.

Bess, F. H., Lichtenstein, M. J., Logan, S. A., Burger, M. C., & Nelson, E. (1989). Hearing impairment as a determinant of function in the elderly. *Journal of the American Geriatrics Society, 37*(2), 123–128.

Bryan, K., & Maxim, J. (2002). Letter to the Editor. *International Journal of Language and Communication Disorders, 37*(2), 215–222.

Caruso, A. J., & Max, L. (1997). Effects of aging on neuromotor processes of swallowing. *Seminars in Speech and Language, 18*(2), 181–192.

Cherney, L. R. (1996). The effects of aging on communication. In C. Bernstein Lewis (Ed.), *Aging: The health care challenge: An interdisciplinary approach to assessment and rehabilitative management of the elderly* (3rd ed., pp. 79–105). Philadelphia: F.A. Davis.

Chodzko-Zajko, W. J., Ringle, R. L., & Vaca, V. L. (1995). Bio-gerontology: Implications for the communication sciences. In R. A. Huntley & K. S. Helfer (Eds.), *Communication in later life* (pp. 3–21). Boston: Butterworth-Heinemann.

Cruice, M. (2002). *Communication and quality of life in older people with aphasia and healthy older people.* Unpublished doctoral thesis. The University of Queensland, Brisbane, Australia.

Hickson, L., & Worrall, L. (1997). Hearing impairment, disability and handicap in older people. *Critical Reviews in Physical and Rehabilitation Medicine, 9*(3 & 4), 219–243.

Hickson, L., & Worrall, L. (2001). Older people with hearing impairment: Application of the new World Health Organization International Classification of Functioning and Disability. *Asia Pacific Journal of Speech, Language, and Hearing, 6,* 129–133.

Hopper, T., & Bayles, K. A. (2001). Management of neurogenic communication disorders associated with dementia. In R. Chapey (Ed.), *Language intervention strategies in aphasia and related neurogenic communication disorders* (pp. 829–846). Philadelphia: Lippincott Williams & Wilkins.

International Federation on Aging. (1996). *Global aging into the 21st century.* Retrieved on September 23, 1999, from the World Wide Web: http://www.ifa-org/page3p.html

Le Dorze, G. & Brassard, C. (1995). A description of the consequences of aphasia on aphasic persons and their relatives and friends, based on the WHO model of chronic diseases. *Aphasiology, 9*(3), 239–255.

Lubinski, R. (1995). State-of-the-art perspectives on communication in nursing homes. *Topics in Language Disorders, 15*(2) 1–19.

Lubinski, R. (1997). Perspectives on aging and communication. In R. Lubinski & D. J. Higginbotham (Eds.), *Communication technologies for the elderly: Vision, hearing, and speech* (pp. 1–22). Clifton Park, NY: Delmar Learning.

McCallum, J., & Geiselhart, K. (1996). *Australia's new aged: Issues for young and old.* Sydney: Allen & Unwin.

Moody, H. R. (2000). *Aging: Concepts and controversies* (3rd ed.). Thousand Oaks, CA: Pine Forge Press.

National Center for Health Statistics. (1995). *Health: United States 1994.* Hyattsville, MD: Author.

National Institute on Aging. (1997). *Disability rate among older Americans declines dramatically.* Retrieved September 22, 1999, from the World Wide Web: http://www.nih.gov:80/nia/new/press/disrate.htm

Ripich, D. (Ed.). (1991). *Geriatric communication disorders.* Austin, TX: Pro-Ed.

Sen, K. (1994). *Aging: Debates on demographic transition and social policy.* London: Zed Books Ltd.

Shadden, B. B. (Ed.). (1988). *Communication behavior and aging: A sourcebook for clinicians.* Baltimore: Williams & Wilkins.

Shadden, B. B., & Toner, M. A. (1997). Introduction: The continuum of life functions. In B. A. Shadden & M. A. Toner (Eds.), *Aging and communication* (pp. 3–17). Austin, TX: Pro-Ed.

Tinker, A. (1996). *Older people in modern society.* London: Longman Ltd.

United Nations. (1992). *Population ageing: Review of national policies and programmes in Asia and the Pacific.* Asian Population Series, 109. New York: United Nations.

United States Census Bureau. (1999). *New census report shows exponential growth in number of centenarians.* Retrieved on September 22, 1999 from the World Wide Web: http://www.nih.gov:80/nia/new/press/growthcent.html

United States Census Bureau. (2000). *National population projections.* Retrieved on October 4, 2000 from the World Wide Web: http://www.census.gov/population/www/projections/natproj.html

Weinstein, B. E. (2000). *Geriatric audiology.* New York: Thieme.

World Health Organization. (1998). *Population aging—a public health challenge.* Fact Sheet No 135. Retrieved January 19, 2000, from the World Wide Web: http://www.who.int/inf-fs/en/fact135.html

World Health Organization. (1999). *Health futures.* Retrieved September 23, 1999, from the World Wide Web: http://www.who.int/hpr/expo/futures0.3.html

World Health Organization. (2001). *International classification of functioning, disability, and health.* Geneva: Author.

Worrall, L., Hickson, L., & Dodd, B. (1993). Screening for communication impairment in nursing homes and hostels. *Australian Journal of Human Communication Disorders, 21,* 53–64.

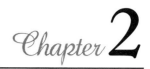

Theoretical Foundations of Communication Disability in Aging

This chapter explains how models of communication, disability, and aging have an impact upon the practice of speech-language pathologists and audiologists who work with older people. Frameworks such as the WHO model, the health-disease continuum, the Communication Accommodation Theory, and underlying constructs of healthy aging are described and their application to practice exemplified.

Gerontology could be considered a separate specialty of speech-language pathology and audiology. The underlying theoretical frameworks for gerontology are different from those that underpin the rehabilitation of younger people with neurogenic communication disability or acquired hearing loss. Just as gerontology is multidisciplinary, the theoretical foundations for communication disability in aging stem from a variety of disciplinary sources. The primary frameworks influencing modern-day practices in communication disability in aging are

- the WHO model: the International Classification of Functioning, Disability and Health
- the health-disease continuum
- healthy aging constructs
- Communication Accommodation Theory (CAT)

Other theoretical frameworks, such as those surrounding the nature of aging, are also important; however, the preceding frameworks are considered to be essential for understanding the premises of this book and for working in the modern practice of gerontological audiology and speech-language pathology.

The WHO Model

One of the fundamental conceptual frameworks for communication disability in aging and one that is used extensively throughout this book is the WHO model. The WHO model, or the ICF, stands for the World Health Organization's International Classification of Functioning, Disability and Health (WHO, 2001a). This well-established model describes the consequences of a health condition on the person and on society as a whole.

Figure 2–1 is a graphic representation of the WHO model. It shows the interaction between a health condition, body functions and structures, activities, and participation. It also illustrates the importance of the effects of environmental and personal factors on functioning. Aging is considered to be a health condition in this framework. In essence, the effects of a health condition are described in the dimensions of body, activities, and/or participation. The definitions of these components are listed here.

In the context of a health condition, (WHO, 2001b)

- Body functions are the physiological functions of body systems (including psychological functions).
- Body structures are anatomic parts of the body such as organs, limbs, and their components.
- Activity is the execution of a task or action by an individual.
- Participation is involvement in a life situation.
- Environmental factors make up the physical, social, and attitudinal environment in which people live and conduct their lives. (WHO, 2001b, p.10)

The negative terms of these three dimensions are impairment, activity limitation, and participation restriction.

The WHO model shows that there are multidirectional interactions among the dimensions; for example, improving participation may help to improve the impairment. The model also shows that contextual (environmental and personal) factors have an influence on the dimensions of body functions and structure, activity, and participation. Contextual factors are the complete background of life. They include environmental factors such as the physical, social, and attitudinal environment, and personal factors such as age, race, gender, edu-

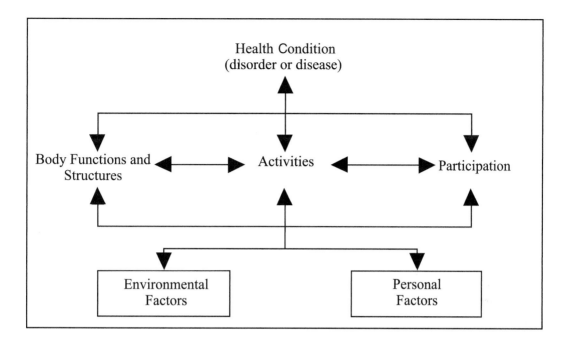

FIGURE 2–1. The WHO (ICF) model (World Health Organization, 2001a). With permission from WHO, Geneva.

cational background, coping styles, and so forth. Although WHO recommends that the dimensions of body, activity, and participation be differentiated from the everyday use of these terms by the capitalization of the first letter, this recommendation has not been widely adopted outside the organization and has, therefore, not been used in this text.

Enderby and John (1997) illustrated how the WHO model works with individuals with a speech or language impairment. Figure 2–2 shows how a mild impairment such as a mild aphasia can produce a devastating participation restriction such as unemployment, social isolation, and nonparticipation in leisure interests or decision making. Figure 2–2 also shows the opposite. It shows that a man (Mr. C) with a severe impairment can have no participation restrictions at all. Figure 2–3 shows an example of two cases from audiology. These cases not only demonstrate how important the three dimensions of the WHO model are, but also serve to illustrate how the model can be used with clients with communication disabilities.

The activity and participation dimensions of the WHO model constitute what traditionally has been called functional communication in speech-language pathology and hearing disability/handicap in audiology. Because many health conditions of older people are chronic in nature, including those affecting communication, rehabilitation efforts need to

Mr. K

Mild Impairment: mild aphasia

↕

Mild-Moderate Activity Limitations: has difficulty making himself understood quickly in groups; has stopped using the telephone; occasionally misunderstands

↕

Severe Participation Restrictions: now unable to be employed in the same job; withdrawn from social occasions; has given up hobbies; no longer contributes to decision making

Mr. C

Severe Impairment: severe athetoid cerebral palsy; quadriplegic and dysarthric

↕

No Activity Limitation: totally independent with adapted wheelchair, adapted accommodation, communication aid, and adaptation to telephone

↕

No Participation Restriction: employed as lawyer, active member of disability movement, full social life

FIGURE 2–2. Illustration of the WHO model in speech-language pathology. Adapted from Enderby and John, 1997.

Mrs. A

Moderate Impairment: moderate bilateral sensorineural

↕

Mild-Moderate Activity Limitations: problems understanding speech in noisy situations, cannot hear telephone ring, cannot hear television at normal volume

↕

Severe Participation Restrictions: withdraws from social situations, has given up her position as secretary of the local bridge club

Mrs. B

Severe Impairment: severe bilateral sensorineural hearing loss

↕

Mild Activity Limitation: minimal difficulties hearing in noise (uses conference microphone, FM system), no problems hearing telephone ring (has flashing light), some problems on telephone even with telecoil and volume control

↕

No Participation Restriction: busy social life, works full time for a disability support agency providing advice to clients about assistive listening devices

FIGURE 2–3. Illustration of the WHO model in audiology.

take a long-term view and attempt to lessen the impact of these chronic conditions on everyday activities and life participation.

The more familiar and earlier WHO model was the International Classification of Impairment, Disability and Handicap (WHO, 1980). There have been several revisions of the WHO model, and the most recent revision, the ICF, was endorsed by the World Health Assembly in May 2001 and is on the Internet at http://www3.who.int/icf/icftemplate.cfm. One of the criticisms of the earlier version of the WHO model was that it was based too much in the medical model of disability. People with disabilities and their advocates who support a social model of disability were outspoken critics of the original WHO framework published in 1980. The current WHO model attempts to achieve a "synthesis in order to provide a coherent view of different perspectives of health from a biological, individual and social perspective" (WHO, 2001b, p. 20). Therefore, it is called a biopsychosocial approach to disability. In speech-language pathology and audiology, this might be interpreted as a holistic approach because it includes all the major approaches to disability. A more detailed description of the medical and social models of disability is contained in Chapter 3.

The overall aim of the new WHO model is to "provide a unified and standard language and framework for the description of health and health-related states" (WHO, 2001b, p. 3). The model and its accompanying extensive classification scheme was developed to

- provide a scientific basis for understanding and studying health and health-related states, outcomes, and determinants

- establish a common language for describing health and health-related states in order to improve communication between different users, such as health care workers, researchers, policy-makers, and the public, including people with disabilities

- permit comparison of data across countries, health care disciplines, services, and time

- provide a systematic coding scheme for health information systems (WHO, 2001b, p. 5)

The WHO model has been used by health professionals, researchers, policy makers, and others as

- a statistical tool, for example, to collect and record data

- a research tool, for example, to measure outcomes

- a clinical tool, for example, in rehabilitation and outcome evaluation

- a social policy tool, for example, in policy design and implementation
- an educational tool, for example, to raise awareness (WHO, 2001b, p.5)

How are these WHO dimensions related to quality of life? Although the WHO dimensions propose to describe the functional states associated with a health condition on a person and on society, the concept of overall quality of life is missing from the model. Cruice, Worrall, and Hickson (2000) interpreted the link between the dimensions used in an earlier version of the WHO model, the ICIDH-2, and quality of life for audiologists and speech-language pathologists (Figure 2–4). In this conceptual model, quality of life is viewed as an entity separate from the WHO dimensions. There is much overlap between the participation dimension and quality of life in particular. These are sometimes considered to be the same concept; however, the two concepts have different origins and are treated quite separately in the scientific literature. Quality of life and participation are considered as two separate but related concepts throughout this text. The model in Figure 2–4 shows that the impairments relevant to speech-language pathologists and audiologists are speech, language, voice, fluency, swallowing, and hearing. The most relevant activity and participation domains listed in the WHO model are communication and interpersonal interaction and relationships; however, because communication enables participation in many life roles, all of the activity/participation domains are relevant. The dimensions of quality of life most relevant to audiologists and speech-language pathologists are social health, mental health, emotional health, and subjective well-being. From a therapeutic perspective, Cruice et al.'s model indicates that improving abilities in the body, activity, and participation dimensions can be expected to make improvements in a number of dimensions of quality of life. This relationship is discussed further in Chapter 6.

The WHO model is important to the practice of audiology and speech-language pathology in the aging area for several reasons.

1. The application of this conceptual framework can lessen the impact of a chronic disability such as a speech, language, or hearing impairment on the everyday life of older people.
2. The model provides a set of internationally recognized terminology for describing the effects of a health condition on functioning. In the multidisciplinary area of aging, where communication has a low profile, the use of recognized terminology is important.
3. The WHO model helps to define to others what can be done for people with communication disabilities (i.e., it shows that audiologists and speech-language pathologists are not only concerned with the impairment but also its effects on everyday activities and participation in life).

The application of this model to the practice of speech-language pathology and audiology with older people is demonstrated by the case studies on pages 26 and 27.

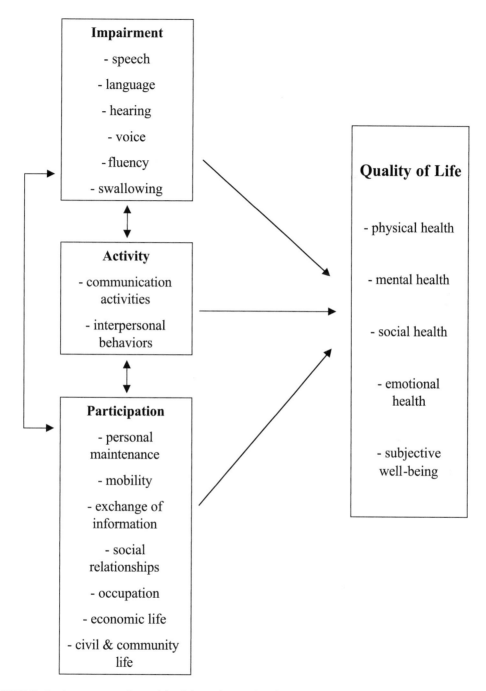

FIGURE 2–4. A conceptual model of the relationship between communication and quality of life: Clinical interpretation for audiologists and speech-language pathologists. Reproduced from Cruice, M., Worrall, L., and Hickson, L. (2000). Quality-of-life measurement in speech pathology and audiology. *Asia Pacific Journal of Speech, Language, and Hearing, 5*(1), 1–20.

Case Study: Speech-Language Pathology

Danielle was a speech-language pathologist employed for 20 hours per week at a large residential care facility for the aged. There were 400 residents at the facility, and 25 residents required ongoing intervention for specific and chronic disease-related speech, language, or swallowing impairments. The communicative environment of the facility was poor as there were few opportunities for residents to interact with each other, and many of the staff-resident interactions were unsatisfactory for both interactants.

Danielle used the WHO framework for a variety of purposes. With the residents who had chronic speech, language, or swallowing impairments, she worked out intervention goals for each client following discussions with the resident (if possible), the family, and the staff. Not only were body-level goals set such as decreasing drooling or improving word retrieval, but activity and participation level goals were established such as keeping track of finances, understanding the craft instructor's directions, conversing with friends at the dinner table, or participating in the church service. The WHO model was used to demonstrate to staff the effect of participation restrictions on impairment and activity levels within the facility (e.g., how a lack of conversational opportunity for residents may contribute to residents' decline in word-retrieval abilities or decreased resident-to-resident interaction). The link between improving a resident's communication at the impairment level (e.g., making sure that the resident's hearing aid is worn and is working well) and the improvement that this can make to the resident's overall participation in the community was well illustrated by the WHO model.

Danielle provided a comprehensive, successful, and meaningful service to the 400-bed residential care facility. The staff understood Danielle's rationale for her service delivery, and residents made gains that were important to their lives in the facility.

In summary, the WHO model was used as a clinical tool and as an educational tool in both cases. It also has the potential to be used as a social policy tool and a research tool with older people with communication disability. Therefore, it forms an important basis for the practice of audiology and speech-language pathology.

The Health-Disease Continuum

In Chapter 1, it was stated that the role of speech-language pathologists and audiologists should be broader than a traditional focus on older people with health conditions such as presbycusis, stroke, dementia, and Parkinson's disease. The health-disease continuum was described to illustrate this. In gerontological speech-language pathology and audiology, ser-

Case Study: Audiology

Brad was an audiologist who worked for the nation's premiere hearing service. He assessed many older people and fitted them with the latest hearing aids; however, a review of 100 of his recent clients found that 8% were not wearing their hearing aids at all, 15% were using them infrequently, and many more were still having difficulty hearing even with the hearing aids. The focus of Brad's service to this point had been on the client's impairments and the fitting of hearing aids to improve hearing levels. Brad used the WHO model to rethink his service to older clients. At the first appointment for each client, he found out more about the problems the client was having by asking questions that related to the activity and participation levels of the WHO framework (e.g., "What are some of the problems you have hearing around the house? How does your hearing restrict your participation in some of the roles you have?"). If the client was having difficulties in these areas, Brad discussed a range of intervention options with the person. These options included hearing aids, assistive listening devices, and communication training. Brad developed a new group program aimed at improving the quality and quantity of his clients' communicative activities and developing strategies for the maintenance of their participation in many of their life roles.

vices are not restricted to people with specific speech, language, or hearing disabilities (e.g., aphasia, dysarthria, sensorineural hearing impairment). These are certainly at one end of the continuum. There is also a subgroup of older individuals with unidentified subclinical communication disabilities (word-retrieval difficulties, cohesion of discourse problems) that pose a risk for that person's ability to maintain independence. There is also the healthy group at the other end of the continuum who are hoping to prevent disability and decline. Davis (1996) describes these three groups as the disabled (the traditional clients of rehabilitation specialists), the worried well who are fighting the daily battle for independent function, and the well elderly who are hoping to prevent disabling conditions. This is the health-disease continuum applied to older people.

Ringel and Chodzko-Zajko have argued the relevance of the health-disease continuum to audiologists and speech-language pathologists on a number of occasions (Chodzko-Zajko, Ringel, & Vaca, 1995; Ringel & Chodzko-Zajko, 1988). Figure 2–5 diagrammatically represents this concept. Ringel and Chodzko-Zajko state that, while there has been a long-standing tradition to categorize aging into two distinct groups, as either primary aging (disease-free) or secondary aging (disease-related), the concept of disease-free aging has become difficult to uphold. They suggest that, rather than dichotomize normal aging and pathological aging, there should be a continuum with exceptional physiological health at one end and overt disease at the other end. In the middle of the continuum, they use the

Health	Disease
Communicative ability	*Communicative disability*
• Hearing loss	• Aphasia
• Word-retrieval difficulties	• Dysarthria
• Pragmatic changes	• Language of dementia

FIGURE 2–5. The health-disease continuum for communication and aging.

term *subclinical* to characterize older people who have significant levels of physiological deterioration, but who cannot be called diseased or unhealthy. Despite understanding that communication forms a continuum from ability to disability, it is often convenient to use the traditional dichotomy of healthy aging and pathological aging. These two terms appear throughout this text. When this dichotomy is used, both healthy older people and subclinical populations are included under the umbrella of healthy aging.

The health-disease continuum also translates into communication ability and disability. People with obvious aphasia, dysarthria, or language of dementia are toward the overt disease end of the continuum. People with overt communication disabilities are the traditional clients of speech-language pathologists and audiologists. However, some people with a mild stroke or early dementia are on the borderline of aphasia and normal language. Moving along the continuum, there is the subclinical group. Large numbers of older people have a multitude of minor communication changes, none of which on their own would constitute a readily identifiable disease-related communication disability, but together they threaten the ability of the person to interact successfully in society. This is the at-risk population or, as Davis names them, the worried well. For example, an 80-year-old person with a mild hearing impairment, mild visual impairment, and mild cognitive changes that are affecting language skills and short-term memory, may still be functioning independently in the community. The social contacts of the person have declined considerably. The person is neither well nor disabled, but probably at risk. The multiple communication changes that have occurred may be the result of other chronic diseases (e.g., diabetes, which can cause visual and/or hearing impairments, or cognitive and communication changes that occur following minor strokes) or are physiological changes related to aging.

Audiologists and speech-language pathologists may have a role in preventing admissions to long-term care facilities; however, the nature of this subclinical communicatively disabled population is not well understood or not well accepted in the audiology and speech-language pathology professions. The link between subclinical communicative disability and social isolation holds a rich vein of scientific inquiry. The following case study illustrates the problems associated with subclinical communication disability.

Case Study: Mr. Hanes

Mr. Hanes is 76 years old and has significant sensory impairments. He wears binaural hearing aids and glasses, but nevertheless has difficulties both seeing and hearing in everyday life. Following an episode where he was hospitalized with a virus 6 months ago, Mr. Hanes developed noticeable word-retrieval difficulties. Although his word-retrieval difficulties are not due to a diagnosed aphasia or dementia, he is not communicatively healthy. He would not traditionally be referred to a speech-language pathologist; however, his word-retrieval abilities (combined with his other sensory impairments) are affecting his social interactions. Some communication strategies and some treatment of his word-retrieval impairment may assist Mr. Hanes to maintain his extensive social network and keep him active in the community.

The funding of speech-language pathologists and audiologists to provide these services varies by location and service provider. In Australia, the Home and Community Care (HACC) program aims to keep people in their own home; therefore, if an older person is eligible for this program, then speech-language pathology and audiology services can be provided. In the United States, the service would be provided by home health care agencies. Currently, the identification of people at risk is primarily based on physical health. Audiologists and speech-language pathologists could develop their roles in this increasingly important and funded area of service delivery.

Speech-language pathologists and audiologists may also have roles to play with the very healthy, well older person. The communication changes associated with age are insidious and occur slowly over a number of years. The older person has time to adapt and accommodate to these gradual changes. Communication changes often go unrecognized, and their effect on life goes unnoticed. Annual checkups at wellness centers are becoming more common for older people, and audiologists in particular have a major role in assessing hearing on an annual basis. Health promotion programs such as the authors' own *Keep on Talking* program (Worrall, Hickson, Barnett, & Yiu, 1998) are being sought by older people. Programs such as this aim to educate older people about some of the communication changes that may occur with aging and help them develop strategies to maintain or enhance their communication skills with increasing age. Further information about health promotion in the community is contained in Chapter 7.

In summary, speech-language pathologists and audiologists could expand their roles with older people across the communication continuum that not only encompasses traditional rehabilitation, but also involves assisting older people to remain in the community. Finally, they have an increasing role in prevention and health promotion. The roles of audiologists and speech-language pathologists may extend from prevention to intervention.

Healthy Aging

Professor Robert Butler, one of the world's leading gerontologists, stated that there are four categories of fitness to maintain with age:

- physical fitness—bodily strength, resilience and agility
- intellectual fitness—keeping the mind active and engaged
- social fitness—forming and maintaining significant personal relationships
- purpose fitness—feelings of self-esteem and control over life (Butler, 1991, p. vii)

These positive concepts of aging are part of the notion of healthy aging. Healthy aging is referred to as successful aging, active aging, positive aging, or aging well. Governments are keen to promote the concept of healthy aging because the approach emphasizes prevention of chronic illnesses and disabilities in older people. The concept of healthy aging, however, is much broader than just prevention of disease. Healthy aging also implies optimal well-being in spite of specific disabilities. The concept of healthy aging for people with disabilities has relevance to audiologists and speech-language pathologists working with older people.

The WHO first coined the term *healthy aging*. The concept takes the view that aging is a developmental or lifelong process and that health promotion is important for maintaining health as people age. The Ottawa Charter for Health Promotion (1986) defined health promotion as a process that enables people to gain more control over their own health. In a policy paper of the Department of Health and Aged Care in Australia (www.health.gov.au/acc/nsaa/hadp/index.htm), healthy aging strategies are designed to achieve the following outcomes.

- prevent, postpone or reverse adverse health conditions
- maintain and/or recover function after health problems

- enhance quality of life through improved physical and emotional well-being
- compress disability to the end of the life span
- minimize the incidence of illness through life
- increase participation in health maintenance and enhancement activities
- increase the contribution by governments, health service providers, researchers, business and the community in a public health approach to aging
- sustain the delivery of health services at a fixed percentage of Gross Domestic Product (Bishop, 1999, p. 6)

Despite being the focus of many governments and international organizations such as the United Nations and the WHO, the concept of healthy aging that emphasizes health promotion is not the predominant view of the audiology and speech-language pathology professions. Why is this? Do speech-language pathologists and audiologists believe that they do not have a role in health promotion or prevention of communication disability? Does the predominantly medical model background of the professions focus solely on the negative, deficit, or impairment-oriented view of aging? How can the concept of healthy aging be relevant to working with older people with communication disabilities? These questions are answered in the next sections.

Importance of Healthy Aging for Audiologists and Speech-Language Pathologists

Healthy aging is potentially an important concept for the professions of audiology and speech-language pathology for two reasons. First, government policy has a profound effect on health care financing, and this ultimately affects the work of speech-language pathologists and audiologists. Healthy aging policies are viewed as governments' answers to reducing the health expenditure explosion associated with increasing numbers of older people. Second, the healthy aging approach makes a lot of sense. If older people adopt a healthy aging approach that is supported by society in general, it may lead to a better quality of life for all older people. There is not only a need for older people to adopt this philosophy, but also for health professionals and society generally to support a healthy aging approach.

The healthy aging approach applies to all older people, whether they are one of the well, worried well, or disabled. For the well older person, it may mean providing education about the importance of maintaining and enhancing communication skills. For the subclinical population or the worried well, it may mean supporting their need for independence by enhancing their communication and social network. For older people with specific communication impairments, it is the maintenance or recovery of function. There is a need to start health promotion activities early, and audiologists and speech-language pathologists could be involved by providing information and services to older people and promoting the healthy communication message to the general public.

Relationship Between Communication and Healthy Aging

Communication has a vital role in healthy aging. Communication is inextricably linked to social health and psychological well-being. Social health is defined as "that dimension of an individual's well-being that concerns how he gets along with other people, how other people react to him, and how he interacts with social institutions and societal mores" (Russell, 1973, p. 75). Social adjustment, social role, and social support measures are all methods of evaluating social health (see McDowell & Newell, 1996, for a critical review of all these categories of measures). Psychological well-being is a complex construct that has been termed emotional well-being or mental health. Measures of life satisfaction, affective state, and psychological distress are all methods of assessing psychological well-being.

Communication is the means by which people adapt to life's stresses. It is the thin thread that can bind it all together, and with its vulnerability, older people (as well as policy makers) need to understand the importance of communication to healthy aging. Figure 1–3 in Chapter 1 summarized the work of Lubinski (1995, 1997) in this area. Why is it that many people other than speech-language pathologists and audiologists do not always understand the importance of communication to healthy aging? Communication disabilities are certainly less visible than physical disabilities; therefore, they are not in the forefront of people's minds. People with communication disabilities, particularly those with expressive difficulties, are generally not outspoken lobbyists because of the very nature of their disability. Finally, communication is a gift that often develops naturally in childhood and then may gradually fade away in older adulthood. Dramatic and sudden changes occur only with the onset of stroke or laryngectomy. The importance of communication to healthy aging is a difficult message to sell to policy makers and older people alike. The link between communication disability and social isolation, however, is an important one; loneliness in older people is a better predictor of death than smoking or cholesterol (Goleman, 1995). The link between communication and healthy aging is an important message to send to policy makers.

The Roles of Audiologists and Speech-Language Pathologists in Healthy Aging

In summary, speech-language pathologists and audiologists may assume roles in health promotion and prevention of communication disability in older people. Audiologists may need to increase the public's awareness of the effects of aging and other factors, such as noise exposure and ototoxic drugs, on hearing. In particular, occupational health and safety programs need to be more effective in ensuring that all people engaged in high-risk noise work wear

ear protectors. Audiologists could also be involved in the identification of hearing impairments throughout the life span. In younger people, preventable diseases that affect hearing need to be targeted; for older people, early identification of hearing loss will lead to aural rehabilitation that provides significant benefit in the long term. If older people wait too long to take action about their hearing impairment, they may find it difficult to adapt to the latest technologies available in hearing aids and other hearing assistance devices.

Speech-language pathologists also have a role in preventing voice, speech, and language difficulties in later life. Vocal hygiene programs for high-risk people are important to maintain a healthy voice in later life. Appropriate dentition is important to maintain clear speech intelligibility, while word-retrieval skills need to be maintained through active use of a person's vocabulary. In addition, purposeful strategies can be put in place for maintaining or enhancing naming of people, places, or objects. In addition, because cognitive skills are closely linked to language skills, speech-language pathologists may choose to promote the notion of intellectual fitness to older people.

Both professions could also promote the importance of maintaining social networks, particularly informal social networks. Effective communication skills are a vital component of maintaining social networks. Well older people should be encouraged to monitor their social and communication fitness through annual checkups. Chapter 4 describes the most suitable test instruments for communication in an annual checkup.

The healthy aging approach also applies to the worried well or those with subclinical communication disability. These people are already experiencing some communication disability and are often fighting to maintain their independence. Intervention by audiologists and speech-language pathologists at this stage may help older people maintain their autonomy in decision making. Many of these people may have already been identified by health and community agencies. There are some older people living in retirement villages who are struggling to maintain their independence. Communication and social fitness may be playing a major role in their loss of independence. Hence, the role of speech-language pathologists and audiologists in optimizing their communication skills and their communication environments is vital.

People with specific and identifiable communication disabilities such as aphasia, dysarthria, or severe hearing loss can also benefit from a healthy aging approach by audiologists and speech-language pathologists. Healthy aging is about maximizing function and allowing the person to age successfully, despite a communication disability. Although this could be construed as a functional approach to rehabilitation, it is more than that. It is stating that speech-language pathologists and audiologists should not reinforce the problems associated with the communication disability by continuing to treat impairments only, such as word retrieval, comprehension, and sentence construction problems for years post-onset. A healthy aging approach suggests the need to actively encourage clients to live their lives, as they would want, despite the communication disability.

In summary, healthy aging is an important philosophy that is being embraced by many countries as a solution to reducing the health effects of population aging (WHO, 2002). Therefore, speech-language pathologists and audiologists need to understand their roles in creating a healthy aging population. Their roles not only include the promotion of maintaining communication and social health to well older people, but may also involve focusing on those with subclinical communication disabilities as well as those with overt communication disabilities.

Communication Accommodation Theory

Audiology and speech-language pathology have primarily used a deficit or impairment approach to aging. That is, older people have a range of communication impairments that increase with age. In this approach, the problem in interactions is seen as resting with the older person with the communication impairment. An alternative approach suggests that the problem lies with both interlocutors (McIntosh, 1996). Communication Accommodation Theory (CAT) (see, for example, Giles, Coupland, & Coupland, 1991) is a model for explaining the processes behind communicative interaction. It has its roots in theories of communication rather than in theories of aging; therefore, it has been applied to interactions with a range of populations. The model is based on the premise that speakers and listeners accommodate to each other's communication patterns.

Although most accommodation is appropriate, there are two major forms of inappropriate accommodation: under- and overaccommodation. Underaccommodation can occur if an interlocutor fails to recognize the cues of his or her partner. For example, if a speaker fails to observe that his conversational partner is having difficulty hearing, underaccommodation will occur if the speaker fails to adjust his or her volume. Overaccommodation occurs when a conversational partner views the other interlocutor in a stereotypical way. This often occurs in intergenerational communication when the younger person automatically assumes an older conversation partner is probably hard of hearing and dependent. A common pattern of overaccommodation for older people, particularly those in residential care facilities for the aged, is a type of communication called either elder speak, patronizing talk, or secondary baby talk (Caporael, 1981). Higher pitch and volume, exaggerated intonation, simplified grammatical structures and vocabulary, greater repetition, and terms of endearment (e.g., dear, love) characterize this form of overaccommodation. This is an agist form of communication because it is based on stereotypical views of older people. It also shows how agism is constructed through communication. Some older people and staff in residential care facilities believe that this form of communication shows affection, support, and warmth; however, the majority of older people do not welcome this type of communication, and it may promote dependency (Ryan, Giles, Bartolucci, & Henwood, 1986).

CAT Applied to Older People

Although CAT has been used to explain cross-cultural miscommunications and other interactions of interest, it has strongly influenced the study of communication in older people. CAT has been used to study intergenerational communication by examining the accommodations made by both younger and older persons to each other's communication. It has also been used to study interactions among people of the same age.

Ryan et al. (1986) introduced the Communication Predicament in Aging model to explain how communication based on stereotypes of aging can create a predicament for older people. The model seeks to explain how a negative cycle is established that ultimately contributes to the reinforcement of age-stereotyped behaviors of the older person. Figure 2–6 shows the negative cycle in the Communication Predicament in Aging model. The cycle begins when the interactant recognizes the social group of the person he or she is about to encounter (i.e., older person) and modifies his or her communication based on stereotypical views of older people. The interactant overaccommodates and uses a patronizing communication style. This restricts the older person's participation in the interaction and can lead to a lowering of self-esteem and confidence by the older person. This in turn may lead to an old identity, which creates more old-age cues in the next communication encounter. Hence, the cycle continues. Inappropriate accommodation in interactions with older people makes older people feel old. They are more likely to have stereotypical accommodations the next time they encounter a younger person. This is the communication predicament of aging.

Another model, the Communication Enhancement in Aging model (Ryan, Meredith, MacLean, & Orange, 1995) (Figure 2–7), shows how this negative cycle can be broken, and older people can be empowered through appropriate accommodation. The cycle begins with the interactant recognizing the individual, rather than the stereotypical cues of the older person. Appropriate accommodation occurs. This might include speaking louder because the other person has cupped a hand behind the ear or simplifying instructions because the other person looks puzzled. It may include no modifications to speaking style or content because the other person is showing every sign of understanding the message. This accommodating communication allows for an appropriate assessment of the older person's needs. With

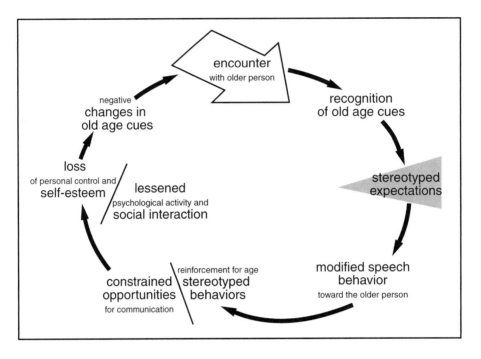

FIGURE 2–6. The Communication Predicament in Aging model. From Ryan, E. B., Meredith, S. D., MacLean, M., and Orange, J. B. (1995). Changing the way we talk with elders: Promoting health using the communication enhancement model. *International Journal of Aging and Human Development*, *41*(2) 89–109. With permission from Baywood Publishing Company, Inc., Amityville, N.Y.

such an appropriate communication pattern and an assessment that demonstrates respect for the older person, increased empowerment occurs through the optimized health and well-being of the older person. This in turn has a positive effect on the communicative opportunities and effectiveness of the older person. Hence, the Communication Enhancement in Aging model is based on the premise that appropriate accommodation must occur and must be based on the recognition of individualized cues.

Both the Communication Predicament in Aging model and the Communication Enhancement in Aging model place a considerable degree of responsibility on the conversational partner of the older person. It emphasizes that the problem may not lie with the older person's communication, but rather with the interaction between the two, based on the appropriateness of the accommodation that occurs.

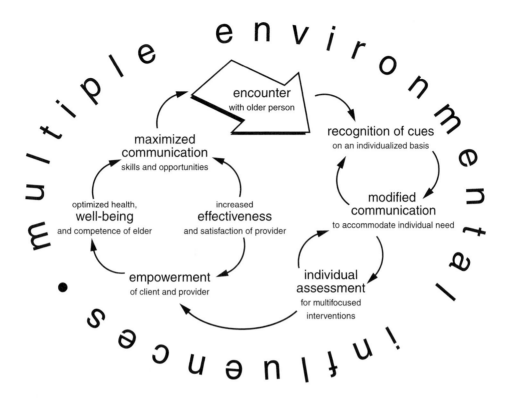

FIGURE 2–7. The Communication Enhancement in Aging model. From Ryan, E. B., Meredith, S. D., MacLean, M., and Orange, J. B. (1995). Changing the way we talk with elders: Promoting health using the communication Enhancement Model. *International Journal of Aging and Human Development, 41*(2), 89–109. With permission from Baywood Publishing Company, Inc., Amityville, N.Y.

CAT Applied to Older People with Communication Disabilities

If older people are disadvantaged by inappropriate accommodation by younger interactants, then this problem is compounded when the older person also has a communication disability. An interpretation of CAT for older people with hearing impairment is shown in Figure 2–8. This figure illustrates that if appropriate accommodation is to occur, interactants need to be able to recognize individual cues of older people with communication disabilities.

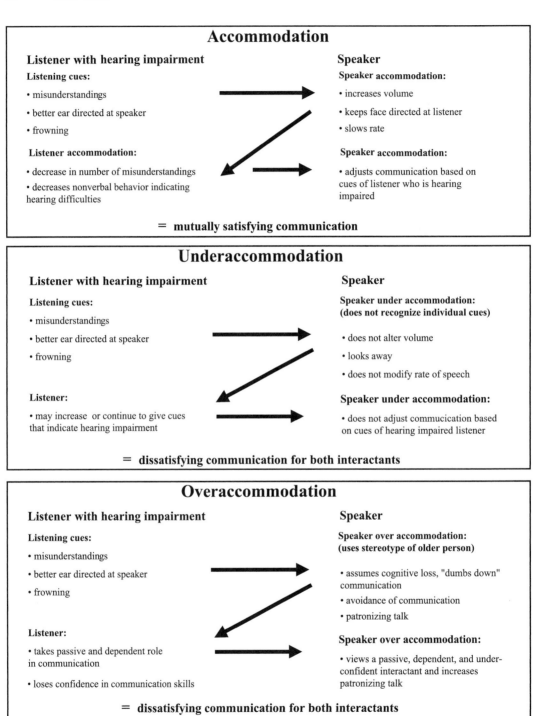

Accommodation

Listener with hearing impairment

Listening cues:

• misunderstandings

• better ear directed at speaker

• frowning

Listener accommodation:

• decrease in number of misunderstandings

• decreases nonverbal behavior indicating hearing difficulties

Speaker

Speaker accommodation:

• increases volume

• keeps face directed at listener

• slows rate

Speaker accommodation:

• adjusts communication based on cues of listener who is hearing impaired

= **mutually satisfying communication**

Underaccommodation

Listener with hearing impairment

Listening cues:

• misunderstandings

• better ear directed at speaker

• frowning

Listener:

• may increase or continue to give cues that indicate hearing impairment

Speaker

Speaker under accommodation:
(does not recognize individual cues)

• does not alter volume

• looks away

• does not modify rate of speech

Speaker under accommodation:

• does not adjust commucication based on cues of hearing impaired listener

= **dissatisfying communication for both interactants**

Overaccommodation

Listener with hearing impairment

Listening cues:

• misunderstandings

• better ear directed at speaker

• frowning

Listener:

• takes passive and dependent role in communication

• loses confidence in communication skills

Speaker

Speaker over accommodation:
(uses stereotype of older person)

• assumes cognitive loss, "dumbs down" communication

• avoidance of communication

• patronizing talk

Speaker over accommodation:

• views a passive, dependent, and under-confident interactant and increases patronizing talk

= **dissatisfying communication for both interactants**

FIGURE 2–8. The Communication Accommodation Theory applied to an older person with hearing impairment.

Implications of CAT for Speech-Language Pathology and Audiology

CAT implies that the problem may not lie solely with the older person. This means that audiologists and speech-language pathologists should pay as much attention to conversational partners as to older people with communication disabilities. It tells the clinician that interactants, particularly health professionals, need to learn to accommodate appropriately to older people's communication. This reinforces the need for education programs that help interactants learn to accommodate appropriately to the communication of older people with communication disabilities.

CAT also indicates that older people with communication disabilities need to learn to accommodate. This is an important factor to consider in direct intervention with the client. It is important to account for the possibility that the conversational partners of older people with communication disabilities are often older persons, maybe with a communication disability. This particularly occurs in older married couples when the primary conversational partners often have hearing impairments themselves. In residential care facilities for the aged, the likelihood of another resident having a communicative disability is high; hence, accommodation is a major factor in these interactions.

CAT suggests that agism will affect communication patterns unless education about the individual nature of communication abilities occurs. This is particularly true for health professionals working with older people. Inappropriate accommodation by care staff needs to be actively discouraged; however, the positive effects of elder speak need to be taken into account. Certainly, the common practice of providing lists of "How to communicate with older people/people with aphasia/people with hearing impairment" needs to be seriously reconsidered. Such materials may promote agist communication patterns by emphasizing the communication impairments of older people.

Finally, speech-language pathologists and audiologists may need to monitor their own interactions with older people, particularly those with communication disabilities. Overaccommodating through use of exaggerated intonation, volume, and articulation is possible, therefore contributing to the communication predicament of aging.

In summary, this chapter described some theories and conceptual models that form the foundation of working with older people with communication disabilities. Most of these constructs are not routinely taught in audiology and speech-language pathology education programs. They belong particularly to the realm of gerontological speech-language pathology and audiology, a separate specialty of the professions that has its own theoretical foundations, drawn predominantly from theories of disability, aging, and communication. In general, these theories convey a positive approach to aging and as such should underpin a new enthusiasm for gerontological audiology and speech-language pathology in the coming years.

KEY POINTS

- Four major theories underpin the practice of speech-language pathology and audiology with older people: the WHO model of functioning and disability, the health-disease continuum, healthy aging, and Communication Accommodation Theory.

- The WHO model describes functional states associated with a health condition. Therefore, it is a basic framework underlying audiology and speech-language pathology.

- The WHO model can be used as a clinical tool in speech-language pathology and audiology, but it can also be used as an educational, social policy, or research tool.

- Health and disease should be seen as points on a continuum, especially with older people.

- Communication ability and disability form a continuum.

- Audiologists and speech-language pathologists could play a role with all older people along this continuum, whether the older person has a recognizable communication disability or not.

- Health promotion with well older people and providing services to those with subclinical communicative disabilities are not traditional roles for audiologists and speech-language pathologists.

- Healthy aging is a major policy trend in many countries.

- Audiologists and speech-language pathologists may have a role in healthy aging, particularly in the maintenance of social and psychological health.

- Communication Accommodation Theory explains the process of how two people accommodate to each other's communicative patterns.

- Under- and overaccommodation during interactions with older people should be a major concern for speech-language pathologists and audiologists.

CLASS ACTIVITIES

- Does your country have an explicit commitment to healthy aging? Look at relevant Web pages. How does this affect services to older people in your country?

- Categorize some of the tests you use in the clinical situation with older people into the WHO dimensions. Describe some rehabilitation goals in each of the WHO dimensions.

- Watch a talk show on television. How do the interactants accommodate to each other? How do you accommodate to an older person? How do you accommodate to an older person with a communication disability? Describe a situation in which you under- or overaccommodated in an interaction.

RECOMMENDED READINGS

Chodzko-Zajko, W. J., Ringel, R. L., & Vaca, V. L. (1995). Biogerontology:

Implications for the communication sciences. In R. A. Huntley & K. S. Helfer (Eds.), *Communication in later life* (pp. 3–21). Boston: Butterworth Heinemann.

Cruice, M., Worrall, L., & Hickson, L. (2000). Measurement of quality-of-life in speech pathology and audiology. *Asia Pacific Journal of Speech, Language and Hearing, 5*(1), 1–20.

Davis, C. M. (1996). Psychosocial aspects of aging. In C. Bernstein Lewis (Ed.), *Aging, the health care challenge: An interdisciplinary approach to assessment and rehabilitative management of the elderly* (3rd ed., pp. 18–44). Philadelphia: F. A. Davis.

McIntosh, I. (1996). Interaction between professionals and older people: Where does the problem lie? *Health Care in Later Life, 1*(1), 29–38.

Ringel, R. L., & Chodzko-Zajko, W. J. (1988). Age, health, and the speech process. *Seminars in Speech and Language, 9*(2), 95–107.

Ryan, E. B., Meredith, S. D., MacLean, M., & Orange, J. B. (1995). Changing the way we talk with elders: Promoting health using the Communication Enhancement Model. *International Journal of Aging and Human Development, 41*(2), 89–107.

World Health Organization. (2001b). *International classification of functioning, disability and health. ICF Introduction.* http://www3.who.int/icf/icftemplate.cfm. Geneva: Author.

REFERENCES

Bishop, B. (1999, March). The National Strategy for an Aging Australia: Healthy Aging Discussion Paper. www.health.gov.au/acc/nsaa/hadp/index.htm

Butler, R. (1991). Foreword. In J. Birren & D. Deutchman, *Guiding autobiography groups for older adults.* Baltimore: John Hopkins University Press.

Caporael, L. R. (1981). The paralanguage of caregiving: Baby talk to the institutionalized aged. *Journal of the Personality and Social Psychology, 40,* 876–884.

Chodzko-Zajko, W. J., Ringel, R. L., & Vaca, V. L. (1995). Biogerontology: Implications for the communication sciences. In R. A. Huntley & K. S. Helfer (Eds.), *Communication in later life* (pp. 3–21). Boston: Butterworth-Heinemann.

Cruice, M., Worrall, L., & Hickson, L. (2000). Measurement of quality-of-life in speech pathology and audiology. *Asia Pacific Journal of Speech, Language and Hearing, 5*(1), 1–20.

Davis, C. M. (1996). Psychosocial aspects of aging. In C. Bernstein Lewis (Ed.), *Aging, the health care challenge: An interdisciplinary approach to assessment and rehabilitative management of the elderly* (3rd ed., pp. 18–44). Philadelphia: F. A. Davis.

Enderby, P., & John, A. (1997). *Therapy outcome measures: Speech-language pathology.* Clifton Park, NY: Delmar Learning.

Giles, H., Coupland, N., & Coupland, J. (Eds.). (1991). *The contexts of accommodation.* New York: Cambridge University Press.

Goleman, D. (1995). *Emotional intelligence.* New York: Bantam.

Lubinski, R. (1995). State-of-the-art perspectives on communication in nursing homes. *Topics in Language Disorders, 15*(2) 1–19.

Lubinski, R. (1997). Perspectives on aging and communication. In R. Lubinski & D. J. Higginbotham (Eds.), *Communication technologies for the elderly* (pp. 1–22). Clifton Park, NY: Delmar Learning.

McDowell, I., & Newell, C. (1996). *Measuring health: A guide to rating scales and questionnaires* (2nd ed.). New York: Oxford University Press.

McIntosh, I. (1996). Interaction between professionals and older people: Where does the problem lie? *Health Care in Later Life, 1*(1), 29–38.

Ottawa Charter for Health Promotion. (1986). First International Conference on Health Promotion. *Health Promotion, 1,* iii–v.

Ringel, R. L., & Chodzko-Zajko, W. J. (1988). Age, health, and the speech process. *Seminars in Speech and Language, 9*(2), 95–107.

Russell, R. D. (1973). Social health: An attempt to clarify this dimension of well-being. *International Journal of Health Education, 16,* 74–82.

Ryan, E. B., Giles, H., Bartolucci, G., & Henwood, K. (1986) Psycholinguistic and social psychological components of communication by and with the elderly. *Language and Communication, 6,* 1–24.

Ryan, E. B., Meredith, S. D., MacLean, M., & Orange, J. B. (1995). Changing the way we talk with elders: Promoting health using the Communication Enhancement Model. *International Journal of Aging and Human Development, 41*(2) 89–107.

Worrall, L., Hickson, L., Barnett, H., & Yiu, E. (1998). An evaluation of the *Keep on Talking* program for maintaining communication skills into old age. *Educational Gerontology, 24*(2), 129–140.

World Health Organization. (1980). *International classification of impairment, disability and handicap.* Geneva: Author.

World Health Organization. (2001a). *International classification of functioning, disability and health.* Geneva: Author.

World Health Organization. (2001b). *International classification of functioning, disability and health. ICF Introduction.* http://www3.who.int/icf/icftemplate.cfm. Geneva: Author.

World Health Organization (2002). *Active ageing: A policy framework.* http://www.who.int/hpr/ageing/ActiveAgeingPolicyFrame.pdf. Geneva: Author.

Chapter 3

Models of Practice in the Management of Older People with Communication Disabilities

Three models of practice can be employed when working with older people who have communication disability: (a) the medical model, which is focused on impairments; (b) the rehabilitation model, which is focused on everyday communication activities; and (c) the social model, which is focused on participation in society. A key difference among these three models is the approach to clinical decision making. The medical model applies a directive approach, whereas the rehabilitation model uses informed decision making, and the social model is based on shared decision making. This chapter describes best practice in terms of a process in which the clinician determines his or her preferred service delivery model, as well as that of the organization in which he or she works, and each client. It is argued that different models are appropriate in different contexts and for different clients and that flexibility is essential to providing the best possible service to older people with communication disability.

It is essential for speech-language pathologists and audiologists to understand the nature of different models of service delivery in health care and the effects of those service delivery models on clients. If these issues are not understood, professionals risk failing their clients and organizational superiors. This risk exists because different models are associated with different value systems and attitudes on the part of the client, the clinician, and the organization. Sometimes the service delivery model is dictated by the organization and/or the payer (e.g., health insurance organizations), sometimes it is a personal choice on the part of the clinician, and sometimes it is dictated by the client, if the clinician and organization are prepared to listen. In the sections that follow, three commonly applied service delivery models are described along with the attitudes and values associated with each. Although presented here as three distinct models, it is recognized that service delivery frequently falls along a continuum with a medical model at one extreme and the social model at the other.

Medical Model

In the medical model of service delivery for people with communication disability the focus is on the person's impairment. The medical model, which has also been called the disease or clinical model, has a long history. In this model, the people who seek services are typically called patients, and the problems they experience are referred to as illnesses, diseases, or pathologies. People are frequently described in terms of their disability (e.g., the aphasic, the deaf girl) rather than being a person first (e.g., the man with aphasia, the girl with hearing impairment). The focus is on the condition, not on the person, or his or her relationship with others and with society. Erdman, Wark, and Montano (1994) pointed out that a key feature of different service delivery models is the communication that occurs between the service provider and the person receiving services. In the medical model, the locus of control of any communicative interaction rests with the clinician. The client's role is as a passive recipient of care.

This directive approach to patient care is most typically used in acute care settings such as hospitals, but it is important to realize that it is not limited to such settings. For example, in many rehabilitation settings, a patient's impairments are determined on entry and a schedule of treatments for those impairments is organized, with little involvement of the client or significant others. Audiologists and speech-language pathologists generally apply the medical model of service delivery in settings in which they encounter older people with communication disability, because this is the model of service delivery with which they are most familiar (Holland, 1994; Madell & Montano, 2000).

Why is this approach so popular? First, it is efficient in terms of time. The course of action (assessment, diagnosis, treatment, discharge) is determined by the clinician with little need for time-consuming discussions with the client. Such efficiency can be extremely popular within an organizational structure suffering from lack of adequate levels of funding. Second, it can be comfortable for the clinician to assume the role of expert and prescribe, without challenge, a course of treatment. Third, agist attitudes of clinicians may prevent them from involving the older individual in the decision-making process. This issue may be difficult for speech-language pathologists and audiologists to acknowledge, but it is one that requires some reflection. Are clients not given choices for intervention because of their age and an assumed level of incompetence? Finally, it is what audiologists and speech-language pathologists have been taught to do and therefore feel most comfortable with. For example, ASHA's scope of practice document for audiologists (ASHA, 1996a) defines audiologists as "autonomous professionals who identify, assess, and manage disorders of the auditory, balance, and other neural systems" (p. 13). The complementary document on scope of practice for speech-language pathologists in that year (ASHA, 1996b) begins with a more participatory statement: "The goal of the profession of speech-language pathology and its members is provision of the highest quality treatment and other services consistent with the fundamental right of those served to participate in decisions that affect their lives" (p. 17). However, the document then goes on to list disabilities that speech-language pathologists treat. The more recent version (ASHA, 2001) describes the scope of practice of speech-language pathologists within the whole WHO model.

Although the medical model has frequently been criticized for its lack of a client-centered focus and not allowing clients more involvement in treatment decisions, it is conceded that there are situations in which this approach is what clients want. For example, in audiology practice, some clients find the decision about which hearing aid to choose overwhelming and will ask the audiologist to make the decision: "You choose, you know what's best." In speech-language pathology practice, a person with dysphagia following stroke is likely to be a passive recipient of care because of the trauma that has just occurred and because of the general effects of the stroke.

However, many older clients have chronic communication disability that requires long-term intervention, and other models of service delivery need to be considered for best practice. Moves away from the traditional medical model are propelled by the needs and expectations of clients, the changing attitudes of clinicians, the advocacy work of consumer groups, and the demands of funding agencies for improved outcomes (Coulter, 1997). For the funding agencies, the issue is that the directive medical approach has been associated with poor treatment compliance (e.g., the patient does not take the prescribed medication because he or she does not understand its importance), leading to questionable functional outcomes (Erdman et al., 1994). Even though the clinician determines the diagnosis and the treatment, in general, it is the client who judges the outcome. "Actively engaging patients in the identification of the problems they wish to address and in the treatment they perceive to be most relevant throughout the provision of services enhances the likelihood that outcome will be successful" (Erdman et al., 1994, p. 48).

The key features of the medical model are summarized in Table 3–1. The table also allows features of the medical model to be compared to those of the rehabilitation and social

TABLE 3–1

FEATURES OF THREE MODELS OF SERVICE DELIVERY FOR WORKING WITH OLDER PEOPLE WITH COMMUNICATION DISABILITY.

	Medical Model	Rehabilitation Model	Social Model
What is the main level of the WHO model?	Impairment	Activity	Participation
What is the source of the person's difficulties?	The person's impairment (i.e., biological or physiological problem)	The person's inability to function in everyday activities	A disabling or non-inclusive society
What is the focus of intervention?	On the communication impairment itself	On the person with communication disability	On the interaction between the person and society and the reduction of barriers to participation
What is the goal of intervention?	To reduce the impairment	To improve ability to function	To enhance quality of life
What is disability?	A problem or illness to be cured	A person to be restored to function	A difference, rather than a problem.
Who mainly determines services provided?	Health professional	Health professional and the client	The client
What is the decision-making process used in intervention?	Directive, top-down	Informed	Shared, collaborative
Where is this model most often used?	Hospital, acute care settings	Rehabilitation unit	Residential care facilities, community centers

models, which are discussed in the following sections. A move along the continuum from the medical to a more social approach requires that audiologists and speech-language pathologists understand the concepts associated with different models and, perhaps most important, have an ability to be flexible and to really listen to what their clients are saying.

Rehabilitation Model

The main differences between the medical and rehabilitation models are related to the management focus and the approach to decision making throughout the therapeutic process (see Table 3–1). In the medical model, the focus of assessment and intervention is on the impairment (i.e., biological or physiological focus); in the rehabilitation model, the focus is shifted to the person with the impairment and his or her ability to function in everyday life. Thus, in addition to measuring impairment, it is necessary to assess the activity limitations associated with impairment. For example, in audiology, application of a rehabilitation model of service delivery demands that the assessment include self-report measures of communication disability as well as standard audiometric tests such as pure-tone and impedance audiometry. In speech-language pathology, an example of a rehabilitation model of service is when aphasia treatment is focused on everyday functional communication activities such as telephoning or chairing a meeting, as well as reducing the language impairment itself.

The focus of the rehabilitation model is on the older person's activity limitations, which is a shift away from the focus on impairments in the medical model. This shift requires an associated attitude change on the part of the speech-language pathologist and the audiologist. It is necessary to acknowledge that tests of clinical impairment do not provide an adequate or complete picture of the difficulties encountered in everyday life by the older person with communication disability. The focus on activity limitations is not a problem for clients, because it is almost always the everyday effects of the impairment that have motivated them to seek assistance. For example, when older people with hearing impairment are asked about the difficulties they are having, they do not reply that their hearing at high frequencies is reduced. They say "I can't understand what people are saying when there is noise in the background" or "I can't hear the telephone ring." Similarly, in speech-language pathology, clients with dysarthria do not complain of restricted articulatory function, but rather of problems they are having being understood by others.

In terms of decision making, the rehabilitation model approach includes more involvement of the client and is best described as informed decision making. The client is provided with information about assessment and management options by the clinician and, following discussion between both parties, a decision is made about how to proceed. This decision is frequently based on a recommendation from the clinician. There is far greater communication between client and clinician than in the medical model, and the communication is more balanced. This change to communication between clinician and client often needs to be initiated by the clinician, who is seen as being in a position of power in the interaction. Many clients, particularly older adults who have operated within the medical model for decades, do not feel comfortable asking for more information, and the clinician needs to be sensitive to this situation and routinely offer information.

Coulter (1997) described a process of informed decision making, called the Patient Partnership strategy, which was recommended for use in the United Kingdom by the National Health Service. This strategy emphasizes "the need to provide patients with the information they need to make informed choices about their treatment" (p. 112). Coulter goes on to address some of the concerns that clinicians have about informed decision making. These concerns are illustrated in Figure 3–1.

It is true that some clients in some circumstances do not want to make decisions. Research suggests that younger people and people with higher education levels are more likely to want to participate in decision making (Cassileth, Zupkis, Sutton-Smith, & March, 1980; Strull, Lo, & Charles, 1984); however, the wishes of a client in this regard should never be assumed based on group effects. For example, a well-educated older woman recently complained to us that she had to insist on participation in decision making about her finan-

---

- Clients do not want to make their own decisions.

- Some things are too complex to explain.

- If we tell people too much about the risks and related factors, this can worry them unnecessarily.

- What do I know, really, about this problem?

- What if they choose the wrong treatment and then blame me because it did not work?

- People will not make the right choices.

- It just takes too much time.

- Clients will be too demanding.

FIGURE 3–1. Concerns clinicians have about involving clients in decision making. Adapted from Coulter (1997).

cial investments, as staff at the bank had assumed she would not want to be so involved because of her age and gender. As to concerns about telling clients too much about medical issues and worrying them unnecessarily, Coulter cited some research studies showing that involving people in decisions improved their health and well-being. Similarly, many of the other perceived obstacles to a change in decision making processes (see Figure 3–1) may be based on incorrect assumptions about what will happen, rather than the reality.

One of the problems in implementing shared decision making is the time required to provide additional information and the need for consumer-friendly forms of information. Coulter (1997) recommended that one way to get around these problems is to develop appropriate resources that can be given to the client to take away and consider. An example of this is a series of interactive video programs (with supporting written information) that has been developed by the U.S.-based Foundation for Informed Decision-Making (Kasper, Mulley, & Wennberg, 1992) illustrating common medical conditions and treatment options. Such materials could also be developed for older people with communication disability and would need to take into account the communication difficulties of this client group, for example,

- large-print text for those with visual difficulties, using bold lettering on clear visual backgrounds,

- simplified text with pictures for those with written comprehension problems,

- captioning on video material for people with hearing impairment and other auditory comprehension problems.

Clients need research-based evidence about treatment options and outcomes provided in a format they can understand and use to make decisions. There is a particular need for this in audiology, where older clients have to make decisions about the selection of hearing aids. Research evidence on the efficacy of different types of hearing aids is available to the public on databases such as PubMed (www.ncbi.nlm.nih.gov/PubMed) and the Cochrane Library (www.cochrane.hcn.net.au); this information may, however, still be difficult for clients to access and understand. Thus, there is a need for relevant and appropriate information to assist clients with communication disability to make informed decisions, and this need will require some considered thought and planning by the clinician. Material would be most appropriately developed in collaboration with relevant consumer organizations; such groups are generally aware of the needs of consumers in this regard.

In summary, the rehabilitation model of service delivery emphasizes the person with the communication impairment (rather than the impairment itself), his or her everyday life activities, and client involvement in the decision-making process. In speech-language pathology, this model has often been termed the functional approach (Worrall, 2000a). The rehabilitation model approach has been recommended many times for use in audiology and is also referred to as a client-centered problem-solving process (Erdman et al., 1994; Gagné, 1998; Madell & Montano, 2000; Stephens, 1996). When considering the person with hearing impairment in a real-life context, some researchers have talked about using an ecological approach to audiological rehabilitation. Ecological audiology considers the client and his or her communication partners in the context of their environment and real-life situations (Gagné, Hétu, Getty, & McDuff, 1995; Noble & Hétu, 1994), although the focus is still firmly on the client. This concept appears to be broader than the rehabilitation model, but not as broad as the social model.

Social Model

In the social model of service delivery, the client is seen, first and foremost, in the context of the society in which he or she lives. Communication is, by nature, interactive and therefore has a social dimension. The problems encountered by individuals with communication disability in everyday life are not just their problems, but are caused by a disabling society. For this reason, the social model has also been called the *social barriers* model (Finkelstein, 1991), the *social oppression* model (Oliver, 1983), and the *accessibility* model (Pichora-Fuller, 1994). The focus of intervention is on the client's effective participation in society, and thus the social model is most closely related to the participation level of the WHO model (2001). The features of the social model as they relate to speech-language pathology and audiology practice are summarized in Table 3–1.

Successful application of the social model requires open communication between client and clinician. Decision making is shared and collaborative, with the pendulum swinging more toward the views of the client than in the informed decision-making process of the rehabilitation model. In the social model, the goal of any intervention is not just to improve function in everyday life, but to improve a person's quality of life. This shift in emphasis is in line with the health care policies for older people of many developed countries, which are aimed at health promotion and enhancing quality of life.

Sometimes, this broader quality-of-life goal can be achieved by working at the levels of impairment and activity in the clinic situation, but sometimes it demands that the clinician and client move out of the clinical situation and address the barriers to participation in society. For example, if a client with a hearing impairment wants to use a public telephone, it may not be enough to ensure that the client has a hearing aid with sufficient amplification and a telecoil and that he or she knows how to use the hearing aid. What if the public telephone system does not include a telecoil? This calls for society and consumer advocacy action: letters to telephone companies and government organizations. As Simmons-Mackie (2000) pointed out, improved ability to communicate does not necessarily mean improved participation in communication situations. Jordan and Kaiser (1996) described a number of societal level projects that have been undertaken in the United Kingdom to allow people with aphasia to participate in everyday life. For example, shops that welcome people with speech and language impairments have been encouraged to place identifying signs in their windows. In another situation, professionals involved in court proceedings in which a witness had aphasia were provided with information about aphasia and the most effective way of communicating with the witness.

Adoption of a social model of service delivery, rather than the more traditional and commonly used medical or rehabilitation models, requires a shift in attitudes and values on the part of speech-language pathologists and audiologists. Because social work was the first profession to take up the social model of disability (Oliver, 1983), Worrall (2000b) argued that values of that profession have application to communication professions in this context (Table 3–2). Hepworth and Larsen (1982) defined the values of a profession as "strongly held beliefs about people, preferred goals for people, preferred means of achiev-

TABLE 3–2

SOCIAL WORK VALUES AND THEIR APPLICATION TO SPEECH-LANGUAGE PATHOLOGY AND AUDIOLOGY PRACTICE.

Social Work Value	Application to Speech-Language Pathology and Audiology
Shared decision making	Can be used from the initial appointment to set goals and determine all management options.
Uniqueness of individuals	Recognition that all clients have unique communication needs and these should be the focus of assessment and intervention.
Strengths perspective	Focus on the client's strengths and work with these. Clients should be encouraged to identify their own strategies and solutions.
Social justice	Audiologists and speech-language pathologists need to influence society to be more inclusive of people with communication disability.
Accountability	It is necessary to be accountable to clients and to organizations.

Note: Adapted from Worrall (2000b).

ing those goals, and preferred conditions of life. Stated simply, values represent selected ideals as to how the world should be and how people should normally act" (p. 20). Curtis (1998) proposed that the four major values in rehabilitation are altruism (i.e., belief in the individual), choice (i.e., the freedom to make choices), empowerment (i.e., the ability to act on choices), and equality (i.e., the belief in each individual's worth and dignity). If audiologists and speech-language pathologists want to apply the social model of service delivery, and it is suggested that in many contexts this model would represent best practice for older people with communication disability, then they need to think about their own value systems.

What are the values of the professions of audiology and speech-language pathology? When students are asked this question, typically they identify three major values.

1. Communication is essential for quality of life.
2. People with communication disability are marginalized and disadvantaged in society.
3. All people with communication disability should have access to speech-language pathology and audiology services.

Aspects of the social model have already been incorporated into some approaches in audiology and speech-language pathology. Ecological audiology, for example, emphasizes the context of the individual client (e.g., the communication environment, communication partners). Intervention for a person with hearing impairment goes beyond the individual and his or her disability and addresses the disabling conditions in the individual's physical and social environments (Noble & Hétu, 1994). If a person with hearing impairment has difficulty understanding in the presence of background noise, many features of the physical environment can be modified to reduce noise and reverberation. If communication with family members is problematic, social environment interventions such as education of family members about appropriate communication strategies may be beneficial.

Another example of application of the social model in audiology follows an approach first described by Green and Kreuter (1991) and is found in Carson and Pichora-Fuller's (1997) description of a health promotion program for older people with hearing impairment in an extended care facility. The program is developed, implemented, and evaluated collaboratively among clinicians and the community participants. The developmental phase includes a detailed analysis of the society in which the older people live, based on questions such as the following.

- What are the community's social priorities?
- What are the specific health goals that contribute to these social priorities?
- What behaviors or environmental factors are linked to the health goals?

- What are the behavioral and educational objectives for the program and the strategies to be used?
- What resources are needed?

On the basis of the responses, specific behavioral, environmental, and educational objectives are formulated. Examples for each of these objectives collaboratively set by residents, family, staff, and administrators include:

Behavioral Objective: After 1 year, there will be a 40% increase in the number of hearing aids worn for part of each day by residents who owned, but did not wear, hearing aids at the start of the program.

Environmental Objective: By the end of the third month, an assessment of the acoustic environment of the extended care facility's group listening areas will be completed.

Educational Objective: By the end of the seventh month, a wide-area infrared assistive listening device will have been installed in one of the group listening areas in the facility.

Although applied in a community context, Carson and Pichora-Fuller maintain that the approach can also be used in planning programs for individuals.

Recently, there has been a move toward the social model of service delivery by speech-language pathologists (e.g., Jordan & Kaiser, 1996), especially by those who are proponents of functional communication approaches (see Worrall & Frattali, 2000). The social model is seen as having broad application to older people with communication disability and to adults with a range of neurogenic communication disability. A groundbreaking example of this is The Aphasia Institute in North York, Ontario, Canada (www.aphasia.on.ca/index.shtml). Kagan and Gailey (1993) described their approach to aphasia as analogous to providing wheelchair ramps for people with physical disability. The ramps in this case are volunteers who are trained to be skilled conversational partners with people with aphasia. Another example of how speech-language pathology is incorporating the social model into practice is the social-environmental approach to traumatic brain injury (Ylvisaker, Feeney, & Urbanczyk, 1993). This approach advocates a positive communication culture within the environment of the person with traumatic brain injury. In rehabilitation facilities, communicative competence is written into the job descriptions of direct care staff, and communication partner training extends beyond the traditional hour or two of in-service training.

To this point, the three major models of service delivery that can be applied when working with older people with communication disability have been described. Each model focuses on a different WHO dimension, and each requires a different approach to decision making. To clarify the differences among these models, the application of each model to particular cases is outlined in the following section.

Models in Action: Case Studies

Mrs. Pryor

Mrs. Pryor is 66 years old and has noticed increasing difficulties understanding what people are saying over the last few years. She decides to make an appointment to see an audiologist.

Medical Model

The audiologist takes a case history relating to presenting problem, onset of loss, right/left ear differences, tinnitus, vertigo, previous ear disease, and medical history. Pure-tone, impedance, and speech audiometry are performed and the results are consistent with a bilateral moderate sensorineural hearing loss with no significant asymmetry. Mrs. Pryor is told that the results show she has a hearing loss in both ears, which is most probably age related. No medical action is required, and Mrs. Pryor is told that binaural in-the-ear hearing aids would be appropriate for her. She agrees and ear impressions are made. An appointment is scheduled in 2 weeks for hearing aid fitting.

Rehabilitation Model

The audiologist takes a case history relating to presenting problem, onset of loss, right/left ear differences, tinnitus, vertigo, previous ear disease, and medical history. The audiologist also asks Mrs. Pryor to outline all of the everyday listening situations that are difficult for her and to describe what motivated her to have a hearing test at the present time. Pure-tone, impedance, and speech audiometry are performed, and results are consistent with a bilateral moderate sensorineural hearing loss with no significant asymmetry. Mrs. Pryor is given a questionnaire to complete that asks her about the degree of difficulty she has in a range of everyday listening situations. She reports always having problems hearing if someone speaks from a distance or if there is noise in the background. She sometimes has difficulty understanding speakers on television. Mrs. Pryor is told that the results show she has a hearing loss in both ears, which is most probably age related. No medical action is required.

The audiologist tells Mrs. Pryor there is a range of audiological services that would benefit her (i.e., hearing aids, assistive listening devices, communication strategies), but that the most beneficial would be the fitting of binaural in-the-ear hearing aids. Mrs. Pryor is asked how she feels about wearing hearing aids. She is a little unsure and wants to know more before making a decision. The audiologist tells her about the hearing aids that are suitable for her and describes how they might help her in the situations that are problematic for her. Mrs. Pryor agrees to the hearing aid fitting, and ear impressions are made. An appointment is scheduled in 2 weeks for hearing aid fitting. Mrs. Pryor is given written information about hearing loss and the hearing aids to take home and read.

Social Model

The audiologist takes a case history relating to presenting problem, onset of loss, right/left ear differences, tinnitus, vertigo, previous ear disease, and medical history. The audiologist also asks Mrs. Pryor to outline all the everyday listening situations that are difficult for her and to describe what motivated her to have a hearing test at the present time. The audiologist also asks Mrs. Pryor if her difficulties understanding what people are saying have limited her social activities in recent years and whether the problem worsened. She is asked if she has any difficulties communicating with certain people in her social network; that is, are some people more difficult for her to communicate with than others? Mrs. Pryor reports she has been having difficulty when communicating with her sister. She is asked about the social activities she was involved in 5 years ago and asked to consider if her hearing problems have caused her to drop out of any activities. If so, is she interested in returning to these activities? She says that she stopped going to the theater a few years ago because she could not understand the actors and that she used to attend art classes, but found these difficult.

Pure-tone, impedance, and speech audiometry are performed, and the results are consistent with a bilateral moderate sensorineural hearing loss with no significant asymmetry. Mrs. Pryor is told that the results show she has a hearing loss in both ears, which is most probably age related. No medical action is required. The audiologist advises Mrs. Pryor there are a number of options from this point on and that it is her decision how to proceed. She is asked to consider what she would like to achieve. Does she want to understand conversations? Does she want to hear the television better? Does she want to go back to the theater and the art classes? Depending on Mrs. Pryor's priorities, goals are set for ongoing rehabilitation. A discussion follows about the range of options that will help her achieve her goals such as hearing aid fitting, auditory training, assistive listening devices, modifications to the physical environment, family counseling, attending a consumer support organization, a communication education program, and so on. Mrs. Pryor says she needs time to consider these options and to discuss them with her family. A follow-up appointment is scheduled in 2 weeks. Mrs. Pryor is given any relevant written information she requests, and she is invited to bring along a friend or family member.

In this example of the application of the social model to audiological assessment, impairment and activity level assessments are included; however, the focus is more on participation than in the medical or rehabilitation model. In addition, there is greater emphasis on shared decision making than in the other two approaches.

Mr. Lawson

Mr. Lawson is a well-educated, 74-year-old who had a stroke 8 months ago. He has a mild-moderate dysarthria accompanied by a mild anomic aphasia. He is seeking ongoing treatment for his speech and language difficulties and has an appointment with the speech-language pathologist in the hospital where he was treated for his stroke.

Medical Model

The speech-language pathologist has the results of Mr. Lawson's most recent Western Aphasia Assessment (Kertesz, 1982) and Frenchay Dysarthria Assessment (Enderby, 1983). These show that naming of objects is poor and that there are significant impairments in tongue and lip strength. The speech-language pathologist agrees to provide weekly therapy and starts directly on tongue and lip exercises in the clinic, including written worksheets for home practice. Naming skills are targeted through word-picture matching in the clinic and sentence completion worksheets for home practice.

Rehabilitation Model

The speech-language pathologist has Mr. Lawson's most recent Western Aphasia Assessment (Kertesz, 1982) and Frenchay Dysarthria Assessment (Enderby, 1983) results. At this appointment, the speech-language pathologist uses a checklist of everyday communication activities, like those provided by Payne (1994) or Worrall (1999), to determine which everyday communication activities should be the focus of treatment. Mr. Lawson and his wife are provided with options about which everyday communicative activities could be the focus of rehabilitation. Mr. Lawson and his wife choose to focus on strategies that Mr. Lawson can use to answer the telephone while his wife is out. Therapy every 2 weeks with Mr. Lawson and his wife enables Mr. Lawson to function more independently at home and allows his wife to leave Mr. Lawson by himself on occasions.

Social Model

In the initial interview with Mr. Lawson and his wife, it became apparent that, although Mr. Lawson wanted to improve his intelligibility and naming, it was important for him to be able to answer the telephone. He was feeling useless, and Mr. and Mrs. Lawson both felt they were not enjoying their retirement years. The speech-language pathologist referred Mr. Lawson to the local Aphasia Center where he became involved in organizing a conference for people with aphasia. Because his aphasia was mild, he was able to register participants at the conference and lead a discussion group about the effect of aphasia on life. His wife was asked to present the spouse's perspective at the conference and in her research for the paper found that many spouses used a variety of methods for enjoying their retirement years despite the presence of aphasia. This experience empowered them to travel the world together and enjoy their retirement years.

Selecting Models of Practice

The question remains: What is the best model for use in gerontological audiology and speech-language pathology? Different models may be appropriately used in different contexts, and the best practice in any particular instance depends on the values and goals of the clinician, of the organization delivering the service, and of the client. The following sections contain a step-by-step description of a process for the clinician to determine best practice, taking into account these factors (Figure 3–2).

Step 1: Self-Reflection

Initially, the clinician should consider what his or her values and beliefs are about provision of services to older people with communication disability.

- Do I believe that all older people are individuals? Do I believe that agism is systemic in society? Are people with communication disability discriminated against?

- Is shared decision making important? Does it work? Will my clients want this? Will my clients benefit? Are they capable of making management decisions? Do I have the time to devote to this?

- What should be the focus of intervention? What kind of treatment will really help them? Who should decide the goals of treatment?

- Should I get involved with the client's family and others in their social group? Is this my role?

Reflection on their responses to these questions should help clinicians become aware of their preferred model of service delivery. Sometimes these preferences are based on clinicians' own values related to therapeutic intervention and familiarity with a particular model (i.e., what they prefer when seeing a health professional), and sometimes preferences have developed from previous work experience. Although an individual clinician may have a clear preference for one particular model of service delivery, it is the clinician's professional responsibility to be flexible about models of service and be able to adapt appropriately to different contexts, that is, to the varying needs of clients and organizations. Thus, working with older people with communication disability requires clinicians to be capable of self-reflection and flexibility.

Step 2: Consider the Organizational Context

Because the culture of an organization has an effect on both the clinician and the client, it is important to determine the preferred model of service delivery of the organization in which

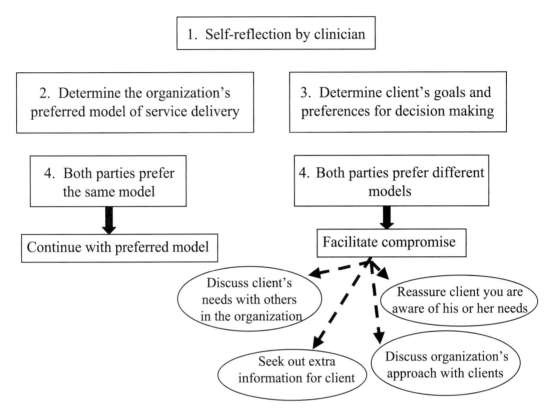

FIGURE 3–2. Process to guide the clinician in best practice of service delivery for older people with communication disability.

the service is being offered. One way to do this is to reflect on the likely responses of colleagues and superiors to Questions 2 through 7 in Table 3–1. Additional questions to consider are

- Do colleagues involve clients in decisions about their management? How do they react if a client wants something other than the recommended treatment? Do they get annoyed with clients who do not take their advice?

- Do they believe that people with communication disability are capable of making choices for themselves?

- Do they actively involve the client's family and significant others in the management process? Do they consider this their role? Is this seen as something only a social worker should do?

- Do they believe that if they fix the client's problem, then all other aspects of their lives will improve?

In terms of generalizations, it seems that the preferred model of service delivery for organizations is linked to the length of time clients are associated with the organization. In acute care settings, such as hospitals and specialist clinics, it is most likely that a medical model will be applied; in centers where people spend more time (e.g., for ongoing rehabilitation following stroke, for aural rehabilitation), it is likely that a rehabilitation model will be applied; and in places where people participate in long-term intervention (e.g., extended care facilities, community centers), it is likely that a social model will be preferred. This preference is not always the case, however, and it is important for clinicians to think about the organizations in which they work and not make assumptions about the model. For example, many residential care facilities for the aged and skilled nursing facilities emphasize nursing care (e.g., bed sore treatment, incontinence management), ignoring the fact that the facility is also the person's home and society.

Step 3: Consider the Individual Client

Once the clinician has determined his or her values and beliefs and the preferred model of service delivery of the organization, a preferred model of practice emerges. This model becomes the platform from which to determine the preferred model of service delivery for each client. Views of the clinician and the organization may alter over time, but are unlikely to change rapidly. The daily changes the clinician has to deal with are those associated with different clients: Each individual client is unique and has his or her own values, beliefs, and preferences for management. There are two major issues the clinician needs to address for each client in order to know how to proceed.

First, the clinician needs to discuss with the client his or her goals for intervention: What would the client like to achieve, what would the client like the speech-language pathologist or audiologist to help him or her with. How these levels relate to the levels of the WHO model (2001) will give the clinician guidance about how to proceed. For example, if a person is mainly concerned with regaining facial symmetry following a unilateral facial paralysis, this goal is at the impairment level. If a person wants to be able to hear the television at a reasonable volume, this goal is at the activity level. If a person wants to be able to join in the community meetings at the retirement village, even with a communication disability, this is a participation level goal. These goals relate to the medical, rehabilitation, and social models, respectively (see Table 3–1). In terms of generalizations again, it is the authors' experience that the goals of clients, like the views of the organizations, are also associated with time. Clients who have an acute illness tend to focus on the impairments that have just occurred. They think about getting back what they have lost and not about how to function in everyday life and in society in the long term. Clients with chronic conditions do think about longer term goals and therefore usually prefer to focus on goals related to everyday activities and participation in society.

Second, the clinician needs to determine the client's preferences regarding decision making. This determination most probably will be evident during the discussion about treatment goals and can be explored further by asking explicit questions about decision making, such as

- Do you want more information to make a decision?
- Would you like to consider these options and let me know your decision next time?
- Do you feel comfortable making decisions about how we should proceed?
- Do you want me to decide what we should do?
- Do you want me to recommend what you should do?

Step 4: Matching of Preferences

In many cases, both the client and the organization will prefer the same model of service delivery, and the speech-language pathologist or audiologist should continue with this approach. However, there will be instances when they do not have the same preferences, and it will be necessary for the clinician to facilitate a compromise. Mismatches between what the organization values and what the client values can be problematic, as the following examples illustrate.

If the organization prefers a medical model or is constrained to the medical model by their economic circumstances, it would be expected that the clinician emphasize short-term management and engage in a set regimen of assessment, diagnosis, and individual treatment for clients. A client, on the other hand, may clearly indicate that he or she is not ready to go ahead with assessment at this stage and wants more information about options (e.g., *Do I really need to see a speech-language pathologist or will I be able to manage by myself? Will this really affect my ability to live my life when I return home? Will treatment work?*). The clinician should try to provide clients with what they need and explain to the organization why client management needs to be different from the usual for this client (see ideas in Figure 3–2). Alternatively, the clinician should put the client in touch with a service provider who can respond to the client's needs.

Another example is when an organization prefers a social model of service delivery and expects clients to be involved in decisions about their management at every stage. It would also be expected that the clinician involve a range of stakeholders (e.g., family members, caregivers) in the communication issues the client wants to address. A client who is more comfortable with a medical model of service delivery may feel pressured by the need to always make choices. The client might also value privacy and be unhappy that caregivers and family members are talking about his or her issues. It is important for the clinician to accept the wishes of the client and advise others in the organization of the client's wishes. In this way, the speech-language pathologist or audiologist is working as an advocate for the client. It is particularly important that clinicians assume this role, as many clients have communication disabilities that prevent them from expressing their needs.

Best practice in any particular situation demands that the goals and concerns of the client are paramount. The clinician may begin by examining his or her own values and beliefs and then realize that to provide the best possible service to older people with communication disability, he or she needs to be flexible and willing to listen to what a client wants. The clinician should consider the values of the organization in which he or she works and try to reconcile the organization's goals with those of the client.

Summary

In summary, this chapter described the principles and values underlying three methods of service delivery for older people with communication disability. These models of practice are not mutually exclusive. There are overlaps among them, and clinicians will often use aspects of all three models for different clients and contexts. In working with older people with communication disability, speech-language pathologists and audiologists need to be familiar with, and be able to apply, each of these models. Being a good health professional is not just about providing good assessments and treatments, it is also about being able to reflect on which approaches work best with each client and in each setting. It is important to be flexible about what is the best way. No one model of service delivery is always best and an understanding of this concept represents a major paradigm shift for some clinicians who happily work in one model only.

KEY POINTS

- Three models of practice are used when working with older people who have communication disability: the medical model, the rehabilitation model, and the social model.
- The medical model is characterized by a focus on impairments and a directive, paternalistic style of clinical decision making.
- The rehabilitation model is characterized by a focus on the person with the impairment and his or her ability to function in everyday life. Typically, a process of informed decision making is used.
- In the social model, the focus is on the person in society, and the problems he or she experiences are seen as being related not only to the client's own performance but also to the disabling society in which he or she lives. Shared decision making generally is applied.

- The use of different models in different settings is linked partly to length of stay. For example, the medical model is most often used in acute health care settings, whereas the social model is more often used in long-term facilities.

- A process for selecting models of practice is described. This process involves self-reflection by the clinician about his or her own professional values, consideration of the organizational context, and, most important, consideration of the wishes of the client.

- Clinicians need to be flexible in their approach in order to provide the most appropriate model of practice in different organizational contexts and with different clients.

CLASS ACTIVITIES

- Speech-language pathology students: Mr. and Mrs. Jamieson ask you for treatment for Mr. Jamieson's speech because Mrs. Jamieson cannot understand him. Mr. Jamieson has the low volume and decrease in articulatory agility that characterizes the hypokinetic dysarthria of Parkinson's disease. Mrs. Jamieson has a bilateral, moderate high-frequency hearing loss and wears bilateral in-the-ear hearing aids. They report difficulty communicating around the home, and it becomes apparent that both are extremely frustrated with each other's communication abilities. How would you go about selecting the best form of treatment for Mr. and Mrs. Jamieson? What treatments would constitute the medical, rehabilitation, and social models of practice?

- Audiology students: Mr. Wilson attends your clinic complaining of difficulty hearing when someone speaks in the car. He also has bilateral tinnitus. He says his hearing loss is related to working as a carpenter when he was younger. He is 78 years old. Outline your process for assessing this client. Explain why you are including each component of the assessment. Your test results indicate that Mr. Wilson has a sloping mild to moderately severe sensorineural hearing loss. What do you do next and why? Think about your recommendations and the model of service delivery they are most closely associated with.

- Outline what you would include in an information pack about treatment options for older people with a particular communication disability (e.g., hearing impairment, aphasia). Remember to include information about the impairment, activity limitations, and participation restrictions as well as management options.

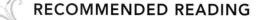

RECOMMENDED READING

Coulter, A. (1997). Partnerships with patients: The pros and cons of shared clinical decision-making. *Journal of Health Service Research and Policy, 2*(2), 112–121.

Erdman, S. A., Wark, D. J., & Montano, J. J. (1994). Implications of service delivery models in audiology. In J. P. Gagné, & N. Tye-Murray (Eds.), Research in audiological rehabilitation: Current trends and future directions. *Journal of the Academy of Rehabilitative Audiology Monograph, 27*(Suppl.), 45–60.

Jordan, L., & Kaiser, W. (1996). *Aphasia—A social approach.* London: Chapman & Hall.

Madell, J. R., & Montano, J. (2000). Audiological rehabilitation in different employment settings. In J. G. Alpiner & P. A. McCarthy (Eds.), *Rehabilitative audiology: Children and adults* (3rd ed. pp. 60–79). Baltimore: Lippincott Williams & Wilkins.

Noble, W., & Hétu, R. (1994). An ecological approach to disability and handicap in relation to impaired hearing. *Audiology, 33*, 117–126.

Worrall, L. E. (2000a). A conceptual framework for a functional approach to acquired neurogenic disorders of communication and swallowing. In L. E. Worrall & C. M. Frattali (Eds.), *Neurogenic communication disorders: A functional approach* (pp. 3–18). New York: Thieme.

Worrall, L. E. (2000b). The influence of professional values on the functional communication approach in aphasia. In L. E. Worrall & C. M. Frattali (Eds.), *Neurogenic communication disorders: A functional approach* (pp. 191–205). New York: Thieme.

Worrall, L. E., & Frattali, C.M. (Eds.). (2000). *Neurogenic communication disorders: A functional approach.* New York: Thieme.

REFERENCES

American Speech-Language-Hearing Association. (1996a). Scope of practice in audiology. *ASHA, 38*(2), 12–15.

American Speech-Language-Hearing Association. (1996b). Scope of practice in speech-language pathology. *ASHA, 38*(2), 16–20.

American Speech-Language-Hearing Association. (2001). *Scope of practice in speech-language pathology.* Rockville, MD: Author.

Carson, A. J., & Pichora-Fuller, M. K. (1997). Health promotion and audiology: The community-clinic link. *Journal of Academy of Rehabilitative Audiology, 30*, 29–51.

Cassileth, B. R., Zupkis, R. V., Sutton-Smith, K., & March, V. (1980). Information and participation preferences among cancer patients. *Annals of Internal Medicine, 92*, 832–836.

Coulter, A. (1997). Partnerships with patients: The pros and cons of shared clinical decision-making. *Journal of Health Service Research and Policy, 2*(2), 112–121.

Curtis, R. S. (1998). Values and valuing in rehabilitation. *Journal of Rehabilitation, 64*(1), 42–47.

Enderby, P. (1983). *Frenchay dysarthria assessment.* San Diego, CA: College-Hill Press.

Erdman, S. A., Wark, D. J., & Montano, J. J. (1994). Implications of service delivery models in audiology. In J. P. Gagné, & N. Tye-Murray (Eds.), Research in audiological rehabilitation: Current trends and future directions. *Journal of the Academy of Rehabilitative Audiology Monograph, 27*(Suppl.), 45–60.

Finkelstein, V. (1991). Disability: An administrative challenge (the health and welfare heritage). In M. Oliver (Ed.), *Social work, disabled people and disabling environments* (pp. 19–39). London: Jessica Kingsley.

Gagné, J-P. (1998). Reflections on evaluative research in audiological rehabilitation. *Scandinavian Audiology, 27*(Suppl. 49), 69–79.

Gagné, J-P., Hétu, R., Getty, L., & McDuff, S. Towards the development of paradigms to conduct functional evaluative research in audiological rehabilitation. *Journal of the Academy of Rehabilitative Audiology, 28*, 7–25.

Green, L. W., & Kreuter, M. W. (1991). *Health promotion planning: An educational and environmental approach* (2nd ed.). Mountain View, CA: Mayfield.

Hepworth, D. H., & Larsen, J. A. (1982). *Direct social work practice: Theory and skills.* Homewood, IL: Dorsey Press.

Holland, A. (1994, September). A look into a cloudy crystal ball for specialists in neurogenic language disorders. *American Journal of Speech-Language Pathology*, 34–36.

Jordan, L., & Kaiser, W. (1996). *Aphasia—A social approach.* London: Chapman & Hall.

Kagan, A., & Gailey, G. F. (1993). Functional is not enough: Training conversational partners for aphasic adults. In A. L. Holland & M. F. Forbes (Eds.), *Aphasia treatment: World perspectives* (pp. 199–226). Clifton Park, NY: Delmar Learning.

Kasper, J. F., Mulley, A. G., & Wennberg, J. E. (1992). Developing shared decision-making programs to improve the quality of health care. *Quality Review Bulletin, 18*, 182–190.

Kertesz, A. (1982). *Western Aphasia Battery.* New York: Grune & Stratton.

Madell, J. R., & Montano, J. (2000). Audiological rehabilitation in different employment settings. In J. G. Alpiner & P. A. McCarthy (Eds.), *Rehabilitative audiology: Children and adults* (3rd ed., pp. 60–79). Baltimore: Lippincott Williams & Wilkins.

Noble, W., & Hétu, R. (1994). An ecological approach to disability and handicap in relation to impaired hearing. *Audiology, 33*, 117–126.

Oliver, M. (1983). *Social work with disabled people.* London: Macmillan.

Payne, J. C. (1994). *Communication profile: A functional skills survey.* Tucson, AZ: Communication Skill Builders.

Pichora-Fuller, K. (1994). Introduction to the special issue on the psycho-social impact of hearing loss in everyday life. *Journal of Speech-Language Pathology and Audiology, 18*(4), 209–211.

Simmons-Mackie, N. (2000). Social approaches to the management of aphasia. In L. E. Worrall & C. M. Frattali (Eds.), *Neurogenic communication disorders: A functional approach* (pp.162–188). New York: Thieme.

Stephens, D. (1996). Hearing rehabilitation in a psychosocial framework. *Scandinavian Audiology, 25*(Suppl. 43), 57–66.

Strull, W. M., Lo, B., & Charles, G. (1984). Do patients want to participate in medical decision making? *Journal of the American Medical Association, 252*, 2990–2994.

World Health Organization. (2001). *International classification of functioning, disability, and health.* Geneva: Author.

Worrall, L. (1999). *Functional communication therapy planner.* Oxon, UK: Winslow Press.

Worrall, L. E. (2000a). A conceptual framework for a functional approach to acquired neurogenic disorders of communication and swallowing. In L. E. Worrall & C. M. Frattali (Eds.), *Neurogenic communication disorders: A functional approach* (pp. 3–18). New York: Thieme.

Worrall, L. E. (2000b). The influence of professional values on the functional communication approach in aphasia. In L. E. Worrall & C. M. Frattali (Eds.), *Neurogenic communication disorders: A functional approach* (pp. 191–205). New York: Thieme.

Worrall, L. E., & Frattali, C.M. (Eds.). (2000). *Neurogenic communication disorders: A functional approach.* New York: Thieme.

Ylvisaker, M., Feeney, T. J., & Urbanczyk, B. (1993). A social-environmental approach to communication and behavior after traumatic brain injury. *Seminars in Speech and Language, 14*(1), 74–86.

Communication Changes With Age

This section uses the WHO's framework of functioning, disability, and health to describe the communication disabilities that occur in older people. Each chapter describes the nature and assessment of communication-related impairments, activity limitations, and participation restrictions. Treatment options are described in Chapters 7, 8, and 9 of this text.

Chapter 4 addresses the hearing, speech, language, and swallowing impairments associated with both healthy and pathological aging. For healthy aging, the major focus is on the areas with which older people are most concerned and that seem to be most vulnerable in aging: hearing and word retrieval. In terms of pathological aging, the effects of diseases such as stroke and dementia of the Alzheimer's type, which are prevalent in older people, are described. Chapter 5 addresses the effects of the impairments on the activity dimension. The everyday communication activities of older people are described, and common assessments that capture the communication activity limitations are listed. The final chapter in this section, Chapter 6, first describes the link between the participation dimension of the WHO model and quality of life. It then describes how healthy older people and older people with communication disabilities describe their participation and quality of life. It also reviews the participation and quality of life measures most suitable for healthy older people and older people with a specific communication disability.

Chapter 4

Communication
and Swallowing
Impairments

Numerous books, reviews, and experimental studies have documented the communication-related impairments associated with both healthy and pathological aging. There are some key areas that the student speech-language pathologist and audiologist can focus on for clinical practice. This chapter presents clinically relevant information in a condensed and simplified format.

The chapter has two main sections. The first section deals with the communication and swallowing impairments that occur in healthy aging, and the second section describes the communication and swallowing impairments associated with pathological aging (i.e., as a result of disease or impairment). The chapter begins with the areas that healthy older people report most difficulty with: hearing and word retrieval. The etiology, prevalence, and measurement of hearing impairment are described, and the process, assessment, changes with age, and differential diagnosis of word retrieval are detailed. Age-related changes in language comprehension, discourse, speech, voice, and swallowing in older people are also summarized. The effects of visual and cognitive impairments on communication in healthy older people are emphasized. In terms of pathological aging, older people are more likely to have pathologies that significantly affect communication and swallowing. In the second section of this chapter, the communication and swallowing impairments associated with stroke, dementia of the Alzheimer's type (DAT), Parkinson's disease, cancer of the head and neck, traumatic brain injury, and amyotrophic lateral sclerosis (ALS) are described. A battery of standardized assessments for these impairments is proposed. The additional challenges that an older client with a communication and/or swallowing disability presents are discussed, and case studies are included that illustrate the complexity of the older client with communication and swallowing impairments.

In this chapter, the communication and swallowing impairments associated with healthy and pathological aging are discussed separately, although it is recognized that aging is in fact a continuum (see Chapter 2). To be consistent with the WHO terminology (2001), the term impairment is used throughout the chapter, although it is important to be aware that the term changes would be more appropriate when discussing healthy older people.

There are numerous documented communication and swallowing impairments in healthy older people. To prioritize these, it is worth considering what older people themselves perceive as the most important communication impairments they experience. What communication changes are older people concerned about? Hickson, Worrall, Yiu, and Barnett (1996) investigated by asking seven groups of healthy older people what they wanted to include in a communication education program about communication impairments with age (see Chapter 7 for details of the program). Using the Nominal Group Technique (Delbecq, Van de Ven, & Gustafson, 1975), the following question was put to each group: "What problems do you have in talking, hearing, understanding, or just generally getting your message across?" The priority areas emerged as: (a) hearing difficulties, (b) memory loss, and (c) word-finding difficulties. Other concerns were lack of concentration, difficulty speaking clearly, feeling isolated, not understanding what is said, problems getting through to people, problems with eyesight, and lack of confidence.

Hearing loss and word-finding difficulties are the main focus of the first section in this chapter because not only are they the key issues of concern for older people, but they are also core areas of gerontological audiology and speech-language pathology practice. Cognitive neuropsychologists and clinicians from other disciplines are perhaps better placed to manage memory problems, although speech-language pathologists have a role in some cases. It should be remembered, however, that memory processes interact with communication, and memory is a key area of concern for older people. Hearing, of course, is the core business of audiologists, although many speech-language pathologists also engage in aural rehabilitation, and all health professionals who work with older people should be aware of hearing impairment in older people. For speech-language pathologists, the frequency and nature of word-finding difficulties are central to the consideration of the differential diagnosis of normal aging, early dementia, and aphasia.

In addition to the focus on these two major areas, the chapter contains a summary of reported impairments in comprehension, conversational discourse, voice, speech, and swallowing associated with healthy aging, as well as a description of the effects of other age-related impairments (i.e., visual and cognitive problems) on communication. The importance of these impairments should not be overlooked, as they have an impact on prevention and intervention programs. Finally, in the section on healthy aging, some assessments that can be used to screen or monitor the communication health of older people are recommended.

In the section of the chapter on pathological aging, the major communication and swallowing impairments associated with age-related diseases are summarized. A core battery of standardized tests for older people with communication impairment is described, and the particular issues about managing older clients with these impairments are discussed. Finally, the chapter presents some case examples that demonstrate the complexity of multiple communication impairments in older people.

Communication and Swallowing Impairments in Healthy Older People

Hearing Impairment

Age-related hearing impairment is generally referred to as presbycusis or presbyacusis. Although a variety of different patterns may occur, the typical audiometric pattern is that of bilateral symmetrical mild to moderate sensorineural hearing loss that is worse in the high frequencies. The onset of hearing difficulties is usually gradual, with many people unaware for some time of the subtle impairments that are occurring. Hearing impairment in healthy older people is highly prevalent, with approximately one in three people over the age of 60 years having a measurable increase in hearing thresholds for pure-tone sounds.

ETIOLOGY

Changes occur in the peripheral and central auditory system with age. A list of the impairments that have been reported is contained in Table 4–1. A number of structural impairments occur to the outer ear with age, and although these are important in the assessment and management of some older clients, they generally have little effect on hearing function. For example, excessive cerumen or wax in the ear canal may need to be removed prior to audiological testing and/or ear impression taking for hearing aid fitting. Changes also occur to the middle ear with age; however, they too have little effect on behavioral test results (Weinstein, 2000).

The loss of pure-tone hearing sensitivity that is characteristic of presbycusis is related to degenerative impairments in the inner ear (see Table 4–1). Although there are changes to many parts of the inner ear with age, it is the degeneration of outer hair cells that most likely accounts for the sloping mild to moderate impairment evident on pure-tone testing (Willott, 1991). Schuknecht (1974) identified different types of presbycusis, based on histological changes and their associated audiometric patterns. For example, strial presbycusis was reportedly characterized by atrophy of the stria vascularis, flat audiometric hearing impairment, and excellent word recognition. Willott (1991) examined these claims of the different presybcusis types in detail and concluded that there is no clear relationship between

TABLE 4–1

AGE-RELATED IMPAIRMENTS TO THE AUDITORY SYSTEM.

Auditory System Component	Description of Impairment
Outer ear	Degeneration of the cartilage Both increased and decreased amounts of cerumen or wax in the canal have been reported Increased hair growth in the ear canal Thinning and loss of elasticity of the skin in the ear canal
Middle ear	Both thickening and thinning of the tympanic membrane have been reported Decreased elasticity and atrophy of the muscles of the middle ear Degenerative changes to the ossicles, including arthritis in the ossicular chain joints and ossification of the bones
Inner ear	Loss of inner and outer hair cells, especially in the basal area of the cochlea Fusing of stereocilia Loss of spiral ganglion cells Decreased elasticity of the basilar membrane Atrophy and vascular changes to the stria vascularis Atrophy of the spiral ligament
Central auditory pathways	Degeneration and decrease in the neurons of the auditory nerve, brainstem, and auditory cortex

Note: From Garstecki and Erler (1997), Hickson and Worrall (1997), Hull (1995), Kricos and Lesner (1995), and Willott (1991). These sources contain reviews that include the original reference citations for each impairment.

pathological age-related changes, which typically occur in a number of different parts of the inner ear, and audiometric patterns.

The effects of central auditory system changes are more complex than a pure-tone hearing loss. Neuronal atrophy may occur in any part of the central nervous system with age, and the central auditory nervous system is no exception. The extent of such changes and the functional manifestations of these on auditory performance is, however, highly variable (Weinstein, 2000). Age-related changes in frequency and temporal resolution, and in binaural processing, have been reported (see Helfer, 1995, for review). These changes may manifest themselves as a reduction in speech perception ability in adverse or difficult listening conditions (e.g., listening in noise, listening to a fast speaker).

The use of the single term presbycusis to describe age-related hearing impairment is problematic, because it implies a single causative factor, that is, age. Age-related hearing impairment is in fact a multifactorial condition involving both endogenous factors related to the aging process per se as listed in Table 4–1, and exogenous factors related to other factors that commonly occur in older people. Exogenous factors include various pathologies known to affect hearing in older people (e.g., diabetes, cardiovascular disease), as well as ototoxicity, noise exposure, and genetic make-up.

Diabetes and cardiovascular disease can occur at any time during a person's life; however, the prevalence is higher among older adults. The relationship between diabetes and hearing impairment is unclear from research findings (Gates, Cobb, D'Agostino, & Wolf, 1993); however, Weinstein (2000) maintains that "clinical experience suggests diabetes that is not properly controlled places older adults at risk of sudden declines in hearing levels that may not be reversible" (p. 76). Stronger relationships have been found between cardiovascular disease and hearing impairment in research studies of older people (Brant et al., 1996; Gates et al., 1993). Interestingly, Brant et al. reported that the risk of hearing impairment increased with rising systolic blood pressure. For example, men with a slightly elevated systolic pressure of 140 have a 32% greater risk of hearing impairment than men with normal blood pressure.

Many of the medications that older people take for the treatment of disease and/or chronic disability are potentially toxic to the auditory system. Some examples are

- antibiotics, for example, gentamycin, neomycin, kanamycin
- pain killers, for example, salicylates
- diuretics, for example, quinine, furosemide
- chemotherapeutic medications, for example, ciplatin

The effects vary depending on dosage and schedule and on the susceptibility of the individual; however, the characteristic effect on hearing is to induce a steeply sloping high-frequency sensorineural hearing impairment.

Noise exposure is a major issue in developed countries. Many older people have a noise-induced hearing loss as well as age-related impairment, and the contribution of each condition is impossible to quantify. Interesting studies of older people living in quieter, nonindustrialized settings such as the Sudan in North Africa and Easter Island in the Pacific Ocean have shown that they have significantly better hearing than older people living in developed countries (Goycoolea et al., 1986; Rosen, Bergman, Plester, El-Mofty, & Satti, 1962). In addition, it has been found that older men have, on average, worse hearing than older women, a fact that is believed to be associated with the greater noise exposure experienced by men both occupationally and recreationally (see review by Hickson & Worrall, 1997). Men are more likely to engage in industrial work and are more likely to participate in noisy recreational pursuits such as shooting and car racing.

The effect of genetic factors is evident in studies of hearing impairment in different ethnic groups. Battle (1993) summarized findings of a number of studies in the United States comparing African-American and Caucasian men. In general, the findings show that African-Americans have better hearing for frequencies above 2000 Hz from about 30 years of age, and the hearing threshold level difference between groups increases with age. Barrenas and Lindgren (1990) postulated that this is because African-Americans are better protected because of a higher melanin content in the inner ear.

PREVALENCE

Prevalence figures reported in the literature for peripheral hearing impairment in older people vary considerably depending on the sample population assessed, the test measures used to determine impairment, and the criteria for impairment. Nevertheless, the figures indicate that some of the facts are

- The prevalence of hearing impairment increases with age (e.g., Davis, 1989).
- The prevalence is higher in males than females (e.g., Moscicki, Elkins, Baum, & McNamara, 1985).
- The prevalence is higher in older people living in residential care than in older people living in the community (e.g., Stumer, Hickson, & Worrall, 1996).
- Although hearing impairment increases with age, thresholds generally plateau at moderate levels (e.g., Harford & Dodds, 1982).
- The rate of deterioration in hearing levels with age is slow, with average decrements of 1 to 2 dB per year reported (e.g., Pedersen, Rosenhall, & Moller, 1989).
- The vast majority of hearing impairment is sensorineural in nature (Gates, Cooper, Kannel, & Miller, 1990).
- Hearing impairment is greatest at the high frequencies (e.g., Gates et al., 1990).

A question often asked is How many older people have a hearing impairment? Different research studies report startlingly different results for this question, depending on the researchers' definition of hearing impairment. For example, Moscicki et al. (1985) used a strict criterion in their evaluation of the Framingham Heart Study Cohort in the United States. A person was categorized as having a hearing impairment if he or she had a hearing threshold level greater than 20 dB at any frequency from 500 to 4000 Hz in the better ear. Not surprisingly, the reported prevalence of hearing impairment was a high 83%. A population study conducted in the United Kingdom by Davis (1989) used a more appropriate criterion. A person was classified as having a hearing impairment if his or her better ear pure-tone average at 500, 1000, 2000, and 4000 Hz was greater than 25 dB. Davis reported that, in the general population, 37% of people in their sixties had a hearing impairment, and 60% of people in their seventies had an impairment. The prevalence of hearing impairment is known to be higher in older people living in residential care facilities for the aged, with approximately 80% reported having a hearing impairment (Mahoney, 1992; Worrall, Hickson, & Dodd, 1993). The prevalence of hearing impairment has also been found to be higher in older people with dementia, a finding that is discussed in more detail later in this chapter.

The prevalence of central auditory impairment is more difficult to quantify. Results depend on the population assessed and the types of assessment of central auditory function that are applied. Cooper and Gates (1991), using speech tests, reported a prevalence of abnormality in 22.6% of 1,026 people aged 64 to 93 years. Stach, Spretnjak, and Jerger (1990) reported a higher prevalence, but this was in a clinical population of 700 patients. The prevalence increased with age and was 72% in those aged 70 to 74 years and 95% in those over 80 years. Newman and Sandridge (2000) reviewed electrophysiological tests of central auditory nervous system function and reported significant age effects on electrocochleography, auditory brainstem response, and higher level responses (i.e., P300 and Mismatch Negativity). Researchers consistently comment on the difficulty of separating peripheral from central effects in the elderly population.

MEASUREMENT OF HEARING IMPAIRMENT

In traditional audiological practice, the assessment of hearing impairment in older adults should be carried out using a standard battery of audiological tests. This assessment typically includes otoscopy, air and bone conduction pure-tone audiometry, immittance audiometry, and speech audiometry. Other procedures, such as auditory brainstem response (ABR) testing and central auditory processing assessment, may be necessary if further investigation is indicated. It is important that audiologists do not fall into the trap of assuming that all hearing impairments observed in older adults are age related and therefore untreatable, or that a person may be too old for treatment. The investigation of other possible etiologies (e.g., otitis media, otosclerosis, acoustic neuroma, Ménière's disease, vascular problems) should not be overlooked. The audiologist should be particularly aware that middle ear disorders are more common in people over 65, a fact that is related to changes in eustachian tube function with age, a less efficient immune system, and a higher prevalence of upper respiratory tract infections that can lead to middle ear infection (Weinstein, 2000). The measurement of the degree and nature of hearing impairment is, therefore, essentially the same as that employed for younger adults and is well documented in many other texts (e.g., Gelfand, 2001; Katz, 2002; Stach, 1998).

There are some age-related impairments to the outer ear that may complicate the use of standard audiometric tests in older people. Changes to the shape of the ear canal and reduced elasticity of the skin in the canal can make it difficult to obtain the airtight seal necessary for immittance audiometry. For pure-tone audiometry, the pressure of standard supra-aural headphones can cause the cartilage of the ear canal to collapse. The effect of this situation is that hearing thresholds are artificially elevated, and inaccurate results are obtained. The typical audiometric pattern associated with collapsing ear canals is a high-frequency conductive loss. This problem is reasonably common in older people, with Schow and Nerbonne (1980) reporting collapsed canals in 10 to 16% of 80 nursing home residents aged 60 to 79 years. The effects of collapsing canals can be reduced by the use of circumaural headphones or insert earphones.

If hearing is to be measured as part of a health-screening program for older adults to identify those who need a complete assessment, there are a number of options for measurement. Pure-tone air conduction audiometry has been used in many instances, and although research indicates that this is indeed the most accurate measure, it is also an expensive option that requires specialized equipment and trained personnel. A simpler option is that of an audioscope (Welch-Allyn Inc., Skaneateles Falls, NY), a handheld otoscope that includes an audiometer that emits pure tones at 40 dB at 500, 1000, 2000, and 4000 Hz. Lichenstein, Bess, and Logan (1988) compared the results obtained with an audioscope with those from conventional pure-tone audiometry in a sample of 178 older clients seen in a primary care practice. They reported the sensitivity (i.e., correct identification of those with significant hearing impairment) to be 94% and the specificity (i.e., correct identification of those with normal hearing or only a mild loss) to be 72%. Since that time, the use of the audioscope has been reported in a number of studies, with similar positive findings about the applicability of this form of testing with older people (Lavizzo-Mourey, Smith, Sims, & Taylor, 1994; Lim & Yap, 2000; McBride, Mulrow, Aguilar, & Tuley, 1994).

Finally, many researchers have investigated the use of self-report questionnaires as screening tools to identify hearing impairment in the older population. This approach is clearly the least expensive option, but it also is the option that identifies the smallest proportion of older people with hearing impairment. Although there are a number of more detailed questionnaires of hearing difficulties (see Chapter 5), Nondahl et al. (1998) found that the single question "Do you feel you have a hearing loss?" is the most sensitive for detecting whether a person has a hearing impairment. They reported a sensitivity of 71% for this question in a sample of 3,556 older Americans. Although this question missed some older people who had hearing impairment as measured with pure-tone air conduction testing, it is argued that such a question is more useful for screening purposes than pure-tone audiometry. People who identify themselves as having a hearing impairment are more likely to be interested in further rehabilitation than those who do not report a hearing problem, irrespective of what pure-tone audiometry shows. Thus, such reflective self-report questions may be useful in the preliminary identification of older adults who might benefit from intervention.

Word-Retrieval Impairments

Word finding is a relatively complex concept that speech-language pathologists need to understand in considerable detail because it is particularly vulnerable to physiological changes to the brain. As already mentioned, it is also something that older people themselves complain about. Older people particularly complain about recalling people's names, but also report difficulty retrieving the names of objects (Albert, Heller, & Milberg, 1988; Cohen & Faulkner, 1986; Goulet, Ska, & Kahn, 1994). The following sections first describe the process of word finding using information-processing models and discourse analyses. Second, the various components of word-finding assessment are outlined, and finally, the use of the Boston Naming Test (BNT; Kaplan, Goodglass, & Weintraub, 1983) to differentially diagnose naming problems associated with normal aging, aphasia, and dementia is described.

THE WORD-RETRIEVAL PROCESS

The stages of word retrieval are described simply by Lesser (1987) (Table 4–2). This table shows that the process of naming can break down at many stages and that the behaviors or symptoms change according to which stage is problematic. Other models of word retrieval that show the complexity of word finding have been proposed by Kay, Lesser, and Coltheart (1996) and Linebaugh (1990). Although these show different routes of the system, they have essentially the same components of (a) a semantic memory or system that is activated by various means, (b) a lexical system that can contain either phonological or orthographic representations, and (c) an output process whereby the words are spoken or written.

Lesser (1987) described the anticipated behavior associated with a breakdown at each level (see Table 4–2). If the breakdown is at the semantic lexicon stage, the person will have difficulty categorizing words and may exhibit semantic paraphasias (e.g., *chair* for *bed*). If the problem is at the phonological lexicon stage, then there is a possibility of anomic circumlocution and neologistic jargon (e.g., "It's a sleeping thing" or "a benowing"). If there are problems within phonological assembly, phonemic paraphasias result (e.g. *bep* for *bed*). Difficulties with phonetic

TABLE 4–2

IMPAIRMENTS IN NAMING INTERPRETED AS RELATED TO STAGES OF WORD-RETRIEVAL.

Stage	Impairment	Behavior
Semantic lexicon	Category loss or degradation Generalized degradation access problem	Failure to define or sort words in specific categories Semantic paraphasia
Phonological lexicon	Impaired word-form representations Impairment of phonological control	Anomic circumlocution Neologistic jargon
Phonological assembly	Impaired phoneme selection and seriation	Phonemic paraphasia
Phonetic planning	Impaired mapping from phonemic to phonetic realization	Verbal dyspraxia
Articulation	Neuromotor damage	Dysarthria

Note: Modified from Lesser, R. (1987). Cognitive neuropsychological influences on aphasia therapy. *Aphasiology, 1*(3), 189–200. Adapted by permission of Psychology Press Ltd., Hove, UK.

planning and articulation result in the motor speech impairments of apraxia and dysarthria, respectively. Word-retrieval errors predominantly occur with impairments such as aphasia or dementia; however, the process also sheds some light on the possible impairments that result from normal aging. It may be that there is some degradation of both the semantic and phonological lexicon in healthy older people, as it is known that occasional semantic paraphasia and anomic circumlocution (including the tip of the tongue phenomenon) occurs in this population.

ASSESSMENTS OF WORD RETRIEVAL

Word retrieval is commonly assessed through confrontation naming tests that require the client to name pictures or objects. Examples of such tests are the

- Boston Naming Test (BNT; Kaplan et al., 1983)
- naming subtest of the Psycholinguistic Assessments of Language Processing in Aphasia (PALPA; Kay, Lesser, & Coltheart, 1997)
- naming subtest of the Western Aphasia Battery (WAB; Kertesz, 1982)
- naming subtest of the Boston Diagnostic Aphasia Examination (BDAE; Goodglass, Kaplan, & Barresi, 2001)

Another common method is the use of divergent naming or generative naming tasks, such as the word fluency subtest of the WAB, in which participants are asked to name as many animals as they can within a minute; or the FAS divergent naming task (Benton & Hamsher, 1976) in which participants are asked to think of any words beginning with F, A, and S, also within a minute. Both divergent naming tasks require the person to retrieve many words within a category. Convergent naming tests on the other hand ask the person to retrieve one specific word. Bowles and Poon (1985) describe a convergent naming task where target words are retrieved from a definition (for example, a vehicle that is able to travel across land and water on a cushion of air: a hovercraft), but this task is not as commonly used in clinical practice.

The BNT is the most popular confrontation picture-naming test (Beele, Davies, & Muller, 1984; Katz et al., 2000; Smith-Worrall & Burtenshaw, 1990). The original version is a 60-item test that uses black-and-white drawn pictures graded for difficulty. Items occurring first in the test are easier because they occur more frequently in English (e.g., *bed*), compared to those that occur later (e.g., *palette*). There are also several shorter versions of the BNT including three 30-item versions (Williams et al., 1989). One version consists of the even- number items, another uses the odd-number items, and there is another empirical version that is based on items that best discriminate between healthy older people and people with dementia (Williams et al., 1989). There are also five 15-item versions of the test. One is part of a brief battery of tests for Alzheimer's disease (Morris et al., 1989); the other four were developed by Mack, Freed, Williams, and Henderson (1992), such that all four versions have equal distribution of word frequency. Shorter versions of the BNT are required because some older people may be unable to attend for long periods of time. March, Worrall, and Hickson (2001) found that the 30-item empirical version had the highest correlation to the original 60-item test and recommended this version as the best alternative to the 60-item version, if time was limited. Table 4–3 lists the 30 items from the empirical version of the shortened BNT.

DOES WORD RETRIEVAL CHANGE WITH AGE?

Although healthy older people report a decline in word-retrieval skills with age (Hickson et al., 1996), there is some conflicting evidence from objective measurement (Cruice Worrall, & Hickson, 2000). Cross-sectional studies have predominantly found a difference between younger and older groups, whereas longitudinal studies have not shown significant change over time (Cruice et al., 2000). Changes observed in the cross-sectional studies may be related to cohort effects (for example, educational differences between young and old subjects) and may not be related to the aging process alone. Age-related change can be examined most effectively in longitudinal studies; however, the longest longitudinal study has only been 4 years, and it may be that significant impairments only occur after a longer period. Some of the variables that affect results of naming tests are visual acuity,

TABLE 4–3

ITEMS FROM THE EMPIRICAL 30-ITEM BNT.

11. Helicopter	40. Knocker
13. Octopus	41. Pelican
18. Mask	43. Pyramid
19. Pretzel	44. Muzzle
23. Volcano	48. Noose
24. Seahorse	49. Asparagus
28. Wreath	50. Compass
30. Harmonica	51. Latch
31. Rhinoceros	52. Tripod
32. Acorn	53. Scroll
33. Igloo	54. Tongs
34. Stilts	55. Sphynx
35. Dominoes	57. Trellis
37. Escalator	58. Palette
39. Hammock	60. Abacus

Note: Modified from Williams et al. (1989).

educational level, cultural differences, and gender, and these may account for the differences between studies (Cruice et al., 2000).

If word-retrieval changes do occur in healthy aging, when do they occur? Accumulated research evidence indicates that in the normal healthy older person decline in performance on a range of psychometric tests is minimal, at least until 70 to 75 years of age (Steuer & Jarvik, 1981). Although there is one study that reported a deterioration in naming on the BNT after 55 years of age (Ivnik, Malec, Smith, Tangalos, & Peterson, 1996), there have been several studies in the naming area that support the so-called "70 years of age hypothesis" (Albert et al., 1988; Borod, Goodglass, & Kaplan, 1980; Mitrushina & Satz, 1995; Nicholas, Obler, Albert, & Goodglass, 1985; Van Gorp, Satz, Kiersch, & Henry, 1986).

Case Study: Mr. Vincent

Mr. Vincent was a successful businessman who, at 84 years of age, was still administering his extensive business interests including share trading on the stock market. He was admitted to the hospital after collapsing at home. While the medical staff queried a mild stroke, Mr. Vincent argued that he had just been working too hard and had a bit of a collapse. The physician asked the speech-language pathologist for an opinion.

Mr. Vincent was adamant that he should not remain long in the hospital. He wanted to return to his business immediately. He had had enough of tests; however, he was persuaded to spend 15 minutes looking at some pictures (the BNT). As the test progressed, he became increasingly agitated with his inability to name the pictures, but refused to acknowledge he was having difficulty, saying, for example, that there was another name for it in his business, and that he never went beyond 7 years of education and therefore did not know the name for *protractor* or *compass*. He scored 37 items correctly from a total of 60, but an analysis of his errors provided the most amount of information. There were 13 semantic errors, and many of these were vague circumlocutions (for example, the person who is going to be murdered, for *noose*), semantic negation (for example, not an easel, for *tripod*). He replied "Don't know" to six items, had three perceptual errors, and had one phonemic error. This pattern is consistent with the errors associated with early dementia, rather than normal aging or aphasia (Chenery, Murdoch, & Ingram, 1996).

Following his performance on the BNT, Mr. Vincent developed a little more insight into his difficulties and agreed to more extensive testing by the neuropsychologist. This testing confirmed that he did have early dementia, and he and his family were able to deal gradually with the issue of handing over business dealings before the dementia progressed too far. In this case, the relative brevity of the BNT and its nonthreatening format were useful in differentially diagnosing a problem and in managing the case to a relatively successful conclusion.

DIFFERENTIAL DIAGNOSIS USING THE BNT

As previously mentioned, the BNT is often used in the differential diagnosis of dementia and normal aging impairments, or dementia and mild aphasia. The case study above describes a clinical scenario in which the BNT was a key tool in differentially diagnosing between healthy age-related impairments, early dementia, and mild aphasia.

Other Communication and Swallowing Impairments

Although hearing impairment and word-finding problems are highly prevalent and cause older people themselves considerable concern, there are a number of other important communication impairments that have been found in healthy older people. Speech-language pathologists and audiologists need to be aware of these subtle impairments for the following reasons:

1. They may affect the clinician's interaction with an older person, for example, if he or she has more difficulty understanding complex and lengthy discourse, complex explanations such as those involving hearing aid use may need to be adapted.

2. Test results may be affected, for example, response on a paragraph comprehension task in an aphasia test may be influenced by normal age-related changes as well as aphasia; alternatively, if the purpose of the assessment is to differentially diagnose early stage dementia and mild aphasia from normal aging, it is important to know the impairments that occur in normal aging.

3. Health promotion programs need to make older people aware of normal communication changes and help them develop strategies to overcome or compensate for these changes (see Chapter 7).

However, a few words of caution are necessary before presenting the research findings in this area. Many studies have examined for impairments and found them. Many studies have not used longitudinal methods, and as mentioned previously, the results of cross-sectional studies may be due to cohort effects, rather than age effects. For example, in cross-sectional studies, differences between a cohort of 70-year-old people, the majority of whom are war veterans with an average of 6 years of formal education and 45 years of working life, and a cohort of 20-year-olds, most of whom are college or university students, may be due to differences in their life experiences rather than age. The possible influence of cohort effects is an important issue to consider when evaluating gerontology research.

LANGUAGE COMPREHENSION

The consensus appears to be that older people are only having difficulties understanding verbal language when the task complexity is increased. At the word level, older people show no decline in their ability to understand words, that is, their comprehension vocabulary remains intact. This ability is in contrast to their ability to retrieve the word, as described in earlier sections. At the sentence level, there is some impairment if the sentence becomes syntactically more complex and longer. At the discourse level, again, the complexity of the material is the main factor. Many authors believe that the basis of the decline in discourse comprehension skills in older people is the demand it places on their declining working memory (Kwong See & Ryan, 1996; Shadden, 1997; Ska & Joanette, 1997). Other factors that affect language comprehension include speech discrimination, response time, attention, distractibility, and redundancy (Cohen, 1979). Gravell (1988) concluded that comprehension difficulties are predominantly found only in language testing situations when the task demands are manipulated, rather than in everyday life.

What are the implications of these changes in language comprehension for audiologists and speech-language pathologists? Clearly, when testing older adults, consideration needs to be given to normal age-related impairments in comprehension, particularly at the discourse level. In interactions with older clients, it should be remembered that comprehension difficulties might occur if the conversation becomes particularly complex or if the background noise is too loud. Health promotion programs may choose to remind older people that their vocabulary remains intact and that their language comprehension is good while the comprehension task is not too complex. Older people could be encouraged to ask for written information to supplement complex verbal explanations, request repetitions of complex information, or ask that information be presented in a simpler format.

Pichora-Fuller (1997) urged rehabilitative audiologists to become involved in making listening easier for older people. Suggestions for rehabilitative audiologists include training talkers to produce clear speech, training people with hearing impairment and their partners to optimize supportive context strategies, and to facilitate their conscious decision making about when to use their mental energy for understanding.

Older people's comprehension of written material (reading) is also important to their well-being. Literacy skills decrease with age (Australian Bureau of Statistics, 1996). Between 41 and 46% of those aged 65 and 74 years in the 1996 Australian Adult Literacy Survey were found to have poor literacy skills, with 75% of these having such poor literacy levels that they would experience difficulty in everyday life (for example, not being able to read newspapers or books and requiring assistance with medicine bottle labels). Speech-language pathologists and audiologists need to remember these statistics when designing patient educational materials for older clients. Patient education materials need to be age-friendly, that is, appropriate for older people.

CONVERSATIONAL DISCOURSE

As Garcia and Orange (1996) noted, speech-language pathologists are often asked to make a judgment about whether the conversational ability of an older person is normal. In most cases, it is in the context of judging whether there are signs of early dementia in the conversational patterns of the individual. Determining whether there are conversational problems in older adults is a complicated process, because the normal older person may have impairments in cognitive, physiological, or sensory abilities; social status and roles; as well as stylistic differences that all impact on conversational ability. Does conversational discourse skill change with age? Are older people more talkative, more focused on past events, more egocentric, more ambiguous, and less efficient and cohesive, as some stereotypes suggest? Age-related impairments in conversational skills have implications for audiologists and speech-language pathologists who interact with, assess, and provide health promotion advice to older clients. These conversational impairments are summarized next, and implications for speech-language pathologists and audiologists are discussed.

Garcia and Orange (1996) provide a comprehensive review of the features of conversational discourse in older people, from linguistic, psychological, sociolinguistic, and psychosocial perspectives. In summary, there are few substantial linguistic impairments in conversational discourse of older people, although some features that have been reported are

- decreased efficiency
- increased ambiguity
- increased degree of topic maintenance
- decreased cohesion
- decreased rate
- increased number of words per clause
- overall increase in number of words.

From a psychological perspective, the influence of cognitive impairments, such as working memory and attention, has been hypothesized to affect conversational discourse (Garcia & Orange, 1996). Of particular interest is a study by Drevenstedt and Bellezza (1993) who asked their participants to generate a story and recall it. Three subgroups of older people emerged: one group was good at storytelling but not good at recalling the story, one group was good at both storytelling and recalling the story, and the third group was poor at both tasks. The last group had generalized memory impairment. This finding implies that memory does have an effect on storytelling as well as story recall.

From a sociolinguistic and psychosocial perspective, Garcia and Orange (1996) described how Communication Accommodation Theory (see Chapter 2) has been used to study the effects of age on conversation. In general, old and young people alike hold negative stereotypical perceptions of older people's conversational abilities. This results in over-accommodated communication that is described as demeaning and patronizing. This, in turn, leads to problems for older people such as loss of social roles and decreased communicative, social, and physical independence. Garcia and Orange (1996) reported on a series of studies by Gould and colleagues who examined the effect of off-topic verbosity (loquaciousness) on the circumstances of older people. Off-topic verbosity was found to be associated with increasing age, an extraverted personality, increased stress (e.g., poor health), and decreased social support. Off-topic verbosity in older people is not well liked by conversational partners, resulting in even lower levels of social support. The cycle continues.

The dilemma for speech-language pathologists is identifying changes associated with normal aging from those associated with diseases such as DAT. There are many similarities between the features of discourse in early Alzheimer's disease and that of normal aging.

However, there are several assessments that assist in this differential diagnostic process (see Garcia and Orange, 1996, for review).

SPEECH AND VOICE

It is relatively easy to tell whether a speaker is young, middle-aged, or old on the telephone. How is this? Most of the clues come from the person's voice and speech characteristics. Benjamin (1997) and Mueller (1997) cited several studies in which the age of the speaker was predicted from speech samples. Even when the sample was a prolonged vowel, the prediction of age was better than chance. This finding suggests that voice and speech characteristics are contributing significantly to people's perception of aging speech patterns.

For speech-language pathologists, the speech and voice characteristics of normally aging adults is important for the reasons stated earlier: for assessment in differential diagnosis, for health promotion activities and, to a lesser extent, for interacting with older people. For audiologists, vocal impairments may occur with hearing loss, and this situation may add another dimension to aural rehabilitation. This section, therefore, describes for speech-language pathologists the speech and voice impairments that occur with normal aging and then discusses for audiologists the vocal impairments that occur with hearing impairment.

Although perceived age-related impairments such as imprecise articulation and slower rate of speech have been well documented through objective measurement, in general these impairments do not affect overall intelligibility of the normally aging older speaker (Benjamin, 1997). Hence, Ryan and Burk's (1974) description of older people's speech being at the mild end of the dysarthria continuum is not surprising. Benjamin (1997) cited several studies in which healthy older speakers were rated as dysarthric during tasks such as diadochokinetic productions and those in the Frenchay Dysarthria Assessment (Enderby, 1983). This finding could be a further example of a subclinical older population (see Chapter 2). Some older people demonstrate differences in areas such as phonemic production, articulatory timing, and rate of speech production when compared with their younger counterparts; however, no change in intelligibility is noted.

What is the cause of these changes in speech production? Ringel and Chodzko-Zajko (1988) discussed these in terms of the "structural and functional integrity of the neural, endocrine, skeletal and muscular system" (p. 95). Sensory, motor, and cognitive behaviors have an impact on the speech mechanism, and age-related impairments occurring at the molecular, cellular, and organ levels all contribute to the decline. Table 4–4 lists the age-related impairments that occur at each stage of the speech mechanism and the associated voice and speech characteristics of healthy older people.

Although speech impairments are not so noticeable in the older adult, vocal impairments in older people are distinctive. Hollien (1995) asked whether an old voice can be normal, because by definition, the older larynx has some sort of pathology. Hollien also warned, however, against the perception that older people should be considered abnormal or sick, simply because they are old. Table 4–4 describes the physiological impairments to the larynx with age and the measured effects that these have on the older voice.

Mueller (1997) reported that 17% of 500 voice cases seen at a university clinic were over 60 years of age. Although the majority had traditional vocal difficulties associated with vocal abuse, vocal fold paralysis, Parkinson's disease, and spasmodic dysphonia, almost a fifth of the cases had problems related to the normal aging process. Kahane and Beckford (1991) remind the voice clinician of common laryngological problems that might also affect the older speaker. These problems include dysphonias with psychogenic etiologies as well as

TABLE 4-4

CHANGES TO THE VOICE AND SPEECH MECHANISM WITH AGE.

Subsystem	Age-Related Physiological Impairments	Changes to Voice and Speech Characteristics
Respiratory function	Senile kyphosis (curvature of the spine) and altered thoracic shape Diminished muscle strength, calcification of rib joints, decreased respiratory efficiency Structural changes in pleura and decreased elastic recoil capacity	*In general, age-related respiratory function changes have little observable effect on voice and speech. Following is the measured difference.* Reduced endurance
Laryngeal function	Bowing from muscle atrophy Cartilaginous calcification and ossification Decreased blood supply Decreased neuromuscular control: neuronal atrophy; neurotransmitter deficiencies; nerve conduction slowing Decreased lubrication of the vocal fold mucosa	*In general, age-related laryngeal impairments have some observable effects on the voice. These are the measured differences.* Increased fundamental frequency for males; reduced or the same fundamental frequency for females Decreased vowel duration time Diminished vocal intensity, except for those with hearing loss Increased jitter, shimmer, and vocal tremor Decreased harmonic/noise ratio Increased hoarseness

Subsystem	Age-Related Physiological Impairments	Changes to Voice and Speech Characteristics
Supralaryngeal function	Structural change to the maxilla and mandible Realignment to the temporomandibular joint associated with loss of teeth leading to altered oral cavity changes and resonatory characteristics Diminished functioning of salivary glands; drying out of tongue and oral mucosa Loss of orofacial and tongue sensitivity Weakening of the pharyngeal musculature and dilation of pharynx Deficiencies in uvula muscles	*In general, age-related supralaryngeal function impairments have little observable effect on speech. These are the measured differences.* Slower speaking rate (increased pauses, slower velocity of articulatory movements, and increased phoneme durations) Articulatory placement for sound production moves to a more neutral position Greater articulatory variability Velopharyngeal insufficiency and increased nasality

Note: From Benjamin (1997), Caruso and Mueller (1997), Hollien (1995), Mueller (1997), and Ringel and Chodzko-Zajko (1988).

those with organic etiologies (e.g., mass lesions, polypoid degeneration, intubation granuloma, leukoplakia or keratosis, or malignant lesions). It is worth noting that the peak incidence of laryngeal cancer is between the ages of 50 and 70 years. Laryngeal cancer is described later in this chapter. Voice difficulties can also occur as a result of systemic problems such as rheumatoid arthritis and hyperthyroidism; vocal symptoms such as laryngitis sicca (i.e., vocal dryness) and reflux laryngitis are also a result of systemic problems in the older person.

Of particular interest to audiologists is the voice of the older speaker who is hearing impaired. People with severe to profound hearing impairment are reported to speak with excessive vocal intensity (Boone & McFarlane, 1988). The type of hearing loss has also been reported to affect vocal intensity, with conductive hearing loss being associated with reduced vocal intensity and sensorineural loss associated with increased vocal intensity (Andrews, 1991; Burzynski, 1987). Weatherley, Worrall, and Hickson (1997) found that older speakers with mild to moderate hearing impairment were increasing their vocal intensity on vowel prolongation but were largely unaware of these changes. Aural rehabilitation programs for older people may, therefore, need to include training on strategies for self-monitoring loudness levels.

SWALLOWING

Although there is some debate about whether age per se impairs swallowing, there is agreement that age-related factors such as pharmacological and medical treatments and poor dentition do affect swallowing. Wheeler (1995) summarized the main aspects of swallowing that are affected as part of the normal aging process as

- decreased efficiency in initiating and completing the oral phase
- increased delay in initiating the pharyngeal stage
- less elevation of the larynx
- decreased duration of cricopharyngeal opening
- decreased oropharyngeal and esophageal peristalsis.

Caruso and Mueller (1997) commented that most of the impairments are temporal in nature, with longer or more variable oral and pharyngeal transit times and slower bolus velocity. Toner (1997) also noted the effect of a decreased sense of taste on the swallowing process. The age-related impairments in swallowing reported above are unlikely to result in noticeable swallowing problems. As with any age-related changes in healthy older people, it is important to remember these changes when assessing swallowing in older people who have had a stroke, have Parkinson's disease, or have other health conditions.

Effects of Visual Impairments on Communication

Visual problems are common in older people. Approximately one third of people over 80 have severe visual acuity problems (Maguire, 1996) that can have significant effects on communication. The effects may include a decreased ability to perceive communication cues such as facial expression or lip movements; difficulties in recognizing people in the near vicinity; and difficulties with watching television, reading, and writing. In addition, the increased social isolation that accompanies a severe visual impairment (e.g., Salive et al., 1992) may also lead to decreased opportunities for communication, thereby creating a spiral of reduced communication opportunity and performance. Although the effects of a severe visual impairment are easier to predict, the effects of mild and moderate visual impairments are less obvious. Older people with mild or moderate visual impairment may not only have reduced visual acuity but they may also have increased sensitivity to glare, reduced sensitivity to colors, reduced ability to perceive depth, poor night vision, and reduced tear flow (leading to increased dryness) (Lubinski & Welland, 1997; Maguire, 1996). In older people with hearing impairment, the ability to compensate for the hearing loss through increased use of visual cues is restricted if the person also has a visual loss.

For the speech-language pathologist, the wide-ranging effects of a visual impairment on communication needs to be well understood, and an audiologist needs to particularly understand the effects of an accompanying visual impairment on receptive communication and aural rehabilitation. Knowledge about the common pathologies associated with visual impairment underlies both disciplines. The most common age-related visual problems are

- Presbyopia or long sightedness: The eye is less able to accommodate from far to near distances. Presbyopia typically starts around 40 years of age, and most people need corrective glasses at age 65. Bifocal lenses are often prescribed once the eye is unable to see both far and near objects. These lenses can create difficulties for the older person when learning to use one lens for near vision and the other for distance vision.

- Cataracts: Opaque regions on the lens affect central vision first. Cataracts are often surgically removed.

- Glaucoma: A rise in pressure in the eyeball puts pressure on the optic nerve. The condition is treatable, and early intervention is recommended.

- Macular degeneration: A condition caused by small hemorrhages to the retina. Gray shadows are seen in the central visual area, and early symptoms include blurring of vision in the affected eye followed by a blind spot.

- Diabetic retinopathy: Occurs when diabetes is not well controlled and micro aneurysms and hemorrhages occur, obstructing the light rays to the retina. (Maguire, 1996)

Many of these conditions may lead to blindness, and audiologists and speech-language pathologists are important advocates for regular eye care in older people. Maguire (1996) stated that annual check-ups are recommended, but cited a study that suggested eye check-ups occur only every 5 to 7 years in residential care facilities for the aged. This situation has important implications for those who work in these facilities.

Weinstein (2000) suggested some useful strategies to employ when assessing older people with visual impairment in the clinical situation.

- Introduce yourself by name.
- Let the older person know when you enter or leave the room.
- Speak before touching the person.
- Approach the older person on the side with better vision.
- Let the person with visual loss do as much as possible as this builds confidence. (p. 31)

Finally, approximately one in five older people have a dual sensory loss, that is, both a visual and a hearing impairment (Hickson et al., 1999). Audiologists need to consider the visual abilities of an older person before prescribing a hearing aid. For example, if a client has a dual sensory impairment, a hearing aid with a remote control and modified battery compartment may be appropriate. In addition, communication education programs that teach listening strategies based on visual cues may also need to be modified for those with dual sensory impairment.

Effect of Cognitive Impairments on Communication

It is important for speech-language pathologists and audiologists to understand cognitive changes with age. For speech-language pathologists, the challenge is to understand the relationship between cognition and language, as they may need to assist with the differential diagnosis of dementia and language disorder. Previous discussions in this chapter about word retrieval and discourse attest to the integral relationship between the two. Likewise, audiologists may have a role in determining the relative effects of a hearing loss from a dementia. For example, staff in a residential care facility may ask the audiologist if the lack of responsiveness of a resident is principally due to hearing impairment or to dementia.

Cognitive age-related changes in both intelligence and memory function have been reported. Intelligence quotients drop by about 1 standard deviation in late 60- and early 70-year-olds (Johnson, 1997). Overall, verbal scores are more stable across time than performance scores (Johnson, 1997). Memory has been widely studied in older people because older people frequently complain of failing memories. Studies have found an age-related decline in both short-term and long-term memory (Garrett, 1992), with long-term memory problems associated with encoding and organization difficulties. Short-term or working memory has been found to be particularly influential in the organization of discourse. Long-term memory is divided into episodic and semantic memory. Semantic memory is a focus for speech-language pathologists and, for once, older people have been shown to have stability or even improvement in one area: passive vocabulary.

To summarize, the communication impairments that occur with increasing age are listed in Table 4–5. Some of these impairments (comprehension, conversational discourse skills, speech) are so subtle they are not reported to be a problem by older people, whereas others, such as hearing, memory, and word-finding problems, are of concern to healthy older people. Age-related changes in vision and cognitive skills also affect communication.

Overall Screening Assessment Battery for Healthy Older People

As noted earlier, there are three reasons why speech-language pathologists and audiologists need to know about communication impairments in healthy aging. The first is to interact appropriately with older people; the second is to determine abnormal patterns associated with pathological impairments; the third relates to monitoring older people's communication health over time as part of a health promotion program.

TABLE 4-5

SUMMARY OF COMMUNICATION IMPAIRMENTS ASSOCIATED WITH AGING.

Communication System	Description of Impairment
Hearing	Decreased sensitivity to pure tones Decreased ability to discriminate speech in adverse listening conditions
Language	Decreased speed and ability to retrieve words Decreased ability to comprehend with increased complexity of the message
Conversational discourse	Difficulty understanding complex and lengthy discourse Decreased efficiency and increased ambiguity in expression Increased degree of topic maintenance, decreased cohesion, decreased rate, increased number of words per clause and overall increase in number of words
Speech	Decreased respiratory support for speech output Imprecise articulation Slower rate of speech
Voice	Increase in pitch for males Decrease in pitch for females Decreased vocal quality

Note: From Caruso and Max (1997), Cherney (1996), Ripich (1991), Shadden (1988), and Shadden and Toner (1997).

There is a need for a comprehensive, yet brief, screening portfolio of communication in all these situations. The screening battery should measure the areas most vulnerable to change, be sensitive to change, and be as brief as possible. The brevity of the measures depends upon the context. For example, in annual health checkups, many areas of functioning may need to be assessed (for example, motor, cognitive, sensory, social, physical, and communication). In many longitudinal studies of aging, communication has generally not been assessed because of the lack of suitable tools. Hearing testing has often been included because of the brevity and objectivity of pure-tone audiometric screening. Figure 4–1 lists suggestions for a simple screening battery for measuring communication impairments in healthy older people. Measures at the impairment, activity, and participation levels are included, and the activity and participation measures are discussed in detail in Chapters 5 and 6, respectively. Although there is lim-

Impairments

- Pure-tone hearing screening (air conduction threshold testing 500 Hz to 4000 Hz)

- Boston Naming Test (30-item empirical version, from Williams et al., 1989)

- Conversational sample (for simple Visual Analogue Scale ratings of voice, speech, and discourse)

  - ○ Vocal quality   Excellent _____ Poor

  - ○ Vocal pitch   Excellent _____ Poor

  - ○ Vocal loudness   Excellent _____ Poor

  - ○ Speech   Excellent _____ Poor

  - ○ Discourse   Excellent _____ Poor

(Visual and cognitive impairments to be measured separately by relevant health professionals, for example, optometry and pyschology.)

Activity (see Chapter 5)

- Hearing Handicap Inventory for the Elderly (Ventry & Weinstein, 1982)

- COMACT (Cruice, 2001)

Participation (see Chapter 6)

- Social networks (Antonucci & Akiyama, 1987)

- Dartmouth COOP Charts (Nelson et al. 1987)

FIGURE 4–1. A simple screening battery for measuring communication impairments in healthy older people.

ited research about the sensitivity of these measures to change over time, the measures have been found to be quick to administer and appropriate to the population (Cruice et al., 2000; Worrall, Hickson, Barnett, & Yiu, 1998; Worrall, Yiu, Hickson, & Barnett, 1995). They also have the advantage of focusing on the communication areas most vulnerable to change. Both the activity and participation level measures are self-report, so although they are best administered in an interview format, they can also be given as written questionnaires. This format decreases the administration time considerably for the entire battery of tests.

Communication and Swallowing Impairments in Pathological Aging

The majority of older clients seen by audiologists fall into the healthy aging group; however, most speech-language pathologists are more likely to be involved in the rehabilitation of older people with identifiable pathologies that have caused a communication or swallowing impairment. This section describes the age-related diseases that commonly result in communication and swallowing impairments The speech, language, hearing, voice, and swallowing impairments that may result from stroke, DAT, Parkinson's disease, cancer of the head and neck, traumatic brain injury, and ALS are summarized (Table 4–6) and the assessments commonly used listed. The particular challenges of working with older people with these impairments are then discussed. Finally, three case studies are described that illustrate the challenge of multiple impairment in this population.

Stroke

Stroke is one of the major causes of chronic disease and the third most frequent cause of mortality in the Western world. In the United States alone, it is estimated that care for people with stroke costs between $5 and $10 billion per year (Mlcoch & Metter, 1994). Seventy percent of strokes occur in people over 65 years of age (Bonita, 1992). Stroke, cerebrovascular accident (CVA), or the increasingly popular term *brain attack* is an interruption of blood supply to the brain. There are two types of strokes: ischemic and hemorrhagic. Ischemic strokes result from a blockage to the arteries supplying blood to the brain. Hemorrhagic stroke occurs when the walls of the blood vessel burst. The blockage in ischemic strokes can be a result of a blood clot that has formed locally in the brain (thrombosis) or that has traveled from elsewhere in the body (embolism). The part of the brain that has been deprived of blood dies as a result. The area around the necrosis also swells and goes into shock (diaschisis). If there is partial or temporary blockage, for example as a result of arteriosclerosis (a thickening of the arterial walls), a transient ischemic attack (TIA) may occur. A TIA is a small stroke lasting less than 24 hours. Multiple strokes can result in multi-infarct or vascular dementia, a different form of dementia from DAT described later. The most common cause of stroke is hypertension or high blood pressure. Other risk factors include obesity, smoking, drinking, and diabetes.

A stroke can cause a multitude of impairments to body function. The major determinant of which impairments remain after a stroke is the location of the stroke in the brain. If the area of the brain that controls the function of the right leg is damaged by the stroke, then paralysis of the right leg will occur. Hemiparesis (a paralysis of half of the body) is a

TABLE 4–6

AGE-RELATED DISEASES THAT MAY CAUSE IMPAIRMENTS OF COMMUNICATION AND SWALLOWING.

Disease	Speech-Language Pathology Implications	Speech-Language Pathology References	Audiology Implications	Audiology References
Cancer of the larynx	Full or partial laryngectomy leading to alaryngeal speech, Dysphagia	Edels (1983); Weinberg, (1980)	May have ototoxic medications prescribed	
Cerebrovascular disease (stroke)	Aphasia, Dysarthria, Dysphagia, Dyspraxia	Carrau & Murray (1999); LaPointe (1990); Murdoch (1990); Yorkston, Beukelman, Strand, & Bell (1999)	Prevalence of hearing impairment is higher in the stroke population than in healthy older people	Formby, Phillips, & Thomas (1987)
Dementia	Language of dementia, Dysphagia	Bayles & Kaszniak (1987); Carrau & Murray (1999); Lubinski (1995)	Prevalence of hearing impairment is higher in older people with dementia than in healthy older people	Palmer, Adams, Bourgeois, Durrant, & Rossi (1999); Uhlmann, Larson, Thomas, Koepsell, & Duckert (1989)
Head injuries (often associated with falls by older people)	Dysarthria, Cognitive-communicative impairment	McDonald, Togher, & Code (1999); Murdoch (1990); Snow & Ponsford (1995)	Hearing impairment is a frequent consequence of head injury, particularly if it is a base of skull fracture	Hofmeister et al. (2000); Fitzgerald (1996); Nosan, Benecke, & Murr (1997)

Disease	Speech-Language Pathology Implications	Speech-Language Pathology References	Audiology Implications	Audiology References
Parkinson's disease	Hypokinetic dysarthria, High level language impairment, Dysphagia	Carrau & Murray (1999); Katz, Davidoff, & Wolfe (1984); Yorkston et al. (1999)	No significant hearing impairments reported	
Amyotrophic lateral sclerosis/ motor neuron disease	Flaccid dysarthria, Dysphagia	Carrau & Murray (1999); Yorkston et al. (1999)	No significant hearing impairments reported	

common sequela of stroke. If the part of the brain that controls visual fields is damaged, a hemianopia may occur. Aphasia and apraxia mostly occur after left hemisphere strokes, whereas a cognitive communication impairment may follow right hemisphere damage. Dysarthria can occur from strokes in many parts of the brain, whereas dysphagia is a common early problem following any stroke.

There are two other problems associated with stroke that are important to consider because they can significantly affect communication with others. They are also behaviors associated with communication disability. First, lability, in which the person cannot inhibit emotional responses (usually crying), is upsetting for both the patient and any conversational partner. Second, perseveration is another behavior associated with aphasia following stroke; it occurs when a word or phrase is repeated inappropriately. This behavior again is often linked with the inability of the person to inhibit a response. Perseveration can lead to recurring utterances such as "Close the door" or "Pain, pain, pain" or "Kevin knife night tonight," which constitute the only remaining language of the client. These are often bizarre pieces of language that are not well understood. The communication and swallowing impairments that result from stroke are described in more detail in the following sections.

APHASIA

Aphasia is caused most often by a stroke in the language processing areas of the left hemisphere. Comprehension and expression of language may be affected, hence a person with aphasia may have difficulty listening, speaking, reading, and writing. A person with the most severe form of aphasia, global aphasia, will have extreme difficulty understanding speech and will have little or no verbal output. He or she may, however, still attempt to communicate and want to be involved in communication, although most communication will be in nonverbal forms such as facial expression, intonation, and eye contact. In the mildest form of aphasia, anomic aphasia, everyday conversation may disguise the word-finding difficulty of the client. On testing, however, word-finding difficulties exist, and the person will often report difficulty in finding the right word in conversation. A person with aphasia once described it as "like having the words wrapped in black plastic in your brain," and another person claimed it was more like clear plastic wrapping because he could see the word but was unable to retrieve it.

There have been attempts to categorize aphasia into syndromes (Geschwind, 1965; Goodglass & Kaplan, 1972). Certainly, there is general consensus that there is a dichotomy between fluent or receptive aphasia and nonfluent or expressive aphasia. It needs to be noted, however, that most people with aphasia have both comprehension and expression problems. The most common classification scheme includes the syndromes of Wernicke's, anomic, conduction transcortical sensory, transcortical motor, global, and Broca's aphasia. Aphasiologists who take a psycholinguistic or cognitive neuropsychological approach, however, argue that aphasia should be considered in terms of the breakdown in language processing rather than in syndromes (see Byng, Kay, Edmundsen, & Scott, 1990). The clinician's view of these two approaches will influence choice of assessment and ultimately choice of treatment. Assessments such as the WAB (Kertesz, 1982) and the BDAE (Goodglass et al., 2001) take a syndrome or localizationist approach, whereas PALPA (Kay et al., 1997) allows the examiner to establish the specific breakdown in the language processing system. Further details of these assessments are included in the assessment section later in this chapter.

Cognitive-Communication Impairment from Right Hemisphere Brain Damage

Damage to the right hemisphere affects the cognitive processes of attention, perception, memory, organization, reasoning, and problem solving, and these, in turn, affect communication skills, particularly pragmatics (Cherney & Halper, 2000). Myers (2001) described the cognitive-communication impairment following right brain damage in terms of three main areas.

1. Linguistic impairments: typically mild impairments at the narrative or discourse level.
2. Nonlinguistic impairments: attention deficits and neglect, in which patients fail to acknowledge the side of the body affected by the stroke.
3. Extralinguistic impairments: monotone pitch, lack of facial expression, literal interpretations of information, poor understanding of humor or irony, and inefficient communication that lacks specificity.

It is the extralinguistic disorders that are the key features of a cognitive-communication impairment following right hemisphere damage.

DYSARTHRIA

Although aphasia is a central disorder of language processing, dysarthria following stroke is caused by damage to the areas of the brain that control the speech muscles. It is, therefore, a speech disorder rather than a language disorder. The most severe form of dysarthria, anarthria, is not common. A client with anarthria is unable to make any intelligible utterances and needs to communicate via writing or with a communication device such as a LightWriter™ (www.zygo-usa.com). In anarthria, lip seal, facial expression, eating, and swallowing are also often severely affected, because the speech muscles are involved in these functions. A mild dysarthria, however, may only manifest itself as slight slurring of speech, particularly when the client is fatigued. There may also be a slight telltale asymmetry of facial muscles in a mild dysarthria. Many people have dysarthria following stroke that is between these two extremes. Table 4–7 summarizes the clinical and perceptual features of different types of dysarthria.

There are two major types of dysarthria following stroke depending on which part of the brain is damaged: spastic dysarthria and flaccid dysarthria. Spastic dysarthria is an upper motor neuron lesion characterized by spastic paralysis, weakness, limited range of motion, and slowness of movement (Yorkston et al., 1999). If the damage is unilateral, there is a substantial amount of compensation by the other half of the brain, and much recovery takes place. On the other hand, if the damage is bilateral, the term used is *pseudobulbar palsy*. In general, pseudobulbar palsy is more severe than a unilateral lesion. There is often an underlying reason why bilateral lesions occur in the motor speech area. The most common is that the client is having multiple strokes or lacunar infarcts, possibly due to diabetes or uncontrolled hypertension. There is, therefore, an increased likelihood of a multi-infarct dementia occurring in conjunction with pseudobulbar palsy. Dysphagia and a condition called pseudobulbar affect, which is a difficulty controlling emotions similar to lability, often accompany pseudobulbar palsy.

The other commonly occurring type of dysarthria is flaccid dysarthria, which is caused by a lesion to the lower motor neuron area. A brainstem stroke can affect the cranial nerves and produce a flaccid dysarthria. The symptoms depend upon which specific cranial nerves have been affected. Damage from stroke can occur in other parts of the brain, leading to other types of dysarthrias. For example, cerebellar stroke is associated with ataxic dysarthria.

Often, strokes result in a person having a mixed dysarthria with characteristics of spastic, flaccid, and ataxic dysarthria, or combinations of these, depending upon the site of lesion. Indeed, Duffy (1995) found that one third of dysarthric cases at the Mayo Clinic over a 3-year

TABLE 4–7

SUMMARY OF CLINICAL AND PERCEPTUAL FEATURES OF DYSARTHRIA.

Type of Dysarthria	Clinical Features[1]	Perceptual Features[2]
Spastic dysarthria	Spastic paralysis Weakness Limited range of motion Slowness of movement	Prosodic excess (excess and equal stress, slow rate) Articulatory-resonatory incompetence (imprecise consonants, distorted vowels, hypernasality) Prosodic insufficiency (monopitch, monoloudness, reduced stress, short phrases) Phonatory stenosis (low pitch, harshness, strained-strangled voice, pitch breaks, short phrases, slow rate)
Flaccid dysarthria	Flaccid paralysis Weakness Hypotonia Muscle atrophy Fasciculations	Phonatory incompetence (breathiness, short phrases, audible inspiration) Resonatory incompetence (hypernasality, imprecise consonants, nasal emission, short phrases) Phonatory-prosodic insufficiency (harsh voice, monoloudness, monopitch)
Ataxic dysarthria	Inaccurate movement Slow movement Hypotonia	Articulatory inaccuracy (imprecise consonants, irregular articulatory breakdowns, distorted vowels) Prosodic excess (excess and equal stress, prolonged phonemes, prolonged intervals, slow rate) Phonatory-prosodic insufficiency (harshness, monopitch, monoloudness)
Hypokinetic dysarthria	Resting tremor Rigidity Bradykinesis Postural instability	Monopitch, reduced stress, monoloudness, imprecise consonants, short rushes of speech, breathiness and harshness, lack of breath support, decreased volume (Darley, Aronson, & Brown, 1975)

Note: [1] From Yorkston et al. (1999); [2] from Duffy (1994).

period were mixed dysarthrias. The perceptual, acoustic, and physiological features of mixed dysarthria vary according to the site of lesion(s). It is for this reason that the assessment of mixed dysarthria "tax the diagnostic skills of the clinician" (Theodoros, 1998, p. 363). Theodoros argues for the inclusion of physiological assessments in these cases to help the diagnostic process.

APRAXIA

When the stroke affects the part of the brain that affects motor planning (the premotor cortex), a dyspraxia occurs. Oral dyspraxia is when the client finds it difficult to complete non-speech oral movements such as "Poke out your tongue." A limb apraxia is demonstrated by an inability to demonstrate simple gestures such as "Make a fist." A verbal dyspraxia is a difficulty with planning speech movements, so there is often groping behavior with the speech muscles as the client tries to say sounds or words. These three types of dyspraxia can occur independently, but often occur together. A severe form of pure verbal dyspraxia renders the person speechless, but language is intact, so the person can write to communicate. These clients become very frustrated and may require many hours of therapy. Verbal dyspraxia, however, often occurs with aphasia, in particular, with a Broca's aphasia.

DYSPHAGIA

Dysphagia is a swallowing impairment, rather than a communication impairment, and is particularly common in the first few days or weeks after a stroke. Over the past decade, swallowing impairments have increasingly become a major focus for speech-language pathologists. In fact, the majority of referrals to speech-language pathologists working in health care settings have been in the area of dysphagia (Sonies, 2000). Groher and Bukatman (1986) found that 13% of patients in two acute care hospitals had swallowing dysfunction, and Trupe and Siebens (1984) reported that 59% of residents in a residential care facility for the aged had dysphagia. The health problems that can result from swallowing dysfunction include dehydration, undernutrition, aspiration pneumonia, depression, or even death (Caruso & Max, 1997).

Many hospitals place all new stroke patients on a nonoral diet (for example, on a nasogastric tube). The patient is at risk of aspiration if an oral intake is started when the swallowing mechanism is not functioning well. In the acute stroke phase, the speech-language pathologist's role is to monitor the functioning of the swallowing mechanism and adjust the patient's diet accordingly. Intervention to improve functioning, such as oromotor exercise or compensatory strategies such as a supraglottic swallow, also may be required.

Dementia of the Alzheimer's Type

DAT is the most common form of dementia. Other types of dementia include Pick's disease, multi-infarct or vascular dementia, primary progressive aphasia, and dementia associated with

Parkinson's disease. Hopper and Bayles (2001) described the criteria for DAT as a gradual onset of cognitive impairments that get worse with time and that are not associated with any other neurological impairments. Hopper and Bayles also reviewed the neuropathological and neurochemical changes responsible for DAT and the risk factors for these changes. The neuropathological changes include an increase in neurofibrillary tangles and neuritic plaques and an overall neuronal atrophy in the brain of people with DAT. Age is the most important risk factor but genetic abnormalities are also related.

Cognitive-Communication Impairment

As in the cognitive-communication disorder associated with right hemisphere damage following stroke, there is a cluster of cognitive processes that are impaired in DAT that have an effect on communication. Memory is the most obvious impairment, and this impairment has an effect on semantics and discourse. Figure 4–2 contains a summary of the conversational features associated with DAT described by Orange and Purves (1996). Hopper and Bayles (2001) summarized the features of communication associated with the progression of DAT. Early in the disease process, people with DAT forget what they have read or heard and become repetitive. As the disease progresses, their discourse becomes fragmented and impoverished, and tangentiality, perseverations, and lack of coherence occur. Formulation and

- Egocentric
- Fewer adherences to conventions of conversation
- Less sensitive to others in conversation
- Shrinking vocabulary
- Fluctuating relevance and accuracy of responses to questions
- Topic maintenance and turn-taking problems, abrupt topic shifting
- Shorter conversational turns
- Intrusions of words and themes, unable to engage in extended discourse
- Partners have difficulty following verbal output
- Disrupted reference and cohesion
- Empty language, primary use of indefinite terms
- Uses more words

FIGURE 4–2. Conversational features of Alzheimer's disease. Adapted from Orange and Purves (1996).

expression of ideas both verbally and in written form become more difficult, as does comprehension ability. Phonology and syntax, however, remain relatively intact throughout.

DYSPHAGIA

The cognitive impairment associated with dementia is also the reason why dysphagia is present in this population. A person with dementia may demonstrate misperception or lack of awareness of food, and distractibility while eating, or may simply forget to swallow. He or she may also exhibit primitive motor patterns, poor bolus preparation, delayed pharyngeal swallow, and reduced laryngeal elevation resulting in possible aspiration (Toner, 1997; Owens, Metz, & Haas, 2000).

Hearing Impairment

The prevalence of hearing impairment in older people with dementia is very high, and research data indicate that hearing impairment may be a risk factor for cognitive decline and that it may exacerbate the symptoms of dementia. Uhlmann et al. (1989) studied 100 older people with DAT matched for age, gender, and educational level with 100 people who did not have dementia. The mean hearing level of the group with dementia was significantly worse (by 3.3 dB) than that of the control group, and the prevalence of hearing impairment was significantly higher in the group with dementia (59% compared with 44% of the control group). Peters, Potter, and Scholer (1988) conducted an interesting longitudinal study of 38 people aged 62 to 89 years who had various forms of dementia. These individuals were assessed on two occasions, separated by 6 to 16 months. Twenty-two of the subjects (55%) were hearing impaired (i.e., better ear pure-tone average at 2000 and 4000 Hz $\geq$ 40 dB HTL). The performance of all subjects on the Mini-Mental State Examination (Folstein, Folstein, & McHugh, 1975) declined over time; however, the decline was significantly greater for the group of subjects with hearing impairment. This difference between subject groups remained after adjustment for the fact that the people with hearing impairment were older.

This indicates the importance of assessing hearing in older people with dementia so that appropriate rehabilitation can be provided. Rehabilitation for older people with dementia and hearing impairment is discussed in Chapter 9. In terms of the assessment of impairment, pure-tone audiometry is typically used to determine hearing levels in this population. Although it is necessary to modify the test procedure somewhat depending on the cognitive abilities of the older person, it has been found that reliable thresholds can be obtained (Uhlmann et al., 1989). The test procedure may be modified as follows:

- Conduct the test in the room with the older person (for example, do not use a client-only test booth).
- Conduct the test at a time when the person is reportedly most alert (arrange a suitable time in consultation with caregivers).

- Repeat instructions slowly a number of times prior to and during the assessment.
- Demonstrate the response required.
- Be prepared to accept a variety of responses (for example, raising a hand, nodding, making a noise, eye blink).
- Start testing at each frequency at a clearly audible presentation level.
- Slow down the rate of stimulus presentation.
- Give substantial encouragement and positive reinforcement during the test.

Parkinson's Disease

Parkinson's disease is a progressive neurological disorder with no known etiology that often occurs in later life. It is characterized by a resting tremor, muscle rigidity, and slowness of movement. A lack of dopamine to the substantia nigra in the subcortex is the cause of the impairments; the drug, L-dopa, is given to redress this imbalance. People with Parkinson's disease have a masklike face, shuffling gait, often have depression, and are at risk for falls. Dementia may also occur. The most significant communication problem associated with Parkinson's disease is hypokinetic dysarthria, but there are also signs of subcortical language impairment and dysphagia.

DYSARTHRIA

The features of hypokinetic dysarthria associated with Parkinson's disease are summarized in Table 4–7. A combination of these features and a paucity of gesture and facial expression lead to significant speech impairment in the later stages of Parkinson's disease.

COGNITIVE-COMMUNICATION IMPAIRMENT

There are a number of cliniconeurological correlation studies that have found language disorders in association with subcortical lesions (Murdoch, 2001). It is not surprising, therefore, that language impairments have been found in people with Parkinson's disease. There has been some controversy, however, about whether these impairments are a product of the dementia associated with Parkinson's disease or a true language impairment. Dementia occurs in approximately 41% of parkinsonian cases (Mayeaux et al., 1992). Lewis, La Pointe, Murdoch, and Chenery (1998) found that people with Parkinson's disease, with and without cognitive impairment, exhibited signs of language impairment. Those with cognitive impairments displayed more extensive language impairments than had been previously acknowledged in the literature. Participants with normal cognitive status had difficulties providing definitions and in sentence construction. All participants had impaired naming and definitional abilities and difficulties interpreting ambiguity and figurative language. In summary, people with Parkinson's disease may show difficulties across a range of complex linguistic functions.

DYSPHAGIA

The most common swallowing difficulty for people with Parkinson's disease is during the transport of the bolus to the back of the tongue in the oral phase. As the disease progresses, the pharyngeal stage may also be affected with delays in the swallowing reflex and laryngeal closure, thereby increasing the risk of aspiration.

Cancer of the Larynx, Pharynx, or Tongue

The incidence of cancer increases with age, and a tumor in the oral cavity, pharynx, or larynx has communication and swallowing consequences. The primary treatment is surgery to remove the tumor and surrounding areas, and the extent of surgery affects the severity of communication and swallowing impairment. For example, a small tongue or lip lesion is unlikely to have a significant effect on communication and swallowing. In contrast, a complete laryngectomy to remove a laryngeal cancer will have a significant effect on communication and, in the initial phases, on swallowing. Chemotherapy and radiotherapy that often accompany the surgery also have an effect on the functioning of the speech musculature, with radiotherapy affecting salivation and causing swelling, and chemotherapy indirectly affecting swallowing through appetite suppression.

APHONIA

The extent of surgery for laryngeal cancer depends upon the site and stage of the tumor. The larynx may be partially or completely removed, resulting in dysphonia or aphonia. If the larynx is removed, the trachea is connected to the outside of the neck through a tracheostomy, and the patient breathes through a stoma (hole) in the neck. The patient has three options for speech.

1. Esophageal voice. This speech is taught by injecting or inhaling air into the esophagus just below the pharyngoesophageal segment. The esophagus can vibrate instead of the larynx. The patient, therefore, speaks by continually injecting air into this space to create sound.

2. A portable electrolarynx. This device uses a battery to vibrate a membrane against the patient's neck to create sound.

3. A voice prosthesis. This speech is currently the most popular and consists of a small one-way valve inserted in the wall between the trachea and the esophagus, which allows air to flow from the trachea to the space below the pharyngoesophageal segment in the esophagus. The one-way valve does not allow fluids or solids to flow back from the esophagus into the trachea and hence into the lungs. A pressure valve may also be used on the stoma to create pressure in the trachea so that adequate air pressure can be channeled into the esophagus for speech. The tracheoesophageal puncture (TEP) for the voice prostheses may be performed at the time of the laryngectomy operation (a primary TEP), or it may be performed in a separate operation sometime after the laryngectomy (a secondary TEP).

DYSPHAGIA

For laryngectomy cases, dysphagia is most likely to occur in the days following surgery. There is a possibility that the surgery has inadvertently created a fistula in the upper esophagus so that liquid escapes through into the trachea or other nearby areas. The fistula is identified and may need to be surgically closed. Dysphagia may be an ongoing impairment in cases where there has been extensive surgery to the oral cavity, for example, in a total glossectomy. The oral phase of the swallow may be affected, and compensatory strategies may need to be implemented.

Traumatic Brain Injury

Traumatic brain injury (TBI) is not normally associated with older people; however, falls, motor vehicle accidents, violent crimes, and failed suicide attempts do occur in this population. It is, therefore, important not to discount TBI as a potential cause of a communication and/or swallowing impairment in an older person. The brain damage associated with TBI is mostly diffuse, but can be focal, and causes a number of cognitive and behavioral changes. These changes include impaired abilities in attention and concentration, initiation and goal direction, judgment and perception, learning, memory, speed of processing, and communication (Prigatano, Roueche, & Fordyce, 1986). Speech, hearing, and swallowing may also be affected by TBI.

COGNITIVE-COMMUNICATION IMPAIRMENT

The cognitive-communication impairment that occurs following TBI is characterized by (ASHA, 1988)

- disorganized, tangential, wandering discourse
- imprecise language and word-retrieval difficulties
- disinhibited, socially inappropriate language
- restricted output
- lack of initiation
- difficulty comprehending extended or rapidly spoken language
- difficulty communicating in distracting or stressful environments
- difficulty reading social cues
- difficulty understanding abstract language
- inefficient verbal learning and verbal reasoning

DYSARTHRIA

The site of lesion and type of injury influences the type of dysarthria following TBI. Diffuse lesions often produce a mixed dysarthria with features of flaccid, spastic, and ataxic dysarthria (see Table 4–7). In severe cases, intelligibility is significantly affected.

HEARING IMPAIRMENT

Hearing impairment may occur following TBI (Fitzgerald, 1996; Nosan et al., 1997). It is most common if the individual has sustained a temporal bone fracture; a longitudinal fracture of this bone is associated with conductive hearing loss, and a transverse fracture is associated with sensorineural loss (Nosan et al., 1997). Hofmeister et al. (2000) pointed out that the clinician will not always be aware that a patient has a temporal bone fracture, however, as the more general description of base of skull fracture is frequently used in medical charts. In summary, it is important for audiologists to be aware that hearing impairment is one of the sequelae of TBI and that older people who have had TBI should receive a comprehensive audiological assessment.

DYSPHAGIA

Dysphagia is a common sequela immediately following TBI. It is often associated with dysarthria, and the cognitive and behavioral consequences of TBI, particularly immediately postinjury, make dysphagia management in this population particularly challenging. In some cases, tracheostomies have been inserted to keep the airway clear. Hence, communication is additionally limited.

Amyotrophic Lateral Sclerosis

ALS is another progressive disease that may begin in midlife but may continue into later life. There are some differences of opinion about the most appropriate terminology; however, motor neuron disease is often the preferred term in countries such as the United Kingdom and Australia, whereas amyotrophic lateral sclerosis (ALS) is commonly used in the United States and Canada. People with ALS gradually lose muscle function; however, cortical functions such as cognition and language remain intact.

DYSARTHRIA

ALS is a disease affecting both the upper and lower motor neurons to varying degrees and results in a mixed dysarthria. If the disease has had a bulbar onset, speech and swallowing functions are often the first affected, and there is rapid deterioration. Maintenance of some form of communication during this period is a vital role for speech-language pathologists. If the disease is primarily corticobulbar and dysarthria is present, there continues to be a role for the speech-language pathologist in the maintenance of speech and swallowing functions, with compensatory and augmentative communication systems initiated at appropriate stages (Theorodos, 1998).

DYSPHAGIA

In bulbar onset cases, swallowing function declines rapidly and there is a need to consider alternative feeding methods (for example, nasogastric tube) relatively early. Perienteral gastrostomy (PEG) feeding is often instituted. The speech-language pathologist again plays an important role in the team management of the client, and end-of-life decisions need to be managed ethically and with sensitivity.

Assessment of Communication and Swallowing Impairments in Pathological Aging

There is a range of standardized assessments available for the impairments described previously (see Figure 4–8). Aphasia, dysarthria, dyspraxia, and tests for right hemisphere damage constitute the basis for much of speech-language pathology practice. More recently, standardized assessments for cognitive-communication impairments associated with dementia have also been developed (see Hopper & Bayles, 2001). The tests in Figure 4–8 are recommended as a starting point for speech-language pathologists working in a clinical setting with older clients.

There are few standardized tests for swallowing. There are, however, numerous scales of general dysphagia severity that have been developed (see Sonies, 2000, for a review). Most consist of a single scale describing the swallowing behavior at each point of the scale. ASHA has been involved in developing many of these scales in the United States (e.g., the Functional Communication Measure scales, the ASHA Functional Outcomes Task Force Matrix or those developed for the National Outcomes Measurement System, see Sonies, 2000). The most popular scale in Australia is the Royal Brisbane Hospital Outcome Measure for Swallowing (Speech Pathology Department, Royal Brisbane Hospital, 1998; Ward & Conroy, 1999) (see Chapter 5). The 10-point rating scale has four stages of oral intake from nil by mouth to maintaining oral intake (see Table 5–8).

There are limitations to techniques such as a modified barium swallow or a fiberoptic endoscopic evaluation of swallowing (FEES) with older people. These measures may not be available in many residential care facilities for the aged or community-based settings; the techniques have questionable repeatability and, in the case of the FEES, the naturalness of the swallow is affected by the procedure, and it is difficult to perform with people who are confused or agitated (Toner, 1997). Observation of mealtime behavior is a source of much information, and cervical auscultation holds promise in providing additional information with less invasiveness and a minimal amount of equipment.

The value of ethnographic methodologies, such as observation of real-life behavior and interviews about everyday behavior, cannot be overstated when assessing older people. For older clients with severe communication and/or cognitive impairments, there may be no other way to assess impairments. Observation of events such as mealtimes or group conversations may be conducted unobtrusively, particularly if the observer is participating in the normal ritual of the event and notes are written up after the event. For older adults with severe impairments, observations of responsiveness or attempts to

TABLE 4–8

SUMMARY OF STANDARDIZED TESTS FOR SPEECH AND LANGUAGE IMPAIRMENTS ASSOCIATED WITH AGING.

Name of Test	Reference	Description
Western Aphasia Battery (WAB)	Kertesz (1982)	One of the most frequently used aphasia tests throughout the world. The oral language section contains 10 subtests that assess spontaneous speech, auditory comprehension, repetition, and naming. The Aphasia Quotient (AQ) is the score calculated from these subtests out of a total of 100. The presence of aphasia is indicated by a score of 93.8 or less. Scores for each of the subtests also guide the determination of the category or type of aphasia. There are seven further subtests that examine reading, writing, praxis, and construction abilities. The scores for all subtests determine the Cortical Quotient or the overall score for the WAB.
Boston Diagnostic Aphasia Examination (BDAE)	Goodglass et al., (2001)	The most recent version of another frequently used aphasia test. Raw scores are converted to percentiles to determine the type of aphasia, but an overall score for the test is not calculated. It includes a 30–45-minute shortened version. Includes assessments of category-specific word comprehension and word production, syntax comprehension, graphophonemic processing, and specific reading disorders.
Rehabilitation Institute of Chicago Evaluation of Right Hemisphere Dysfunction-Revised (RICE-R)	Halper, Cherney, Burns, & Mogil, (1996)	Assists in differentially diagnosing right hemisphere dysfunction as well as determining the severity of the impairment. Includes a behavior observation profile, a pragmatic communication skills rating, a visual scanning and tracking assessment, and an analysis of writing and metaphorical language.

continues

TABLE 4–8 CONTINUED

Name of Test	Reference	Description
Arizona Battery for Communication in Dementia (ABCD)	Bayles & Tomoeda (1993)	Designed for the assessment of people with mild and moderate dementia. Consists of 14 subtests that assess the areas of linguistic expression, linguistic comprehension, verbal episodic memory, mental status, and visuospatial construction. The examiner can determine an overall score for the test as well as break down the scores to analyze the profile of skills across the test.
Frenchay Dysarthria Assessment (FDA)	Enderby (1983)	A frequently used test in the United Kingdom and other British Commonwealth countries. Can be administered to individuals with different types of dysarthria and different etiologies. Examines reflexes, respiration, lips, jaw, soft palate, tongue, and laryngeal function, and includes a simple measure of overall intelligibility. Each task is rated on a 9-point scale. Provides a graphic display of the overall strengths and weaknesses of the client's speech function.
Apraxia Battery for Adults (ABA)	Dabul (1979)	A useful test to detect and determine the severity of apraxia. Has six subtests including diadochokinetic rate, imitation of words of increasing length, picture naming, three repetitions of multisyllabic words, oral and limb apraxia tasks, and an inventory of behaviors that are associated with apraxia.

interact with other people may be noted. The modality and success of communication attempts may also be of therapeutic interest. Talking with clients, their family members, and professional caregivers is also another source of valuable information about the client's communication and/or swallowing abilities. Talking with the client and his or her caregivers may be an informal conversation or a more structured interview, during which responses to specific questions are sought.

Challenge of Older Clients With Communication and Swallowing Impairments

When clinicians consider the impairments associated with pathological aging, some additional challenges that the older client presents to the clinician are worth noting. These challenges are discussed below in relation to nature of the impairment, the assessment, and the treatment of older clients with a communication disability.

EFFECT OF AGE ON THE NATURE OF THE IMPAIRMENT AND ASSESSMENT

1. *Type and severity of impairment*. Older people are not only more prone to diseases that affect communication and swallowing, but increasing age may also have an impact on the type and severity of the impairment. Chapman (1988) and Chapman and Ulatowska (1991) noted, for example, that the older person has greater susceptibility to different types of stroke than a younger person has. This produces an increased prevalence of posterior type lesions, leading to a higher incidence of Wernicke's aphasia. The severity of the aphasia is often greater, and this, combined with more posterior lesion sites, results in a higher incidence of global aphasia. Hence, older people often present with more severe aphasia that is often global or Wernicke's type.

   Multiple strokes are also more common with age, and this multiplicity may have an effect on the type of dysarthria and dysphagia. For example, multiple strokes are more likely to give rise to a bilateral spastic dysarthria (pseudobulbar palsy) or a mixed dysarthria, combining elements of spastic, flaccid, and ataxic dysarthria. Multiple strokes may also mean that several stages of the swallowing process are affected more severely.

   Early or late onsets of diseases such as Alzheimer's or Parkinson's disease also affect the nature of impairment in the older person. In general, an earlier onset of the disease indicates a more aggressive disease. Increasing age also increases the likelihood that an insidious disease, such as cancer of the larynx, may have progressed further. Therefore, the disease may well be more severe in an older person than in a younger person.

2. *Increased co-morbidity*. As noted on many occasions, multiple impairments are a feature of aging. Hence, the probability that other communication-related impairments exist increases with age. For example, Holland and Bartlett (1985) found that 23% of their sample of participants with aphasia over 70 years of age showed signs of dementia, whereas none of the participants less than 60 years of age showed any signs. Aphasia test results in older people may, therefore, be influenced by the presence of cognitive impairments. The increased prevalence of hearing and visual impairments in older people will also affect assessment and treatment of any client with another communication disability, and the co-occurrence of other health problems such as heart or respiratory diseases will also influence assessment and treatment.

3. *Lack of normative data*. Many communication and swallowing assessments have limited normative data for older people, particularly for those in the oldest groups.

Because people are living longer now than when many tests were developed, normative data may be unavailable for current older age groups. The lack of normative data for older clients limits the interpretation of test results, as age-related impairments are not taken into account. The Boston Naming Test (BNT; Kaplan et al., 1983), for example, was originally normed for people aged 59 years and younger, with no normative data provided for those over 59 years.

4. *Complexity of medical history*. Obtaining an accurate medical history of the client is an important first step in any assessment process in speech-language pathology and audiology. Chapman (1988) and Chapman and Ulatowska (1991) noted that the medical history of older clients is often longer and more complex than younger clients. It can sometimes be difficult to obtain a good case history when it is so complex. It may also be difficult because the spouse who may be providing the history is usually an older person. Lack of specific medical information is particularly problematic in residential care facilities for the aged where limited information is passed on to the facility via the client's chart (Pye, Worrall, & Hickson, 2000).

Effect of Age on Treatment and Recovery

1. *Consent to treatment*. The decision about whether to treat is a complex one. Shared decision making (Coulter, 1997; Worrall, 2000) in which joint responsibility for deciding a course of action is shared among the client, the family, and the clinician is recommended. Although age is not a barrier to successful rehabilitation for many people with communication disabilities, there are some older people who choose not to invest too many of their limited mental, physical, and financial resources into rehabilitation. They may decide to live with what life has dealt them. The decision to treat or not to treat is not the clinician's alone. In addition, it must be remembered that to deny treatment on the basis of age alone is a form of age discrimination.

2. *Recovery rate*. Chapman and Ulatowska (1991) noted that recovery from aphasia is often slower in older people than younger people in the initial stages, but there is evidence to suggest that older people make as many gains as younger people in the long term. There is no evidence that age alone slows recovery, but the increased chances of co-morbidity and other factors discussed in this section may have an effect on recovery rate in older people.

3. *Energy levels*. Older people have less stamina and may fatigue more easily. Hence, assessment and treatment sessions need to be shorter. This is particularly the case in the acute stages of stroke or sudden onset of disease when the client is still in the hospital. Apart from the physical, mental, and emotional effects of the disease that he or she is coping with, there is also the issue of coping with the hospital environment in the acute phase (see Chapter 8). The older person is frequently having physical and occupational therapy as well as speech-language therapy. These treatments take a particularly heavy toll on the older patient who has had a stroke who may have been relatively sedentary before the stroke.

4. *Social support and counseling*. The social situation of an older person is different from that of a younger person. His or her role in the family is different, and adult

sons, daughters, and sometimes grandchildren want to know how the communication disability will affect their father, mother, grandmother, or grandfather. These are important considerations, and family sessions are frequently an essential component of the audiology or speech-language pathology program. The spouse is often older and may be fearful of the caregiver role he or she is thrust into. Some older clients have limited family support and limited social networks generally. If the older person has communication disability, it may be necessary for the speech-language pathologist or audiologist to assist the client when discussing treatment options with other health professionals. For example, the clinician may attend a session with a social worker to discuss viable accommodation or home services for the client.

In summary, older people are susceptible to a number of diseases that cause communication or swallowing impairments. This section has summarized the diseases, their possible effects on communication and swallowing, described a test battery for this population, and described the additional clinical challenges of an older client with a communication disability.

Case Studies

Many of the communication and swallowing impairments associated with age have been described in this chapter. It has been emphasized that it is often difficult to differentiate between normal and abnormal communication impairments. In some cases, it is also difficult to differentiate between coexisting impairments. Many of the effects of the impairments are interrelated, creating a synergy between impairments; hence, the presence of multiple impairments is different from the sum of several impairments. The reality of clinical life is that many older people, particularly those who are frail, very old, and living in residential care facilities for the aged, have multiple impairments that are affected by the environment in which they live. Three case studies are described below that exemplify the complexity of gerontological audiology and speech-language pathology and the challenges clinicians face in the assessment of impairments.

In summary, these case studies demonstrate that many older people have multiple impairments, and the assessment process and differential diagnosis is often complex. Standardized tests of impairment have been supplemented by informal evaluations and trial-and-error interventions. Even then, it is not always possible to determine the exact nature of the underlying impairments of older people. It may be more useful, therefore, for clinicians to seek information about the effects of the impairment on everyday life. The clinician could look to the client to determine what everyday communication is important to him or her and what effect the impairments are having on communicative

Case Study: Stroke and Hearing Impairment

Mr. Baker was a 79-year-old war veteran who had conduction aphasia following a stroke 14 weeks previously. His Aphasia Quotient on the WAB was 67.6. Pure-tone audiometry showed that Mr. Baker had a bilateral sensorineural hearing impairment, moderate in one ear and severe in the other. Speech discrimination was attempted but could not be assessed because Mr. Baker's aphasia made it impossible for him to repeat the test words. Prior to the stroke he had been fitted with a behind-the-ear hearing aid in his better ear. His comprehension of speech was poor, partly due to the aphasia and partly due to the hearing loss. His speech was loud and characterized by phonemic errors and anomia. Mrs. Baker was also hearing impaired but did not wear hearing aids, and both Mr. and Mrs. Baker were becoming increasingly frustrated by their conversation attempts. Mr. Baker struggled to hear and understand his wife. When he attempted to reply or initiate conversation, his wife could not guess what the intended mispronounced words were and often asked him to repeat a word that he had struggled to say.

The diagnostic problem lay in differentiating whether it was his aphasia or his hearing difficulties that were predominantly contributing to the communication breakdowns. New hearing aids were fitted for both Mr. and Mrs. Baker, and strategies were put in place to facilitate communication attempts between them. A quiet room was found for them in the rehabilitation center and, with the help of the audiologist and speech-language pathologist, both participants learned communication repair strategies that improved the flow of conversation. The improved hearing status of the couple clarified that Mr. Baker's comprehension difficulties were mostly due to his hearing difficulties but that his phonemic paraphasias were mostly due to aphasia. In the context of Mr. Baker's hearing impairment, aphasia treatment did not target phonological decoding and encoding. Instead, conversational coaching with the couple (see Chapter 9 and Ylvisaker & Holland, 1985) remained the primary focus of speech-language pathology intervention.

and social life. In turn, the clinician could examine the impact of contextual factors, activity, and participation levels on the impairment. The emergence of activity- and participation-based descriptions of older people's communication difficulties is the focus of the next two chapters. The effect of contextual factors is discussed in the following three chapters that focus on the clinical settings of the community, hospital, and residential care facility for the aged.

Case Study: Early Dementia

Mrs. James was an 81-year-old widow living in her own home. Three years ago she had moved from a rural area to the city to be near her son and daughter. She also moved to be closer to specialist health care facilities because she had severe asthma. The move away from her long-time friends in the country, the loss of her husband 18 months previously, and several hospitalizations following asthma attacks led to a reactive depression that was treated with antidepressants. She had developed cataracts and was soon to have them surgically removed. Following her admission for cataract removal, she was referred to the rehabilitation team at the hospital for upgrading of her independence prior to being discharged home. Mrs. James scored poorly on the Mini-Mental State Exam (Folstein et al., 1975), and the geriatric physician referred her to the speech-language pathologist with a query of early dementia. The case history taken by the speech-language pathologist revealed that Mrs. James' vision was restricting her mobility and independence at home, she was taking a cocktail of 11 medications, she had only 5 years of formal education, and she had become socially isolated with only her son and daughter visiting once a week. On the BNT, she scored 28 from a total of 60 with 16 instances of semantic cues (because she could not see the pictures well enough), 11 "Don't know" responses, and the rest were correct following a phonemic cue. Pure-tone screening audiometry found a mild to moderate bilateral sensorineural hearing loss. Her voice was hoarse and low pitched and when she did speak, which was not often, her language and discourse appeared relatively intact. She appeared depressed with little animation in her speech and little initiation of conversation.

In this case, the primary impairments were visual loss and depression. Coupled with social isolation and the interaction of medications, it was difficult to unravel the web of factors contributing to this client's declining independence. Although some cognitive loss was not ruled out, the impression of the team was that the combined effect of the continuing depression and sensory deprivation from the dual sensory loss and social isolation meant that Mrs. James would not be able to cope at home for much longer. A change in her antidepressant medication and the removal of her cataracts led to a significant improvement in Mrs. James' mood and communicative behavior. She was subsequently assessed more fully for any cognitive impairments that might indicate the presence of dementia. The results confirmed the team's initial opinion that the depression and the sensory losses were masking her generally good cognitive and communication skills. She and her family decided to move her to a nearby retirement village so that she would have some company and have her ongoing health needs monitored more closely. This move was successful for Mrs. James who continues to live relatively independently in the retirement village, attending many of the social events that are offered. She is now considering hearing aid fitting and has requested an audiological appointment.

Case Study: Hearing Impairment and Dementia

Mrs. Mason has been a resident of the Hometown Nursing Home for 8 years. She has a moderate-severe dementia and a moderate-severe mixed hearing loss. She has two behind-the-ear hearing aids, but they have remained in the bottom drawer of her bedside cabinet for most of the past year. The visiting audiologist has been asked to review Mrs. Mason's case to determine if anything can be done. The nursing staff have resorted to shouting in her ear to relay instructions, but this is usually not very successful. The audiologist decides to try a binaural listening device to see if Mrs. Mason responds in a specific communicative situation. The primary caregiver is asked to sit opposite Mrs. Mason in a quiet, well-lit room. When the caregiver speaks into the microphone of the amplifier, Mrs. Mason's eyes light up and she looks directly at the caregiver and responds appropriately. Other attempts are not so successful, with some responses being tangential. Nevertheless, the caregiver reports that this is the most Mrs. Mason has said during her time at the nursing home. It appears that Mrs. Mason's dementia is not as severe as previously thought. The amplifier is used more regularly, and because it has been successful, the audiologist and nursing staff decide to try new hearing aids. The hearing aids are managed by the nursing staff, and although Mrs. Mason only wears them for 3 to 4 hours a day, nursing staff report that Mrs. Mason is easier to care for and communicate with during that time.

 KEY POINTS

- Speech-language pathologists and audiologists need to be aware of the communication impairments associated with healthy aging so that they can consider these when interacting with older clients, so that they can understand the effects of these impairments on assessment tasks, and so that they can develop appropriate communication education programs for older people.

- Hearing impairment, memory problems, and word-finding difficulties are the major areas of communication that concern healthy older people.

- Other less significant impairments have been found in comprehension, conversational discourse, speech, voice, and swallowing.

- Hearing impairment and word-finding difficulties are the key areas of practice for audiologists and speech-language pathologists working with healthy older people.

- Numerous changes occur to the peripheral and central auditory system with age (refer to Table 4–1); the most significant of these is the damage to the inner ear that gives rise to the bilateral sloping mild to moderate sensorineural hearing impairment typically found in older people.

- Hearing impairment in older people is measured with a standard adult audiological assessment test battery, although some modifications to procedures may be necessary for the older adult.

- Hearing impairment is highly prevalent in older people, and the prevalence increases with age.

- The prevalence of hearing impairment is even higher in older people living in residential care facilities for the aged and in older people with dementia.

- There is mixed evidence about word-retrieval impairments with age, depending on whether cross-sectional or longitudinal research methodology has been employed.

- The BNT is a popular means of assessing word retrieval in older people and can assist with the differential diagnosis of dementia, aphasia, and normal aging processes.

- A number of shortened versions of the BNT are available.

- Cognitive impairments associated with healthy aging can complicate the differential diagnosis of conditions such as hearing loss, dementia, and aphasia.

- Visual impairments are common in older people and can affect communication.

- A screening communication assessment for healthy older people is recommended (see Figure 4–1).

- The major pathological conditions that occur in old age and are associated with communication and swallowing impairments are stroke; dementia of the Alzheimer's type (DAT); Parkinson's disease; cancer of the larynx, pharynx, or tongue; traumatic brain injury (TBI); and amyotrophic lateral sclerosis (ALS).

- Both standardized (see Figure 4–8) and nonstandardized assessments may be necessary to differentially diagnose the communication and swallowing impairments of older people.

- Successful clinical management of the older client depends on the clinician's understanding of the fact that older clients are different from younger clients in a number of ways and that this will affect assessment and intervention strategies.

CLASS ACTIVITIES

- Interview a healthy older person and ask about any changes he or she has experienced in communication over the years (i.e., about any difficulties in hearing, speaking, reading, or writing).

- Administer the BNT to a healthy older person. What errors did the person make? Can you identify any factors that may have contributed to these errors (e.g., visual difficulties, educational background)?

- Divide the class into small groups and ask them to consider the following case example:

  > You are asked by the nurse in charge of a dementia ward at a residential care facility for the aged to assess Mr. Booth in bed 7. When you go to see him and try to communicate with him, he does not respond in any way. His eyes are open and he looks at you. What could you do to determine the nature of Mr. Booth's communication difficulties? Ask each group to develop an assessment plan and then present it to the class for discussion.

RECOMMENDED READING

Bayles, K. A., & Kaszniak, A. W. (1987). *Communication and cognition in normal aging and dementia*. San Diego: College-Hill Press.

Chapman, S. B., & Ulatowska, H. K. (1991). Aphasia and aging. In D. N. Ripich (Ed.), *Handbook of geriatric communication* (pp. 241–254). Austin, TX: Pro-Ed.

Hickson, L., & Worrall, L. (1997). Hearing impairment, disability, and handicap in older people. *Critical Reviews in Physical and Rehabilitation Medicine, 9* (3 & 4), 219–243.

Hull, R. (1995). *Hearing in aging*. Clifton Park, NY: Delmar Learning.

Huntley, R. A., & Helfer, K. S.(Eds.). (1995). *Communication in later life*. Newton, MA: Butterworth-Heinemann.

Lubinski, R. (Ed.). (1995). *Dementia and communication*. Clifton Park, NY: Delmar Learning.

Mueller, P. B. (Ed.). (1997). Normal aging and communication processes [Special issue]. *Seminars in Speech and Language, 18*(2).

Orange, J. B., & Purves, B. (Ed.). (1996). Discourse and aging [Special issue]. *Journal of Speech-Language Pathology and Audiology, 20*(2).

Ripich, D. N. (Ed.). (1991). *Handbook of geriatric communication*. Austin, TX: Pro-Ed.

Shadden B. B., & Toner M. A. (Eds.). (1997). *Aging and communication: For clinicians by clinicians*. Austin, TX: Pro-Ed.

Weinstein, B. E. (2000). *Geriatric audiology*. New York: Thieme.

REFERENCES

Albert, M. S., Heller, H. S., & Milberg, W. (1988). Changes in naming ability with age. *Psychology and Aging, 3*(2), 173–178.

American Speech-Language-Hearing Association. (1988). The role of the speech-language pathologist in the identification, diagnosis, and treatment of individuals with cognitive-communication impairments. *ASHA, 30,* 79.

Andrews, M. L. (1991). *Voice therapy for children: The elementary school years*. (3rd ed.). Clifton Park, NY: Delmar Learning.

Antonucci, T. C., & Akiyama, H. (1987). Social networks in adult life and a preliminary examination of the Convoy Model. *Journal of Gerontology, 42,* 519–527.

Australian Bureau of Statistics. (1996). *Aspects of literacy: Assessed skills levels*. Canberra: Australian Bureau of Statistics.

Barrenas, M. L., & Lindgren, F. (1990). The influence of inner ear melanin on susceptibility to TTS in humans. *Scandinavian Audiology, 19,* 97–102.

Battle, D. E. (1993). *Communication disorders in multicultural populations*. Boston: Butterworth-Heinemann.

Bayles, K. A., & Kaszniak, A. W. (1987). *Communication and cognition in normal aging and dementia*. San Diego, CA: College-Hill Press.

Bayles, K. A., & Tomoeda, C. K. (1993). *Arizona battery for communication disorders of dementia*. Tucson, AZ: Canyonlands Publishing.

Beele, K. A., Davies, E., & Muller, D. J. (1984). Therapists's views on the clinical usefulness of four aphasia tests. *British Journal of Disorders of Communication, 19,* 169–178.

Benjamin, B. J. (1997). Speech production of normally aging adults. *Seminars in Speech and Language, 18*(2), 135–141.

Benton, A. L., & Hamsher, K. (1976). *Multilingual aphasia examination*. Iowa City: University of Iowa Press.

Bonita, R. (1992). Epidemiology of stroke. *Lancet, 339,* 342-344.

Boone, D. R., & McFarlane, S. C. (1988). *The voice and voice therapy*. (4th ed). Englewood Cliffs, NJ: Prentice Hall.

Borod, J. C., Goodglass, H., & Kaplan, E. (1980). Normative data on the Boston Diagnostic Aphasia Examination, Parietal Lobe Battery, and the Boston Naming Test. *Journal of Clinical Neuropsychology, 2*(3) 209–215.

Bowles, N. L., & Poon, L. W. (1985). Ageing and retrieval of words in semantic memory. *Journal of Gerontology, 40*(1) 71–77.

Brant, L. J., Gordon Salant, S., Pearson, J. D., Klein, L. L., Morrell, C. H., Metter, E. J., & Fozard, J. L. (1996). Risk factors related to age-associated hearing loss in the speech frequencies. *Journal of the American Academy of Audiology, 7*(3), 152–160.

Burzynski, C. M. (1987). The voice. In H. G. Mueller & V. C. Geoffrey (Eds.), *Communication disorders in aging: Assessment and management* (pp. 214–237). Washington, DC: Gallaudet University Press.

Byng, S., Kay, J., Edmundson, A., & Scott, C. (1990) Aphasia tests reconsidered. *Aphasiology, 4,* 67–91.

Carrau, R. L., & Murray, T. (1999). *Comprehensive management of swallowing disorders.* Clifton Park, NY: Delmar Learning.

Caruso, A. J., & Max, L. M. (1997). Effects of aging on neuromotor processes of swallowing. *Seminars in Speech and Language, 18*(2) 181–191.

Caruso, A. J., & Mueller, P. B. (1997). Age-related changes in speech, voice and swallowing. In B. B. Shadden & M. A. Toner (Eds.), *Aging and communication: For clinicians by clinicians* (pp. 117–134). Austin, TX: Pro-Ed.

Chapman, S. B. (1988). The older aphasic patient: The problems and the potential. *Seminars in Speech and Language, 9*(2), 135–147.

Chapman, S. B., & Ulatowska, H. K. (1991). Aphasia and aging. In D. N. Ripich (Ed.), *Handbook of geriatric communication* (pp. 241–254). Austin, TX: Pro-Ed.

Chenery, H. J., Murdoch, B. E., & Ingram, J. C. L. (1996). An investigation of confrontation naming performance in Alzheimer's dementia as a function of disease severity. *Aphasiology, 10,* 423–441.

Cherney, L. R. (1996). The effects of aging on communication. In C. Bernstein Lewis (Ed.), *Aging: The health care challenge* (3rd ed.). (pp.79–105). Philadelphia: F.A. Davis.

Cherney, L. R., & Halper, A. S. (2000). Assessment and treatment of functional communication following right hemisphere damage. In L. E. Worrall & C. M. Frattali (Eds.), *Neurogenic communication disorders: A functional approach* (pp. 276–293). New York: Thieme.

Cohen, G. (1979). Language comprehension in old age. *Cognitive Psychology, 11,* 412–429.

Cohen, G., & Faulkner, D. (1986). Memory for proper names: Age differences in retrieval. *British Journal of Developmental Psychology, 4,* 187–197.

Cooper, J. C., Jr., & Gates, G. A. (1991). Hearing in the elderly—the Framingham cohort, 1983–1985: Part II. Prevalence of central auditory processing disorders. *Ear and Hearing, 12*(5), 304–311.

Coulter, A. (1997). Partnerships with patients: The pros and cons of shared decision making. *Journal of Health Services Research and Policy, 2*(2) 112–121.

Cruice, M. (2001). *The effect of communication in quality of life in older adults with aphasia and healthy older adults.* Unpublished doctoral thesis, The University of Queensland, Brisbane, Australia.

Cruice, M., Worrall, L., & Hickson, L. (2000). Boston Naming Test results for healthy older Australians: A longitudinal and cross-sectional study. *Aphasiology, 14*(2), 143–155.

Dabul, B. (1979). *Apraxia battery for adults.* Tigard, OR: CC Publications.

Darley, F. L., Aronson, A. E., & Brown, J. R. (1975). *Motor speech disorders.* Philadelphia: Saunders.

Davis, A. C. (1989). The prevalence of hearing impairment and reported hearing disability among adults in Great Britain. *International Journal of Epidemiology, 18,* 911–917.

Delbecq, A. L., Van de Ven, A. H., & Gustafson, D. H. (1975). *Group techniques for program planning.* Glenview, IL: Scott, Foresman.

Drevenstedt, J., & Bellezza, F. S. (1993). Memory for self-generated narration in the elderly. *Psychology and Aging, 8*(2) 187–196.

Duffy, J. R. (1995). *Motor speech disorders: Substrates, differential diagnosis and management.* Baltimore: Mosby.

Edels, Y. (Ed.). (1983). *Laryngectomy: Diagnosis to rehabilitation.* London: Croom Helm.

Enderby, P. (1983). *Frenchay Dysarthria Assessment.* San Diego, CA: College-Hill Press.

Fitzgerald, D. (1996). Head trauma: Hearing loss and dizziness. *The Journal of Trauma: Injury, Infection and Critical Care, 40*(3), 488–497.

Folstein, M. F., Folstein, S. E., & McHugh, P. R. (1975). Mini-Mental State: A practical method for grading the cognitive state of patients for the clinician. *Journal of Psychiatric Research, 12,* 189–198.

Formby, C., Phillips, D. E., & Thomas, R. G. (1987). Hearing loss among stroke patients. *Ear and Hearing, 8*(6), 326–332.

Garcia, L., & Orange, J. B. (1996). The analysis of conversation skills of older adults: Current research and clinical approaches. *Journal of Speech-Language Pathology and Audiology, 20*(2), 123–138.

Garrett, B. (1992). Gerontology and communication disorders: A model for training clinicians. *Educational Gerontology, 18,* 231–243.

Garstecki, D.C., & Erler, S.F. (1997). Hearing in older adults. In B.B. Shadden & M.A. Toner (Eds.), *Aging and communication: For clinicians, by clinicians* (pp. 97–116). Austin, TX: Pro-Ed.

Gates, G. A., Cobb, J. L., D'Agostino, R. B., & Wolf, P. A. (1993). The relation of hearing in the elderly to the presence of cardiovascular disease and cardiovascular risk factors. *Archives of Otolaryngology Head and Neck Surgery, 119*(2), 156–161.

Gates, G. A., Cooper, J. C., Kannel, W. B., & Miller, N. J. (1990). Hearing in the elderly: The Framingham cohort, 1983–1985. I. Basic audiometric results. *Ear and Hearing, 11,* 247–256.

Gelfand, S. A. (2001). *Essentials of audiology* (2nd ed.). New York: Thieme.

Geschwind, N. (1965). Disconnection syndromes in animals and man. *Brain, 88,* 237–294, 585–644.

Goodglass, H., & Kaplan, E. (1972). *The assessment of aphasia and related disorders.* Philadelphia: Lea & Febiger.

Goodglass, H., Kaplan, E., & Barresi, B. (2001). *Boston Diagnostic Aphasia Examination* (3rd ed.). Philadelphia: Lippincott Williams & Wilkins.

Goulet, P., Ska, B., & Kahn, H. J. (1994). Is there a decline in picture naming with advancing age? *Journal of Speech and Hearing Research, 37,* 629–644.

Goycoolea, M. V., Goycoolea, H. G., Rodriquez, L. G., Farfan, C. R., Martinez, G. C., & Vidal, R. (1986). Effect of life in industrialized societies on hearing in natives of Easter Island. *Laryngoscope, 96,* 1391–1396.

Gravell, R. (1988). *Communication problems in elderly people: Practical approaches to management.* Beckenham, UK: Croom Helm.

Groher, M. E., & Bukatman, R. (1986). The prevalence of swallowing disorders in two teaching hospitals. *Dysphagia, 1,* 3–6.

Halper, A. S., Cherney, L. R., Burns, M. S., & Mogil, S. I. (1996). RIC evaluation of communication problems in right hemisphere dysfunction—revised (RICE-R). In A. S. Halper, L. R. Cherney, & M. S. Burns (Eds.), *Clinical management of right hemisphere damage.* (2nd ed., pp. 99–132). Gaithersburg, MD: Aspen Publishers.

Harford, E. R., & Dodds, E. (1982). Hearing status of ambulatory senior citizens. *Ear and Hearing, 3*(3), 105–109.

Helfer, K. S. (1995). Auditory perception by older adults. In R. A. Huntley & K. S. Helfer (Eds.), *Communication in later life* (pp. 41–84). Newton, MA: Butterworth Heinemann.

Hickson, L., Lind, C., Worrall, L., Yiu, E., Barnett, H., & Lovie-Kitchin, J. (1999). Hearing and vision in healthy older Australians: Objective and self-report measures. *Advances in Speech-Language Pathology, 1*(2), 95–105.

Hickson, L., & Worrall, L. (1997). Hearing impairment, disability, and handicap in older people. *Critical Reviews in Physical and Rehabilitation Medicine, 9*(3 & 4), 219–243.

Hickson, L., Worrall, L., Yiu, E., & Barnett, H. (1996). Planning a communication education program for older people. *Educational Gerontology, 22*, 257–269.

Hofmeister, B., Hickson, L., Macivor, C., Towers, E., Brown-Rothwell, D., Sockalingam, R., & Hazelton, R. (2000). Audiological outcomes of severe traumatic brain injury with base of skull fracture. *Australian and New Zealand Journal of Audiology, 22*(2), 59–75.

Hollien, H. (1995). The normal aging voice. In R.A. Huntley & K.S. Helfer (Eds.), *Communication in later life* (pp. 23–40). Newton, MA: Butterworth-Heinemann.

Holland, A. L., & Bartlett, C. L. (1985). Some differential effects of age on stroke-produced aphasia. In H. K. Ulatowska (Ed.), *The aging brain: Communication in the elderly* (pp. 141–155). Austin, TX: Pro-Ed.

Hopper, T., & Bayles, K. A. (2001). Management of neurogenic communication disorders associated with dementia. In R. Chapey (Ed.), *Language intervention strategies in aphasia and related neurogenic communication disorders.* (4th ed, pp. 829–847). Philadelphia: Lippincott Williams & Wilkins.

Hull, R. (1995). *Hearing in aging.* Clifton Park: Delmar Learning.

Ivnik, R. J., Malec, J. F., Smith, G. E., Tangalos, E. G., & Peterson, R. C. (1996). Neuropsychological tests' norms above age 55: COWAT, BNT, MAE Token, WRAT-R Reading, AMNART, STROOP, TMT, and JLO. *The Clinical Neuropsychologist, 10,* 262–278.

Johnson, D. J. (1997). Mental status and aging: Cognition and affect. In B. B. Shadden & M. A. Toner (Eds.), *Aging and communication: For clinicians by clinicians* (pp. 67–96). Austin, TX: Pro-Ed.

Kahane, J. C., & Beckford, N. S. (1991). The aging larynx and voice. In D. N. Ripich (Ed.), *Handbook of geriatric communication disorders.* (pp. 165–186). Austin, TX: Pro-Ed.

Kaplan, E.F., Goodglass, H., & Weintraub, S. (1983). *The Boston Naming Test* (2nd ed.). Philadelphia: Lea & Febiger.

Katz, J. (2002). *Handbook of clinical audiology* (5th ed.). Philadelphia: Lippincott Williams & Wilkins.

Katz, R., Davidoff, M., & Wolfe, G. (1984). *Improving communication in Parkinson's disease: A guide for patient, family and friends.* Danville, IL: The Interstate Printers and Publishers.

Katz, R. C., Hallowell, B., Code, C., Armstrong, E., Roberts, P., Pound, C., & Katz, L. (2000). A multinational comparison of aphasia management practices. *International Journal of Language & Communication Disorders, 35*(2), 303–314.

Kay, J., Lesser, R., & Coltheart, M. (1996). Psycholinguistic assessments of language processing in aphasia (PALPA): An introduction. *Aphasiology, 10,* 159–179.

Kay, J., Lesser, R., & Coltheart, M. (1997). *Psycholinguistic assessments of language processing in aphasia.* Hove, UK: Psychology Press.

Kertesz, A. (1982). *Western Aphasia Battery.* New York: Grune & Stratton.

Kricos, P. B., & Lesner, S. A. (1995). *Hearing care for the older adult.* Boston: Butterworth-Heinemann.

Kwong See, S. T., & Ryan, E. B. (1996). Cognitive mediation of discourse processing in later life. *Journal of Speech-Language Pathology and Audiology, 20,* 109–117.

LaPointe, L. L. (Ed.). (1990). *Aphasia and related neurogenic language disorders.* New York: Thieme.

Lavizzo-Mourey, R., Smith, V., Sims, R., & Taylor, L. (1994). Hearing loss: An educational and screening program for African-American and Latino elderly. *Journal of the National Medical Association, 86*(1), 53–59.

Lesser, R. (1987). Cognitive neuropsychological influences on aphasia therapy. *Aphasiology, 1*(3) 189–200.

Lewis, F. M., LaPointe L. L., Murdoch, B.E., & Chenery, H. J. (1998). Language impairment in Parkinson's disease. *Aphasiology, 12*(3), 193–206.

Lichtenstein, M. J., Bess, F. H. & Logan, S. A. (1988). Validation of screening tools for identifying hearing-impaired elderly in primary care. *Journal of American Medical Association, 259,* 2875–2878.

Lim, J. K., & Yap, K. B. (2000). Screening for hearing impairment in hospitalized elderly. *Annals of the Academy of Medicine Singapore, 29*(2), 237–241.

Linebaugh, C. A. (1990). Lexical retrieval problems: Anomia. In L. L. La Pointe (Ed.), *Aphasia and related neurogenic language disorders* (pp. 96–112). New York: Thieme.

Lubinski, R. (Ed.). (1995). *Dementia and communication.* Clifton Park: Delmar Learning.

Lubinski, R., & Welland, R. J. (1997). Normal aging and environmental effects on communication. *Seminars in Speech and Language, 18*(2), 107–126.

Mack, W. J., Freed, D. M., Williams, B. W., & Henderson, V. W. (1992). Boston Naming Test: Shortened versions for use in Alzheimer's disease. *Journal of Gerontology: Psychological Sciences, 47,* 154–158.

Maguire, G. H. (1996). The changing realm of the senses. In C. Bernstein-Lewis (Ed.), *Aging: The health care challenge* (3rd ed., pp.126–146). Philadelphia: F. A. Davis Company.

Mahoney, D. F. (1992). Hearing loss among nursing home residents: Perceptions and realities. *Clinical Nursing Research, 1*(4), 317–332; discussion 333–315.

March, E. G., Worrall, L. E., & Hickson, L. M. H. (2001). Performance of an Australian older sample on the Boston Naming Test and comparability of short-form test versions. *Cognitive Neuropsychological Assessment 3,* 179–192.

Mayeux, R., Denaro, J., Hemenegildo, N., Marder, K., Tang, M. X., Cote, L. J., & Stern, Y. (1992). A population-based investigation of Parkinson's disease with and without dementia. Relationship to age and gender. *Archives of Neurology, 49*(5), 492–497.

McBride, W. S., Mulrow, C. D., Aguilar, C., & Tuley, M. R. (1994). Methods for screening for hearing loss in older adults. *American Journal of Medical Science, 307*(1), 40–42.

McDonald, S., Togher, L., & Code, C. (1999). *Communication disorders following traumatic brain injury.* Hove, UK: Psychology Press.

Mitrushina, M., & Satz, P. (1995). Repeating testing of normal elderly with the Boston Naming Test. *Aging, 7*(2) 123–127.

Mlcoch, A. G., & Metter, E. J. (1994). Medical aspects of stroke rehabilitation. In R. Chapey (Ed.), *Language intervention strategies in adult aphasia.* (3rd ed., pp. 27–46). Philadelphia: Lippincott Williams & Wilkins.

Morris, J. C., Heyman, A., Mohs, R. C., Hughes, J. P., van Belle, G., Fillenbaum, G., Mellits, E. D., Clark, C., & the CERAD Investigators. (1989). The consortium to establish a registry for Alzheimer's disease (CERAD). Part I. Clinical and neuropsychological assessment of Alzheimer's disease. *Neurology, 39,* 1159–1165.

Moscicki, E. K., Elkins, E. F., Baum, H. M., & McNamara, P. M. (1985). Hearing loss in the elderly: An epidemiologic study of the Framingham heart study cohort. *Ear and Hearing, 6,* 184–190.

Mueller, P. B. (1997). The aging voice. *Seminars in Speech and Language, 18*(2) 159–169.

Murdoch, B. E. (1990). *Acquired speech and language disorders: A neuroanatomical and functional neurological approach.* Cheltenham, UK: Stanley Thornes (Publishers) Ltd.

Murdoch, B. E. (2001). Subcortical brain mechanisms in speech and language. *Folia Phoniatrica et Logopaedica, 53,* 233–251.

Myers, P. S. (2001). Communication disorders associated with right hemisphere damage. In R. Chapey (Ed.), *Language intervention strategies in aphasia and related neurogenic communication disorders.* (4th ed., pp. 809–827). Philadelphia: Lippincott Williams & Wilkins.

Nelson E., Wasson, J., Kirk, J., Keller, A., Clark, D., Dietrich, A., Stewart, A., & Zubkoff, M. (1987). Assessment of function in routine clinical practice: Description of the COOP chart method and preliminary findings. *Journal of Chronic Diseases, 40*(1), 55S–63S.

Newman, C. W., & Sandridge, S. A. (2000). Performance on electrophysiologic tests of central auditory nervous system function. In B. E. Weinstein (Ed.), *Geriatric audiology* (pp. 115–140). New York: Thieme.

Nicholas, M., Obler, L., Albert, M., & Goodglass, H. (1985). Lexical retrieval in healthy aging. *Cortex, 21,* 595–606.

Nondahl, D. M., Cruickshanks, K. J., Wiley, T. L., Tweed, T. S., Klein, R., & Klein, B. E. K. (1998). Accuracy of self-reported hearing loss. *Audiology, 37,* 295–301.

Nosan, D., Benecke, J., & Murr, A. (1997). Current perspective on temporal bone trauma. *Otolaryngology—Head and Neck Surgery, 117,* 67–71.

Orange, J. B., & Purves, B. (1996). Conversational discourse and cognitive impairment: Implications for Alzheimer's disease. *Journal of Speech-Language Pathology and Audiology, 20*(2), 139–154.

Owens, R. E., Metz, D. E. & Haas, A. (2000). *Introduction to communication disorders: A life-span perspective.* Boston: Allyn & Bacon.

Palmer, C. V., Adams, S.W., Bourgeois, M., Durrant, J., & Rossi, M. (1999). Reduction in caregiver-identified problem behaviors in patients with Alzheimer disease in post-hearing-aid fitting. *Journal of Speech, Language, and Hearing Research, 42*(2), 312-328.

Pedersen, K. E., Rosenhall, U., & Moller, M. B. (1989). Changes in pure-tone thresholds in individuals aged 70–81: Results form a longitudinal study. *Audiology, 28,* 194–204.

Peters, C. A., Potter, J. F., & Scholer, S. G. (1988). Hearing impairment as a predictor of cognitive decline in dementia. *Journal of the American Geriatrics Society, 36,* 981–986.

Pichora-Fuller, M. K. (1997). Language comprehension in older listeners. *Journal of Speech-Language Pathology and Audiology, 21*(2), 125–142.

Prigatano, G., Roueche, J., & Fordyce, D. (1986). Nonaphasic language disturbances after brain injury. In G. P. Prigatano (Ed.), *Neuropsychological rehabilitation after brain injury* (pp. 18–28). Baltimore: Johns Hopkins University Press.

Pye, D. J, Worrall, L. E, & Hickson, L. M. H. (2000). Assessing and treating functional communication in an extended care facility. In L. Worrall & C. Frattali (Eds.), *Neurogenic communication disorders: A functional approach* (pp. 312–328). New York: Thieme.

Ringel, R. L., & Chodzko-Zajko, W. J. (1988). Age, health and the speech process. *Seminars in Speech and Language, 9*(2), 95–107.

Ripich, D. N. (Ed.). (1991). *Handbook of geriatric communication.* Austin, TX: Pro-Ed.

Rosen, S., Bergman, M., Plester, D., El-Mofty, A., & Satti, M. H. (1962). Presbycusis study of a relatively noise-free population in the Sudan. *Annals of Otology, Rhinology and Laryngology, 71,* 727–743.

Ryan, W., & Burk, K. (1974). Perceptual and acoustic correlates of aging in the speech of males. *Journal of Communication Disorders, 7,* 181–192.

Salive, M. E., Guralnik, J., Christen, W., Glynn, R. J., Colsher, P., & Ostfeld, A. M. (1992). Functional blindness and visual impairment in older adults from three communities. *Opthalmology, 99*(12), 1840–1847.

Schow, R. L., & Nerbonne, M. A. (1980). Hearing levels among elderly nursing home residents. *Journal of Speech and Hearing Disorders, 45,* 124–132.

Schuknecht, H. F. (1974). *Pathology of the ear.* Cambridge, MA: Harvard University Press.

Shadden, B. B. (Ed). (1988). *Communication behavior and aging: A sourcebook for clinicians* Baltimore: Williams & Wilkins.

Shadden, B. B. (1997). Language and communication changes with aging. In B. B. Shadden & M. A. Toner (Eds.), *Aging and communication: For clinicians by clinicians* (pp. 135–170). Austin, TX: Pro Ed.

Shadden B. B., & Toner M. A. (Eds.). (1997). *Aging and communication: For clinicians by clinicians.* Austin, TX: Pro-Ed.

Ska, B., & Joannette, Y. (1996). Discourse in older adults: Influence of text, task, and participants characteristics. *Journal of Speech-Language Pathology and Audiology, 20,* 101–108.

Smith-Worrall, L., & Burtenshaw, E. J. (1990). Frequency of use and utility of aphasia tests. *Australian Journal of Human Communication Disorders, 18*(2), 53-67.

Snow, P., & Ponsford, J. (1995). Assessing and managing changes in communication and interpersonal skills following traumatic brain injury. In J. Ponsford (Ed.), *Traumatic brain injury: Rehabilitation for everyday adaptive living* (pp. 137–164). Hove, UK: Lawrence Erlbaum Associates.

Sonies, B.C. (2000). Assessment and treatment of functional communication in dysphagia. In L. E. Worrall & C. M. Frattali (Eds.), *Neurogenic communication disorders: A functional approach* (pp. 262–275). New York: Thieme.

Speech Pathology Department, Royal Brisbane Hospital. (1998). *Royal Brisbane Hospital Outcome Measure for Swallowing.* Available from Speech Pathology Department, Royal Brisbane Hospital, Herston 4029, QLD, Australia.

Stach, B. A. (1998). *Clinical audiology: An introduction.* Clifton Park, NY: Delmar Learning.

Stach, B. A., Spretnjak, M. L., & Jerger, J. (1990). The prevalence of central presbycusis in a clinical population. *Journal of the American Academy of Audiology, 1*(2), 109–115.

Steuer, J., & Jarvik, L. F. (1981). Cognitive function in the elderly: Influence of physical health. In J. L. McGaugh & S. B. Kiesler (Eds.), *Aging: Biology and behavior* (pp. 231–253). New York: Academic Press.

Stumer, J., Hickson, L., & Worrall, L. (1996). Hearing impairment, disability and handicap in elderly people living in residential care and in the community. *Disability and Rehabilitation, 18*(2), 76–82.

Theodoros, D. G. (1998). Mixed dysarthria. In B. E. Murdoch (Ed.), *Dysarthria: A physiological approach to assessment and treatment* (pp. 337–372). Cheltenham, UK: Stanley Thornes (Publishers) Ltd.

Toner, M. A. (1997). Treating dysphagia in the elderly: Prevention, assessment and intervention. In B. B. Shadden & M. A. Toner (Eds.), *Aging and communication: For clinicians by clinicians* (pp. 379–408). Austin, TX: Pro-Ed.

Trupe, R., & Siebens, A. (1984). Prevalence of feeding and swallowing problems in nursing homes. *Archives of Physical Medicine, 65,* 651–652.

Uhlmann, R. F., Larson, E. B., Thomas, S. R., Koepsell, T. D., & Duckert, L. G. (1989). Relationship of hearing impairment to dementia and cognitive dysfunction in older adults. *Journal of American Medical Association, 261,* 2875–2878.

Van Gorp, W. G., Satz, P., Kiersch, M. E., & Henry, R. (1986). Normative data on the Boston Naming Test for a group of normal older adults. *Journal of Clinical and Experimental Neuropsychology, 8*(6) 702–705.

Ventry, I. M., & Weinstein, B. E. (1982). The Hearing Handicap Inventory for the Elderly: A new tool. *Ear & Hearing, 3,* 128–134.

Ward, E. C., & Conroy, A-L. (1999). Validity, reliability and responsivity of the Royal Brisbane Hospital Outcome Measure for Swallowing. *Asia Pacific Journal of Speech, Language and Hearing, 4,* 109–129.

Weatherley, C., Worrall, L., & Hickson, L. (1997). The effect of hearing impairment on the vocal characteristics of older people. *Folia Phoniatrica et Logopaedica, 49,* 53–62.

Weinberg, B. (Ed.). (1980). *Readings in speech following total laryngectomy.* Baltimore: University Park Press.

Weinstein, B. E. (2000). *Geriatric audiology.* New York: Thieme.

Wheeler, D. G. (1995). Communication and swallowing problems in the frail older person. *Topics in Geriatric Rehabilitation, 11*(2), 11–25.

Williams, B. W., Mack, W., & Henderson, V. W. (1989). Boston Naming Test in Alzheimer's disease. *Neuropsychologia, 27,* 1073–1079.

Willott, J. F. (1991). *Aging and the auditory system: Anatomy, physiology and psychophysics.* Clifton Park, NY: Delmar Learning.

World Health Organization. (2001). *International classification of functioning, disability and health.* Geneva: Author.

Worrall, L. (2000). The influence of professional values on the functional communication approach in aphasia. In L. Worrall & C. Frattali (Eds.), *Neurogenic communication disorders: A functional approach* (pp. 191–205). New York: Thieme.

Worrall, L., Hickson, L., Barnett, H., & Yiu, E. (1998). An evaluation of the Keep on Talking program for maintaining communication skills into old age. *Educational Gerontology, 24*(2), 129–140.

Worrall, L., Hickson, L., & Dodd, B. (1993). Screening for communication impairment in nursing homes and hostels. *Australian Journal of Human Communication Disorders, 21,* 53–64.

Worrall, L. E., Yiu, E., M-L., Hickson, L. M. H., & Barnett, H. M. (1995). Normative data for the Boston Naming Test for Australian elderly. *Aphasiology, 9,* 541–551.

Ylvisaker, M., & Holland, A. L. (1985). Coaching, self coaching and rehabilitation of head injury. In D. F. Johns (Ed.), *Clinical management of neurogenic communication disorders* (pp. 243–227). Boston: Little, Brown.

Yorkston, K. M., Beukelman, D. R., Strand, E. A., & Bell, K. R. (1999). *Management of motor speech disorders in children and adults.* Austin, TX: Pro-Ed.

Chapter 5

Communication Activity Limitations

It is important that speech-language pathologists and audiologists understand the effects of communication impairments on the lives of older people. This chapter describes the activity dimension of the WHO model (2001), the everyday activities of older people, and then, specifically, the everyday communication activities of older people. This is followed by a review of studies that have determined the activity limitations of older people with hearing, speech, and language impairments. Finally, assessments that target the communication activity dimension in healthy older people and people with specific communication impairments are presented.

Chapter 4 described the myriad of communication impairments that may occur as people age (e.g., hearing impairment, word-finding difficulties) or when they develop a health condition such as stroke dementia or Parkinson's disease. Obviously, this information is important for audiologists and speech-language pathologists. However, it is also important to understand the practical implications of such impairments on the everyday lives of older people, both healthy older people and those with known communication disability. It is the everyday effects, not the impairments themselves, that will motivate the older person to seek assistance and that will subsequently become the goals for intervention. The everyday effects can be considered in terms of communication activity limitations, which are discussed in this chapter, and communication participation restrictions and quality of life changes, which are discussed in Chapter 6. For example, an older person with hearing impairment might have difficulty understanding conversation (an activity limitation), and this difficulty may mean that he or she no longer attends social gatherings (a participation restriction), and therefore may have a poor quality of life. The questions addressed in this chapter are: What are the communication activities of older people? What communication activity limitations do they experience? How can the speech-language pathologist or audiologist assess these?

Activities in the WHO model

An activity is defined by WHO as the execution of a task or action by an individual (WHO, 2001). The activity dimension of the WHO model provides a useful framework for considering the everyday activities of older people. The dimension contains a list of major everyday activities, as well as a detailed coding scheme and set of qualifiers for data collectors. The list of activities is not specific to communication (i.e., it includes the whole range of daily activities) and it is not specific to older people (i.e., it is for people of all ages). So, why should speech-language pathologists and audiologists working with older people look at the WHO activity list?

The first reason is that the list can serve to broaden the clinician's perspective about the everyday activities of clients, and that is why this list is presented initially in this chapter. The second reason is that it offers a possible framework for the comprehensive assessment of communication activities in daily life, a topic that is discussed later in the chapter. The sections that follow discuss research that has evaluated activities of older people specifically and communication activities in particular.

The activity level of the WHO model contains nine domains. Each domain describes a range of activities from the simple to the complex. Participation has the same list of domains. The nine domains are

1. Learning and Applying Knowledge
2. General Tasks and Demands
3. Communication
4. Mobility
5. Self Care
6. Domestic Life
7. Interpersonal Interactions and Relationships
8. Major Life Areas
9. Community, Social, and Civic Life

Clearly, the two domains that relate most closely to communication are domain 3, Communication, and domain 7, Interpersonal Interactions and Relationships. The Communication domain is divided into three main areas.

1. Receiving
2. Producing
3. Conversation and the Use of Communication Devices and Techniques

The Interpersonal Interactions and Relationships domain is divided into general and particular categories. A detailed breakdown of activities included in these two domains is shown in Table 5–1. In addition to these, there are numerous activities listed in other domains of the WHO model that involve communication (see examples in Table 5–2). Communication is involved in activities such as learning and applying knowledge, self-care and domestic activities, mobility, and most of the other activity domains in the ICF. This spectrum illustrates the notion that communication underpins many of the everyday activities of life. It is an excellent argument for an interdisciplinary approach to communication disability by audiologists and speech-language pathologists. It is also an argument against relying solely on traditional standardized communication assessments that may not tap into important areas of everyday activity that involve communication.

Everyday Activities of Older People

In this section, the research evidence about the everyday activities of older people is described. The aim of this section is to increase awareness about what older people do. Do they sit around all day doing nothing (as agist stereotypes suggest)? Do they engage in the same kinds of activities as younger people?

In this section, the results of one of the few comprehensive studies of the everyday activities of older people are described. Horgas, Wilms, and Baltes (1998) investigated the nature and frequency of everyday activities in a representative sample of 485 individuals aged 70 to 105 years (Mean age = 84.9 years) who took part in the Berlin Aging Study. The majority of the participants (86.4%) were living in the community, and 13.6% lived in extended care facilities.

Horgas et al. (1998) used the Yesterday Interview developed by Moss and Lawton (1982) to study the everyday activities of the participants. In this interview, the participant is asked to give details about what he or she had done the previous day, from waking up to going to sleep at night. Details about the type, frequency, and duration of activities are collected, as well as where the activity took place and who else was involved in the activity. The

TABLE 5–1

LIST OF ACTIVITIES FROM THE COMMUNICATION AND INTERPERSONAL INTERACTIONS AND RELATIONSHIPS DOMAINS OF THE WHO (2001) MODEL .

Communication

Communicating–receiving	Spoken messages
	Nonverbal messages
	Formal sign language messages
	Written messages
	Other specified and unspecified activities of receiving communication
Communicating–producing	Speaking
	Producing nonverbal messages
	Producing messages in formal sign language
	Writing messages
	Other specified and unspecified activities of producing messages
Conversation and use of communication devices and techniques	Conversation
	Discussion
	Using communication devices and techniques
	Other specified and unspecified conversation activities and use of communication devices and techniques

Interpersonal Interactions and Relationships

General interpersonal interactions	Basic interpersonal interactions
	Respect and warmth in relationships
	Appreciation in relationships
	Tolerance in relationships
	Criticism in relationships
	Social cues in relationships
	Physical contact in relationships
	Complex interpersonal interactions
	Forming relationships
	Terminating relationships
	Regulating behaviors within interactions
	Interacting according to social rules
	Maintaining social space
	Other specified and unspecified general interpersonal interactions

Interpersonal Interactions and Relationships

Particular interpersonal relationships	Relating with strangers Formal relationships Informal social relationships Family relationships Intimate relationships Other specified and unspecified particular interpersonal relationships

Note: Reprinted with permission from WHO.

researchers coded activities into 44 different types and, from these, identified eight main activity domains. The activity domains, in descending order, beginning with the most frequently occurring were

1. Basic personal maintenance (e.g., eating, preparing for bed)
2. Instrumental activities of daily living (IADL) (e.g., shopping, household chores)
3. Resting
4. Other leisure activities (e.g., sport, gardening)
5. Leisure activities: television watching
6. Leisure activities: reading
7. Social activities (e.g., talking to people, telephoning)
8. Paid work

TABLE 5–2

EXAMPLES OF ACTIVITIES FROM OTHER SECTIONS OF THE WHO (2001) MODEL THAT ALSO INVOLVE COMMUNICATION.

Learning and applying knowledge	Purposeful sensory experiences Basic learning Applying knowledge
Self-care	Looking after one's health
Domestic life	Acquisition of necessities Household tasks Caring for household objects and assisting others
Major life areas	Education Work and employment Economic life

Comparison of the domains from the Horgas et al. (1998) study with those listed in the WHO model shows a great deal of similarity. There are only two major activity domains reported by Horgas et al. that are not included in the WHO model, and these are resting and television watching. It may be that these two activities have a more major role in the everyday lives of older people than in the general population. From a communication perspective, the most important finding of this study was that the activity of watching television is a major everyday activity of older people and is one that is not included in the WHO activities. Audiologists and speech-language pathologists need to be aware that the ability to hear and understand television may be an important everyday activity for many clients and one that may need to be a focus of assessment and intervention.

In terms of the time spent doing the activities each day, the pattern of results reported by Horgas et al. (1998) was somewhat different. For example, although basic personal maintenance was the most frequently reported activity, it was not the major time consumer, accounting for approximately 2.5 hours per day. Activities coded as basic personal maintenance were arising, personal care, eating, and preparing for bed. The average day was 16 hours long, and Figure 5–1 shows the average amount of time in each of the major activities. Most time was spent engaging in instrumental activities of daily living (e.g., shopping, household chores), watching television, and resting. When all the leisure domains of watching television, reading, and other leisure activities are considered together, they take up about one third of a person's day.

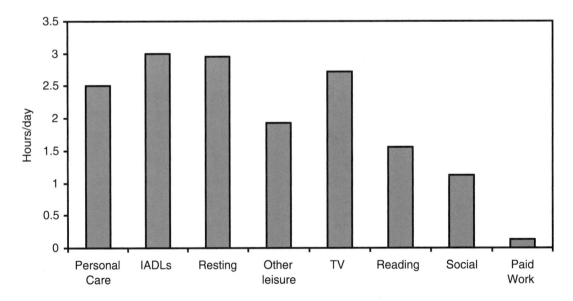

FIGURE 5–1. Average amount of time per day spent by older people in a range of activities, n = 485. Adapted from Horgas, Wilms, and Baltes (1998).

Participants were also asked whom they were with during the day, and the results indicated that the vast majority of the day, approximately 10.5 hours, was spent alone. About 3 hours were spent with the spouse or partner. Other people, with whom the older people had contact, were roommates, groups, professional caregivers, children, relatives, and friends. The fact that Horgas et al. (1998) included participants who were living in the community and those in residential care settings may help to explain the findings to some degree. Only 31% were married; the remaining 69% were widowed, divorced, or never married.

Horgas et al. (1998) also analyzed the relationships between older people's everyday activities and the participants' personal attributes. They noted some interesting relationships among everyday activities, age, and residential status. People living in long-term care facilities engaged in IADL tasks and leisure activities less often, and for less time, than people living in the community, and they spent more time resting. The same pattern was observed with increasing age. This may occur because older people and those living in residential care facilities are less able to engage in more strenuous activities with age or because the environment provides them with fewer opportunities to do so. The effect of gender was discussed in another report on the activities of older people in the Berlin Aging Study (Smith & Baltes, 1998). Women spent significantly more time than men in IADLs, and men reported spending more time in the leisure activity of watching television. Such differences appear to be due to traditional role distributions in the household.

In summary, the results of Horgas et al.'s (1998) study showed that older people were engaged in a wide range of activities, that they spent about one third of their day pursuing leisure activities, that they spent a substantial amount of time alone each day, and that increasing age and residential status were associated with more sedentary activities. The question remains, do younger people do the same things? An Australian Bureau of Statistics (1999) study compared the daily activities of people aged 15 to 64 years with those aged 65 and over. It was reported that older people spent more hours per week on personal care, housework, and social and leisure activities; younger people spent more time on employment and education. Both groups spent the same amount of time sleeping.

Everyday Communication Activities of Older People

Many of the everyday activities that the older people in the Horgas et al. (1998) study engaged in were essentially communication activities. For example, many of the IADLs (e.g., shopping, banking), the leisure activities (e.g., watching television, reading, writing), and all of the social activities involved communication. However, Horgas et al. did not study communication activities in detail. Two investigations that have undertaken this study are described here (Davidson, Worrall, & Hickson, in press; Shadden, 1988).

As part of an interview about communication and communication problems, Shadden (1988) asked 18 people ranging in age from 68 to 89 years whom they most commonly communicate with, how often, and what was the topic of communication. The most common communication partners are presented in Table 5–3. The participants reported they talk most often to other older people. In addition, 94% of the participants stated they believed they had fewer people to speak with than younger people. The individuals reported the major reasons for this are that friends or family have either died or moved away and the older person's ability to move around and make contacts was restricted. The most common topics of conversation reported by the older people in this study are shown in Table 5–4; these focused mainly on the past, on family, and on health problems. Although Shadden's study indicates communication partners and topics are rather restricted, it should be noted she did not assess the range of communication partners and topics, but looked only at those reported to be most common. For speech-language pathologists and audiologists to determine if the communication activities of older people with disabilities such as hearing

TABLE 5–3

OLDER PEOPLE'S REPORTS OF THEIR MOST COMMON COMMUNICATION PARTNERS

Communication Partner	Number of Participants Reporting (Total N = 18)
Other older people, peers	9
Family	4
Neighbors	2
Health professionals	2
Community service people (e.g., at banks, restaurants, etc.)	2
Other professionals (e.g., minister)	1
Church acquaintances	1
People at special centers for the elderly	1

Note: (Participants could choose more than one). Adapted from Shadden, 1988.

TABLE 5–4

OLDER PEOPLE'S REPORTS OF THEIR MOST COMMON TOPICS OF CONVERSATION

Topic	Number of Participants Reporting (Total N = 18)
Past, life experiences, successes, jobs, and so forth	10
Family (particularly children and grandchildren)	6
Health, ailments, illnesses, dying, and death	5
Gossip/talk about immediate environment and people in that environment, unusual happenings	4
Religion, spiritual concerns	3
Topics of everyday interest (general observations)	2
Weather	2
Gardening	1
Politics, social concerns, ideas, news	1
Financial concerns	1
Expressions of gratitude	1

Note: (Participants could choose more than one). Adapted from Shadden (1988).

impairment and aphasia are limited because of the disabilities, it is necessary to know more about the range of communication activities in which healthy older people are engaged.

More detailed evidence is available from the work of Davidson et al. (in press) who observed the communication activities of healthy older people in real-life settings. Such naturalistic observations allow the researcher to record the complexities and subtleties of everyday communication. The participant group consisted of 15 people (8 women and 7 men) ranging in age from 63 to 80 years. Fourteen participants lived with family members, and one lived alone.

Each participant was observed during his or her regular daily activities for 8 hours, over three time periods, within a week's time frame. Coding of communication activity episodes detailed the complexity and interacting factors inherent in social communication. Coding included place and time, duration of communication activity, communication partners, and topics of communication. Communication activities were grouped under eight major headings, and the frequency of each is depicted in Figure 5–2. It can be seen from this data that the most common communication activity is conversation. The participants had many different communication partners; in fact, the total was 371 partners for the 15 participants. All communicated with spouses and other family members, as well as friends and neighbors, health professionals, services/trades people, and a wide range of acquaintances. There were 84 topics of conversation discussed during the observation periods, and although the common topics were similar to that of Shadden's (1988) study (i.e., family, health, friends and neighbors, hobbies and interests, everyday activities, and plans), there were also detailed discussions about complex issues such as differences between generations, competitiveness, stress, cost of living, cost of childcare, drug use in the community, gasoline prices, and so forth.

The results of these studies on the communication activities of healthy older people have significant implications for the assessment of activity limitations in this population. Older people engage in a wide range of communication activities, with conversation being the most

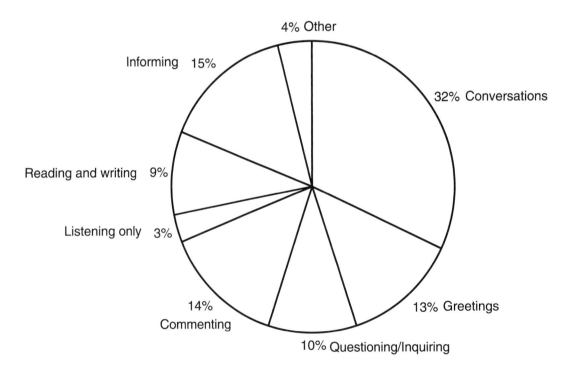

FIGURE 5–2. Frequency of different types of communication activities engaged in by older people. Adapted from Davidson, Worrall, and Hickson (1998).

common activity. They have a broad range of communication partners and topics of communication. Standardized assessments that include a restricted list of communication activities may not tap into the breadth of activities or the uniqueness of each older person's communication patterns. Assessments of activity limitations should be client centered and focus on the individual's everyday experiences.

Everyday Communication Activity Limitations of Older People With Communication Impairments

In this section, the activity limitations that have been reported for older people who have communication disabilities associated with hearing impairment and aphasia are described. The discussion here is restricted to these two conditions, because the literature on activity limitations in other communication disabilities is extremely limited.

Effects of Hearing Impairment

The effects of hearing impairment on the communication activities of older people have been examined extensively using self-report measures, that is, by asking older people about the activity limitations they experience in everyday life. The difficulties experienced by older individuals vary and depend on a number of factors related to context, for example, where they live, whom they communicate with, and their attitude toward communication. Difficulties also relate to degree of impairment, but the relationship is not straightforward (e.g., Stumer, Hickson, & Worrall, 1996). Although an older person with a moderate degree of hearing impairment is more likely to report more activity limitations than a person with a mild hearing impairment, the person does not necessarily do so. In fact, many people with significant hearing impairment do not report any communication activity limitations. Despite this individual variation, Hickson and Worrall (1997) summarize some common patterns that emerge, and these are described in the following paragraphs.

Difficulty hearing speech is the most frequently reported problem of adults of all ages with hearing impairment (Davis, 1989), and older adults are no exception. It should be pointed out here that when people say they can't "hear," frequently they qualify this by saying "I can hear it, but I just can't understand it." The high frequency of reported difficulty understanding conversation is not surprising in view of the evidence reported earlier in this chapter that showed conversation is the most common communication activity of older adults. Following difficulties in hearing conversation, the next most commonly reported problem is that of hearing television and/or radio (Stephens, 1980; Stephens & Zhao, 1996). Again, this is in line with the findings of research about the activities of older people reported previously (Horgas et al., 1998) that showed the average older person watched almost 3 hours of television per day. Although there are some commonalties, there are also many differences in the activity limitations reported by people with hearing impairment. Figure 5–3 shows the activity limitations identified by a group of seven older people with hearing impairment who attended the authors' clinic. Some of the limitations were common to more than one group member (e.g., difficulty hearing people with soft voices), whereas others were unique (e.g., hearing instructions of the band master).

As noted earlier, there are differences between the everyday activity patterns of older people living in residential care facilities for the aged and those living in the community. Similarly, the effects of hearing impairment on the everyday lives of older people living in these facilities are different from those who live in the community. The research indicates that older residents engage in fewer communication activities than community-based people, and in line with this finding, they report fewer communication activity limitations. Stumer et al. (1996) compared the hearing impairment and disability/handicap of two groups of

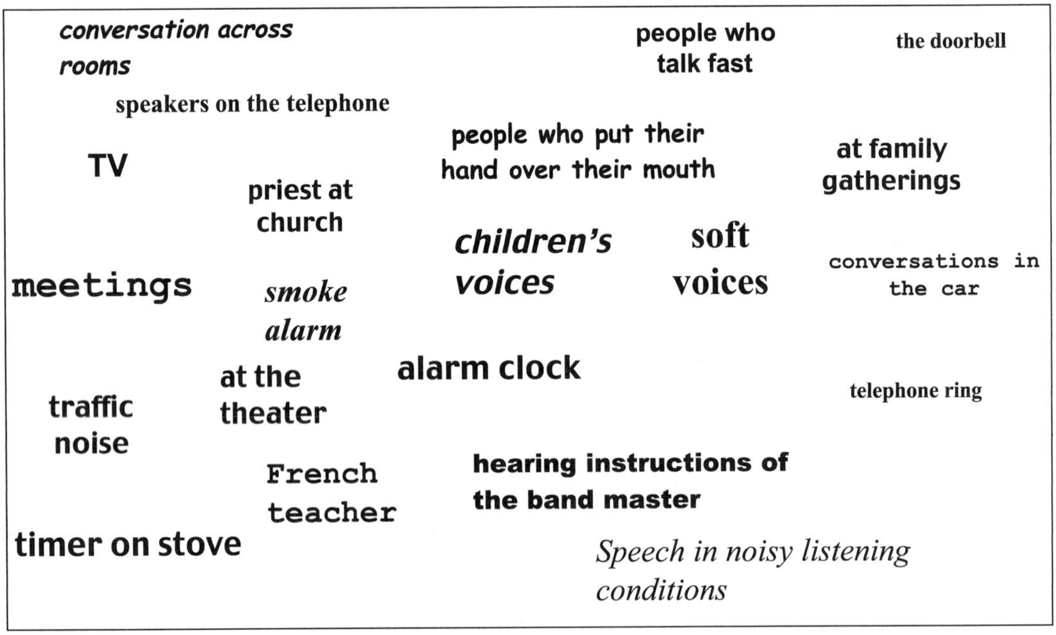

FIGURE 5–3. Some difficulties in hearing and understanding described by seven older people with hearing impairment.

older participants: one living in the community and one in extended care. Results showed that 95% of residents and 70% of community-based older people had a measured hearing impairment; however, 27% of residents and 42% of community-based people reported difficulties hearing in everyday life. Thus, despite having a higher prevalence of hearing impairment than their community-based counterparts, the residents of extended care facilities reported fewer limitations in everyday life. This finding may occur for a number of reasons. For example, residents may have fewer opportunities to communicate and are, therefore, less aware of their communication difficulties, or they may have other health problems that take priority over any communication problems.

Effects of Aphasia

In one of the only studies to examine the effects of a language impairment (in this case, aphasia) on the everyday communication activities of older people, Davidson et al. (in press) compared the communication activities of 15 healthy older people with a matched sample of 15 older people with aphasia. The activities of the 15 healthy older people, described earlier in this chapter, were compared to the activities of 15 people with chronic aphasia. The participant groups were matched for age, gender, level of education, and living situation.

Comparing the results for the two groups gives an indication of the activity limitations experienced by people with chronic aphasia. The major findings were

- People with aphasia were involved in fewer communication activities and for less time.
- The types of communication activities were the same for both groups (see Figure 5–2).
- People with aphasia watched television more often than healthy older people.
- People with aphasia had fewer communication partners.
- The types of communication partners were the same for both groups.
- People with aphasia communicated with more health professionals than did healthy older people.

People with aphasia may not perform well in everyday communicative activities, but the relationship between their severity of impairment and their difficulties in everyday communication is not as strong as some people think. Some people with aphasia do far better than would be predicted based on a traditional clinical assessment of everyday communication. They have learned to compensate (e.g., by increasing their use of nonverbal cues, looking to their conversational partners for help) and have developed compensatory strategies to circumvent their difficulties (e.g., writing notes or a script before making a telephone call, using an answering machine to screen telephone calls). In contrast, some individuals with a mild aphasia may perform poorly in everyday tasks because of their lack of compensatory strategies. Individuals generally perform better in their own home than in the hospital. The familiarity of the types of communication topics and the conversational partners appears to enhance their communicative success in the home. Sometimes this is because there is not as much demand placed on communication in the home, and, in general, the individual with aphasia is more relaxed in his or her own environment. In communicative situations outside the home, however, additional demands may be placed on the individual with aphasia (e.g., requesting an item in a shop when there is a long line or conversing with someone who does not know how to accommodate the speaker with aphasia). The importance of natural context on communicative performance cannot be underestimated.

Assessments of Communication Activities

This section begins with an overview of the different methods that can be used in the assessment of communication activities and is followed by a discussion of assessment procedures for both healthy older people and people with specific communication disabilities (i.e., people with hearing impairment, aphasia, dementia, dysphagia, and dysarthria).

The assessment of everyday communication activity limitations can be undertaken in one of three ways: (a) by direct observation, (b) by simulating a real life activity in the clinic, and (c) by asking the client and/or the significant other about his or her abilities or difficulties in real life (Davidson & Worrall, 2000). Although it is clear that direct observation would yield the most valid results, it is also clear that, because of time and financial constraints, this is not always the most practical means of assessment. Opportunities for this do arise at times however, for example, when the speech-language pathologist or audiologist works in the residential care facility for the aged where the client lives. In this situation it may well be practical and most appropriate for the clinician to observe the client's performance in real-life daily activities (e.g., during lunch, at social events).

Assessment of Healthy Older People

The recommended method of communication activity assessment for healthy older people living in the community is self-report. There are two interview protocols that could be applied for the determination of communication activity limitations. The first one in Table 5–5 is based on the Yesterday Interview protocol; the second one in Appendix A is the Communicative Activities (COMACT) Checklist by Cruice (2001). The COMACT Checklist is based on aphasia research (Davidson et al., in press; LeDorze & Brassard, 1995;

TABLE 5–5

YESTERDAY INTERVIEW PROTOCOL FOR THE ASSESSMENT OF THE COMMUNICATION ACTIVITY LIMITATIONS OF HEALTHY OLDER PEOPLE.

The aim of this interview is to find out if you are having any difficulties with communication in your everyday life. Can you tell me what you did yesterday, from waking up in the morning to going to sleep at night? Write down a list of the activities as the person says them.

Some these activities involve communication: talking, listening, reading, or writing. Let's go through the list together and mark those that involved communication.

Now we will go through the marked activities again, and I want you to tell me if you were having any difficulties with these activities and why you think the difficulties occurred. Let the person explain the activity and write down any difficulties. Prompt the person to consider why the difficulties might have occurred.

Was yesterday a typical day for you? If yes, then proceed to question 6. If no, record the reasons why the person thinks the day is atypical.

Since yesterday was not typical for you, can you tell me if there are any communication activities that you engage in on a typical day that I have missed here? If yes, then record the activity and any difficulties experienced as in question 3.

Do you have any other difficulties in talking, listening, reading, or writing that you can tell me about?

Note: Reproduced by permission from the Speech Pathology Department, Royal Bisbane Hospital, Queensland, Australia.

Oxenham, Sheard, & Adams, 1995; Parr, 1995), with consideration of item content from the ASHA-FACS (Frattali et al., 1995), the CETI (Lomas et al., 1989), as well as other informal communication activity checklists. Information is elicited through an interview format and takes approximately 20 minutes to complete. Each participant is asked how often he or she undertakes the given communicative activities. This questioning could be expanded to include a question about whether any difficulties arise in any of the activities. The Yesterday Interview protocol is more time consuming than the checklist, but provides greater detail about the individual. Although recommended here for use with healthy older people, such measures could also be used for the assessment of older people with communication disability.

Assessment of Older People With Communication and Swallowing Disability

The concept of functional assessment (i.e., based on everyday activities) has been established within the fields of hearing impairment and aphasiology for a number of years. Attempts have been made to standardize many of the functional assessments used in aphasia on related populations such as dementia and TBI. Functional assessment, however, has become so important in rehabilitation that impairment-specific functional assessments are being developed. The next section reviews the established activity level assessments suitable for older people with hearing impairment and aphasia, as well as the developing areas of dementia and dysarthria. Disorders such as cognitive-communication disorders following right hemisphere damage, TBI, and voice and fluency disorders do occur in older people (see Chapter 4), but are not as central to gerontological practice and are not covered in this section. Rating scales rather than detailed functional assessments are being used for dysphagia. Because dysphagia is a major concern for speech-language pathologists, particularly those who work in residential care settings for the aged, functional rating scales for dysphagia are also reviewed in this section.

HEARING IMPAIRMENT

In the clinical situation in which an older person from the community seeks audiological assessment, the most appropriate and efficient way to evaluate his or her activity limitations is again self-report. There are a number of questionnaires that have been designed specifically for the older population (see Appendixes B to F). Although many of these measures include the old WHO term (i.e., *handicap*) for participation in their titles, they do, in fact, assess activity limitations as well as handicap. This confusion of terminology has arisen in the United States, because of the early ASHA (ASHA, 1981), which advocated the use of the general term handicap to encompass all of the everyday effects of impairment. That is, no distinction was made between disability (activity limitations) and handicap (participation restrictions). Examples of self-report measures of hearing activities are

- Appendix B contains the full version of the Hearing Handicap Inventory for the Elderly (HHIE; Ventry & Weinstein, 1982). It has 25 items and includes some items that assess activity limitations (e.g., *Does a hearing problem cause you difficulty when listening to TV or radio?*). Response categories are *Yes, Sometimes, and No.* There is also a screening version of this test (HHIE-S; Ventry & Weinstein, 1983) that has 10 items.

- Appendix C contains the Self Assessment of Communication (SAC; Schow & Nerbonne, 1982), another screening questionnaire designed for use with older people. It has 10 items, 6 of which assess hearing activity limitations (e.g., *Do you experi-*

ence communication difficulties in situations when speaking with one other person?). Response categories are more complex than the HHIE, and five choices are: *Almost Never (or Never)*, *Occasionally (About a quarter of the time)*, *About Half the Time*, *Frequently (About three-quarters of the time)*, and *Practically Always (or Always)*. The SAC can be used in conjunction with the Significant Other Assessment of Communication (SOAC; Schow & Nerbonne, 1982), as the comparison of the two results can give insight into the level of awareness of both parties. This comparison may be important in subsequent rehabilitation.

- The Nursing Home Hearing Handicap Index (NHHHI; Schow & Nerbonne, 1977) was designed specifically for older people living in extended care facilities (see Appendix D). It has 10 items, 4 of which assess activity limitations (e.g., *Do you have trouble hearing the radio or TV?*). The older person is asked to respond using a 5-point rating scale, from *Very Often* (5) to *Almost Never* (1). The NHHHI has a self and staff version and, as with the SAC and the SOAC, the comparison of results between the two can assist with planning further rehabilitation. For example, if the resident reports no hearing difficulties, yet the staff member reports a number of problems, this issue needs to be addressed. It may be that the resident is unaware that he or she is having problems (e.g., the person does not know that his or her television is turned up very loud) or that the staff member has mistaken a client's communication problems for hearing impairment when there is another cause (e.g., early dementia).

- Another questionnaire that can be used with older people living in residential care is the Denver Scale of Communication Function—Modified (DSSC-M; Kaplan, Feely, & Brown, 1978; see Appendix E). This 34-item test has one section that focuses on activity limitations. This section, called *Specific Difficulty Listening Situations*, has 11 items (e.g., *When someone calls me from another room, I have much trouble hearing*). Response categories range from *Definitely Agree* to *Definitely Disagree*, with a neutral response of *Irrelevant*. This last category can be very useful from a rehabilitation point of view, as it provides information about the range of communication activities that a client is involved in, as well as his or her difficulties in different situations.

In addition to the questionnaires described here, there are numerous others that have been developed for the adult population that may be able to be applied to older adults (see Noble, 1999, for review).

One of the problems with standard questionnaires is that they restrict the client to describing difficulties on a closed set of activities. Admittedly, the activities included in the questionnaires are those that many older people are known to engage in, but nevertheless the items are general and, therefore, may not be relevant to the everyday life of individual clients. For example, clients might describe activity limitations when playing card games, when listening to a French teacher, or when trying to follow the choir master's instructions, to mention just a few of the many and varied possibilities. For this reason, it may well be more appropriate to ask individual clients open-ended questions about everyday communication and the difficulties faced. The Client Oriented Scale of Improvement (COSI; Dillon, James, & Ginis, 1997) is an assessment instrument that has been developed for use in rehabilitative audiology that applies this approach (see Appendix F). It allows the clinician and the client to prioritize the goals as well. At the very least, standard closed-set questionnaires should be supplemented with open-ended questions to ensure the clinician has the full picture of a client's difficulties and that nothing has been missed.

APHASIA

Aphasiology has a long tradition of functional communication assessment. The Functional Communication Therapy Planner (Worrall, 1999) contains an assessment component, which is described in Chapter 7. There are several other assessments that can be employed to assess communication activities of older people with aphasia:

- ASHA's Functional Assessments of Communication Skills for Adults (ASHA FACS; Frattali, Thompson, Holland, Wohl, & Ferketic, 1995) is one of the few standardized assessments based on real-life observations of communication. The authors recommend that the clinician observe the client on at least three occasions prior to scoring the ASHA FACS. The clinician then rates all 43 items (Table 5–6) on a 7-point scale of communication independence. The client does not need to be present for the scoring of the assessment. The 43 items are grouped into four domains: (a) social communication, (b) communication of basic needs, (c) reading, writing, and number concepts, and (d) daily planning. Each domain is then rated on the four qualitative dimensions of adequacy, appropriateness, promptness, and communication sharing. If there has been no opportunity to observe the activity, the clinician may base the rating on information obtained from other sources (e.g., family members, nurses). The ASHA FACS was piloted and standardized on people with aphasia and TBI and is currently being standardized on additional populations.

- The Communicative Abilities in Daily Living (CADL; Holland, 1980) and the more recent version, the Communication Activities of Daily Living—second edition (CADL-2; Holland, Frattali, & Fromm, 1999) are measures that use simulation of everyday tasks, such as going to the doctor, to directly assess performance in communication activities. The CADL-2 begins when the client enters the room. The first item rates the client's ability to greet and then to hand the examiner a pencil. Most items are

TABLE 5–6

EXAMPLES OF COMMUNICATION ACTIVITIES IN THREE FUNCTIONAL COMMUNICATION ASSESSMENTS FOR APHASIA.

ASHA FACS	CADL-2	CETI
Social communication (e.g., refers to familiar people by name, requests information of others, explains how to do things, exchanges information on the phone)	Social interactions (e.g., greeting, correcting, inferring, explaining, requesting)	Getting someone's attention
	Reading, writing, using numbers (e.g., indicating time, selecting from a menu, reading bus timetables, using a calendar, calculating time, reading signs, reading numbers)	Getting involved in group conversations that are about him or her
Communication of basic needs (e.g., recognizes familiar faces, makes strong likes or dislikes known, expresses feelings, requests help when necessary, makes needs or wants known, responds in an emergency numbers)		Giving yes and no answers appropriately
		Communicating his or her emotions
		Indicating that he or she understands what is being said to him or her
Reading, writing, number concepts (e.g., understands simple signs, uses common reference materials, follows written directions, understands basic printed material, prints/writes/types name, fills out short forms, writes messages)	Divergent communication	Having coffee-time visits and conversations with friends and neighbors
	Contextual communication	Having a one-to-one conversation with you
	Nonverbal communication	Saying the name of someone whose face is in front of him or her
	Sequential relationships	Communicating physical problems such as aches and pains
	Humor/metaphor/ absurdity	Having a spontaneous conversation
Daily planning (e.g., knows what time it is, dials telephone numbers, keeps scheduled appointments, uses a calendar for time-related activities)		Responding to or communicating anything without words

Note: ASHA FACS (Frattali et al., 1995), CADL-2 (Holland et al., 1999), CETI (Lomas et al., 1989).

responses to questions asked about photographed or drawn stimuli; for example, when the client is shown a menu, the person is asked to choose an item for lunch. If the client finds the lunch section of the menu and chooses an item for lunch, the highest rating of 2 is given; if the client locates the lunch menu but does not choose an item, a rating of 1 is given; and, if, for example, items from all three menus are chosen, then a 0 rating is given. There are five scenarios that span several items through the 50-item test: the initial greeting and interview, a visit to a doctor's office, driving a car, shopping for groceries, and reporting a fire (see examples of items in Table 5–6). Hence, the ratings of functional communication are given once the clinician has observed the patient in simulated tasks.

■ The Communicative Effectiveness Index (CETI; Lomas et al., 1989) is a good example of a speech-language pathology measure that uses reported performance. The CETI contains 16 items that are rated by the partner of the person with aphasia on a Visual Analogue Scale (see Table 5–6 for list of items.) The test items were developed by the partners of people with aphasia using group analysis and, therefore, reflect the perceptions of significant others. Lomas et al. (1989) argued that significant others are in the best position to observe everyday communication of aphasic people and that their perceptions of functional communication ability are important. Hence, this is a measure of reported performance by the partners of people with aphasia.

■ The Functional Communication Profile (FCP; Sarno, 1969) was the first of its kind. It is an observational tool where the examiner rates the 45 items on a 9-point scale. The rating scale compares the client's performance on each activity to premorbid levels of functioning.

■ The Assessment of Language-Related Functional Activities (ALFA; Baines, Martin, & McMartin Heeringa, 1999) is a recent addition to the range of functional communication assessments for aphasia. This test uses simulated tasks within 10 subtests: telling time, counting money, addressing an envelope, solving daily math problems, writing a check and balancing a checkbook, understanding medicine labels, using a calendar, reading instructions, using a telephone, and writing a telephone message.

DEMENTIA

Dementia is a particular concern when working with the older population. Interventions may seek to slow down the rate of decline in everyday communication skills and, hence, functional communication assessments are becoming an important part of dementia care. Lubinski and Orange (2000) described a functional assessment and a number of discourse analysis tools developed specifically for dementia. These include

- The Functional Linguistic Communication Inventory (FLCI; Bayles & Tomoeda, 1994), a 30-minute assessment designed for middle and late stage dementia. The assessment has 10 parts covering greetings and naming, answering questions, writing, understanding signs, object-picture matching, reading comprehension, reminiscing, following spoken commands, gesture, and participating in a conversation.

- The Discourse Assessment Profile (Terrell & Ripich, 1989), the Rating Scale of Communication in Cognitive Decline (Bollinger & Hardiman, 1991), and the Pragmatic Assessment of Communication—Dementia (England, O'Neill & Simpson, 1996) are three discourse analysis tools developed for dementia. Various behaviors such as turn taking and using and understanding nonverbal behavior are rated or scored.

DYSARTHRIA

Many age-related diseases have dysarthria as a common sequela. Stroke, Parkinson's disease, motor neuron disease, Huntington's disease, and multiple sclerosis are some of the specific conditions associated with dysarthria. It is possible that the variety of etiologies has dispersed the research effort in developing standardized measures of functional outcome in dysarthria. As Beukelman, Mathy, and Yorkston (1998) reported, the emphasis in motor speech disorders has been on the pathology and impairment. The conceptualization of activity-level assessments appropriate for people with motor speech disorders is also not well developed. There is one commonly used functional measure in the literature, the Assessment of Intelligibility in Dysarthric Speakers (AIDS; Yorkston & Beukelman, 1984). This is a test of single word intelligibility, sentence intelligibility, and speaking rate. At the single word level, dysarthric speakers are recorded as they say 50 words. The judge selects the word that has been spoken using a multiple-choice format or transcribes the word. At the sentence level, intelligibility is judged using a word-by-word transcription. Although the complexity of the message is varied and listener familiarity may be varied, the standardized AIDS does little to include natural context. Although it is more probably based at the impairment level, there are few assessments that measure more complex communicative activities, particularly those that incorporate natural contexts.

One promising measure is the Communicative Effectiveness Survey (Sullivan, Beukelman, & Gaebler, 1997, cited in Yorkston, Beukelman, Strand, Bell, & Hustad, 1999). The survey consists of 15 everyday communication activities that are rated on a 7-point effectiveness scale by the dysarthric speaker, a family member, or a friend. Items include *Having a conversation with a few friends (at home or bedside)*, *Speaking in front of a small group without a microphone*, and *Conversing through the outdoor speaker system with an employee at a fast food restaurant or at a gas station*. There are three blank items at the end of the survey for the participants to add their specific context. Although there is no reported rationale for the items, or evidence of psychometric studies, the concept of choosing relevant everyday communicative items for the assessment of people with dysarthria is clinically important. This tool would be useful to gain an impression of some of the communicative activity limitations experienced by individuals with dysarthria.

DYSPHAGIA

Sonies (2000) described 17 functional outcomes scales for people with dysphagia. The proliferation of simple scales of functional swallowing reflects the increasing attention to dysphagia by the speech-language pathology profession and the need to monitor outcomes within this expanding service area. Many scales still assess swallowing impairments rather than activity limitations or participation restrictions. The consensus appears to be that dysphagia can be rated at the activity level through the type of modified diet the person needs to maintain safety and nutritional status. The terminology of diet modification varies across facilities, so a standard rating scale, or the most popular rating scale, is difficult to find. Because many of the rating scales are new and developed specifically for clinicians by clinicians, many do not have psychometric data.

One scale that has been widely accepted across Australia (Worrall & Egan, in press) and has extensive psychometric data (Ward & Conroy, 1999) is the Royal Brisbane Hospital Outcome Measure for Swallowing (Speech Pathology Department, Royal Brisbane Hospital, 1998). The 10-point rating scale has four stages of oral intake from Nil by Mouth to Maintaining Oral Intake (see Figure 5–4). Each level has a number of characteristics that have to be present to make the rating. For example, to assign a rating of 4 in the Commencing Oral Intake stage, the patient must be tolerating small amounts of thickened/thin fluids only (e.g., posthead/neck surgery having sips of water), and should not be at a stage where the speech-language pathologist only conducts the swallowing trial. The patient may or may not have nonoral supplementation for food and/or fluid requirements (e.g., nasogastric, intravenous) supervision with regard to safety of swallow and may or may not meet all fluid and/or food requirements orally.

The Future: The WHO Model as a Communication Activity Assessment Tool?

In this chapter, a number of activity-level assessments for healthy older people and people with specific communication and swallowing impairments have been described. In general, these assessments have relied on quite a restricted list of communicative activities, and the

NIL BY MOUTH
Level 1 Patient aspirates secretions
Level 2 Difficulty managing secretions but patient protecting airway
Level 3 Coping with secretions

COMMENCING ORAL INTAKE
Level 4 Tolerates small amounts of thickened/thin fluids only

ESTABLISHING ORAL INTAKE
Level 5 Commencing/continuing modified diet—is being provided supplementation
Level 6 Commencing/continuing modified diet—no supplementation required
Level 7 Upgrading modified diet

MAINTAINING ORAL INTAKE
Level 8 Swallowing function at patient's optimal level
Level 9 Swallowing function at premorbid/preadmission level
Level 10 Swallowing function at better than premorbid/preadmission level

FIGURE 5–4. Royal Brisbane Hospital Outcome Measure for Swallowing. Reproduced with permission from Speech Pathology Department, Royal Brisbane Hospital, Australia.

limitations of these standardized functional assessments need to be recognized. It would be valuable to include supplements to these assessments, such as additional observation in natural contexts, and interviews of key stakeholders (e.g., family members, friends, caregivers).

As mentioned at the start of this chapter, the activity list contained in the WHO model could be used as a framework for the assessment of communication activities in older people. Admittedly, it too contains another set list, as many of the conventional speech-language pathology and audiology assessments do; however, the list is far more comprehensive. For example, the WHO model includes both simple and complex activities. Sometimes clinicians limit assessments and, therefore, interventions, to simple activities related to communication, such as receiving and understanding messages, and fail to consider the effect of communication problems on more complex activities, such as performing at work. Indeed, the WHO list serves to remind us that communication underpins and is a prerequisite for most activities of everyday life. A further advantage to using the WHO model as a basis for activity assessment in the future is that, because its usage is broader than just for audiologists and speech-language pathologists, it may help the professions become more consistent with other professions in conceptual frameworks and terminology.

Older people are involved in a wide range of everyday communication activities, and it is essential that audiologists and speech-language pathologists consider the effects of communication impairments on these everyday activities. Traditionally, clinicians have assessed impairments and have included some measures at the activity level. In speech-language pathology, such measures have been called functional communication assessments; in audiology, they have been termed disability/handicap measures. A number of activity-level assessments for healthy older people and people with communication and swallowing disabilities have been reviewed in this chapter, and the possibility of assessments based on the WHO model has been suggested.

Activity-based assessments are an important part of measuring the overall communication disabilities of older people. Clinicians need to be able to select the assessment that most suits their client in order to plan intervention and measure the outcomes. When selecting a standardized assessment, the parameters the clinician should consider include the purpose of the assessment (e.g., diagnosis, discharge planning), the setting (e.g., hospital, residential care facility for the aged, community), the type of impairment (e.g., aphasia, dysarthria, dementia), and the extent of item sampling in the assessment (basic or extensive) (Davidson & Worrall, 2000). Alternatively, clinicians may choose an individualized approach and simply assess the everyday communicative activities that are the focus of rehabilitation (see Worrall, 1999). Self-report, direct observation, and interviews with significant others should be used, if possible, to supplement clinical assessment. Intervention subsequent to assessment of communication activities is discussed in the next section of the book.

 ## KEY POINTS

- For comprehensive rehabilitation, it is important to consider not just the impairments that a person suffers, but the effects of those communication impairments on the individual's everyday life.
- The everyday effects can be considered in terms of communication activity limitations as per the WHO model.
- Leisure activities form a large part of older people's everyday activities.
- Older people spend a lot of time alone or with a spouse and other older people.
- Difficulty hearing conversation and hearing the radio and television are the most commonly reported activity limitations of older people with hearing impairment.

- Residents with hearing impairment in residential care facilities for the aged report fewer communication activity limitations than community-based older people with hearing impairment because of fewer opportunities to engage in communication in residential care.

- People with aphasia have been observed to engage in fewer communicative activities and have fewer communication partners. Their performance in everyday communicative tasks varies across settings and is usually better in the home environment than in the clinic setting.

- Assessment of everyday communication can be accomplished through direct observation, observation of a simulated task, or by asking the client and/or a significant other about the client's abilities in real life.

- Communication activities of older people can be assessed using the Yesterday Interview or the Communication Activities Checklist.

- Communication activities of community-based older people with hearing impairment can be assessed by the Hearing Handicap Inventory for the Elderly or the Self Assessment of Communication.

- Older people with hearing impairment living in residential care facilities for the aged can be assessed by the Nursing Home Hearing Handicap Index or the Denver Scale of Communication Function.

- Older people with aphasia can be assessed on either the ASHA Functional Communication Skills for Adults, the Communication Activities in Daily Living (second edition), the Communicative Effectiveness Index, the Functional Communication Profile, or the Assessment of Language Related Functional Activities.

- Communicative activity level functions can be assessed in people with dementia using the Functional Linguistic Communication Inventory or a discourse analysis tool.

- Functional effects of dysarthric speakers are often assessed using the Assessment of Intelligibility of Dysarthric Speakers.

- The effects of dysphagia are often measured using an outcome scale such as the Royal Brisbane Hospital Outcome Measure for Swallowing.

- The activity list included in the WHO model can be useful as a framework for more detailed assessment at the activity level because it includes a wider range of everyday activities than traditional audiology and speech-language pathology assessments.

- To find out more about the everyday effects of communication problems, traditional standardized activity level assessments should be supplemented by extended observation in natural contexts and/or interviews with key stakeholders.

CLASS ACTIVITIES

1. Break the class into small groups of three to four students and ask each group to consider one of the activities in Table 5–2 and to describe
   - how communication is involved in the activity,
   - how a communication impairment (e.g., hearing impairment, dysarthria) might limit a person's ability to perform the activity, and
   - how to assess the person's ability to perform the activity.

2. Ask students to complete the Yesterday Interview themselves. They should write down the activities they were involved in and how much time was spent on each. At the end ask the students to compare their activities to those in Figure 5–1 for older people. Discuss differences and similarities.

3. Each student should interview one older person using both procedures in Table 5–5 and in Chapter 5 Appendix A. They should summarize the results from both and compare and contrast the findings. Did the older person experience any communication difficulties? What did the person cite as the cause for the difficulties? Did both measures provide the same information? If not, how were they different?

RECOMMENDED READING

Davidson, B., & Worrall, L. (2000). The assessment of activity limitation in functional communication: Challenges and choices. In L. E. Worrall & C. M. Frattali (Eds.), *Neurogenic communication disorders: A functional approach* (pp.19–34). New York: Thieme.

Hickson, L., & Worrall, L. (1997). Hearing impairment, disability and handicap in older people. *Critical Reviews in Physical and Rehabilitation Medicine*, 9(3 & 4), 219–243.

Horgas, A. L., Wilms, H-U., & Baltes, M. M. (1998). Daily life in very old age: Everyday activities as expression of successful aging. *The Gerontologist*, 38(5), 556–568.

Noble, W. (1999). *Self-assessment of hearing and related functions*. London: Whurr Publishers Ltd.

Shadden, B. (1988). Perceptions of daily communicative interactions with older persons. In B. B. Shadden (Ed.), *Communication behavior and aging: A sourcebook for clinicians* (pp. 12–40). Baltimore: Williams & Wilkins.

Stumer, J., Hickson, L. & Worrall, L. (1996). Hearing impairment, disability and handicap in elderly people living in residential care and in the community. *Disability and Rehabilitation, 18*(2), 76–82.

REFERENCES

Australian Bureau of Statistics. (1999). *Year book Australia*. Canberra: Australian Bureau of Statistics.

American Speech-Language-Hearing Association. (1981). Task force on the definition of hearing handicap. *ASHA, 23*, 293–297.

Baines, K. A., Martin, A. W., & McMartin Heeringa, H. (1999). *Assessment of language-related functional activities*. Austin, TX: Pro-Ed

Bayles, K. A., & Tomoeda, C. K. (1994). *Functional Linguistic Communication Inventory*. Tucson, AZ: Canyonlands Publishing.

Beukelman, D. R., Mathy, P., & Yorkston, K. (1998). Outcomes measurement in motor speech disorders. In C. M. Frattali (Ed.), *Measuring outcomes in speech-language pathology* (pp. 334–353). New York: Thieme.

Bollinger, R., & Hardiman, C. J. (1991). *Rating scale of communication in cognitive decline*. Buffalo, NY: United Educational Services.

Cruice, M. (2001) *The effect of communication in quality of life in older adults with aphasia and healthy older adults*. Unpublished doctoral thesis. The University of Queensland, Brisbane, Australia.

Davidson, B., & Worrall, L. (2000). The assessment of activity limitation in functional communication: Challenges and choices. In L. E. Worrall & C. M. Frattali (Eds.), *Neurogenic communication disorders: A functional approach*. (pp. 19–34). New York: Thieme.

Davidson, B., Worrall, L., & Hickson, L. (in press). *Observed communication activities of people with aphasia and healthy older people*. Manuscript submitted for publication.

Davis, A. C. (1989). The prevalence of hearing impairment and reported hearing disability among adults in Great Britain. *International Journal of Epidemiology, 18*, 911–917.

Dillon, H., James, A., & Ginis, J. (1997). Client Oriented Scale of Improvement (COSI) and its relationship to several other measures of benefit and satisfaction provided by hearing aids. *Journal of the American Academy of Audiology, 8*(1), 27–43.

England, J. E., O'Neil, J. J., & Simpson, R. K. (1996). Pragmatic assessment of communication in dementia (PAC-D). *American Journal of Alzheimer's Disease, 11*, 7–10.

Frattali, C., Thompson, C., Holland, A., Wohl, C., & Ferketic, M. (1995). *American Speech-Language-Hearing Association Functional Assessment of Communication Skills for Adults.* Rockville, MD: ASHA.

Hickson, L., & Worrall, L. (1997). Hearing impairment, disability and handicap in older people. *Critical Reviews in Physical and Rehabilitation Medicine, 9*(3 & 4), 219–243.

Holland, A. L. (1980). *Communicative abilities in daily living.* Baltimore: University Park Press.

Holland, A., Frattali, C., & Fromm, D. (1999). *Communication activities of daily living* (2nd ed.). Austin, TX: Pro-Ed.

Horgas, A. L., Wilms, H-U., & Baltes, M. M. (1998). Daily life in very old age: Everyday activities as expression of successful aging. *The Gerontologist, 38*(5), 556–568.

Kaplan, H., Feely, J., & Brown, J. (1978). A modified Denver scale: Test-retest reliability. *Journal of the Academy of Rehabilitative Audiology, 11,* 11–32.

Le Dorze, G., & Brassard, C. (1995). A description of the consequences of aphasia on aphasic persons and their relatives and friends, based on the WHO model of chronic diseases. *Aphasiology, 9*(3), 239–255.

Lomas, J., Pickard, L., Bester, S., Elbard, H., Finlayson, A., & Zoghaib, C. (1989). The Communicative Effectiveness Index: Development and pyschometric evaluation of a functional communication measure for adult aphasia. *Journal of Speech and Hearing Disorders, 54,* 113–124.

Lubinski, R., & Orange, J. B. (2000). A framework for the assessment and treatment of functional communication in dementia. In L. E. Worrall & C. M. Frattali (Eds.), *Neurogenic communication disorders: A functional approach* (pp. 220–246). New York: Thieme.

Moss, M., & Lawton, M. P. (1982). Time budgets of older people: A window on four lifestyles. *Journal of Gerontology, 35,* 576–582.

Noble, W. (1999). *Self-assessment of hearing and related functions.* London: Whurr Publishers Ltd.

Oxenham, D., Sheard, C., & Adams, R. (1995). Comparison of clinician and spouse perceptions of the handicap of aphasia: Everybody understands "understanding." *Aphasiology, 9*(5), 477–493.

Parr, S. (1995). Everyday reading and writing in aphasia: Role change and the influence of premorbid literacy practice. *Aphasiology, 9*(3), 223–238.

Sarno, M. T. (1969). *The functional communication profile: Manual of directions.* New York: Institute of Rehabilitation Medicine.

Schow, R. L., & Nerbonne, M. A. (1977). Assessments of hearing handicaps by nursing home residents and staff. *Journal of the Academy of Rehabilitative Audiology, 10,* 2–12.

Schow, R. L., & Nerbonne, M. A. (1982). Communication screening profile: Use with elderly clients. *Ear and Hearing, 3*(3), 135-147.

Shadden, B. (1988). Perceptions of daily communicative interactions with older persons. In B. B. Shadden (Ed.), *Communication behavior and aging: A sourcebook for clinicians.* (pp. 12–40). Baltimore: Williams & Wilkins.

Smith. J., & Baltes, M. (1998). The role of gender in very old age: Profiles of functioning and everyday life patterns. *Psychology and Aging, 13*(4), 676–695.

Sonies, B. C. (2000). Assessment and treatment of functional swallowing in dysphagia. In L. E. Worrall & C. M. Frattali (Eds.), *Neurogenic communication disorders: A functional approach.* (pp. 262–275). New York: Thieme.

Speech Pathology Department, Royal Brisbane Hospital. (1998). *Royal Brisbane Hospital Outcome Measure for Swallowing.* Available from Speech Pathology Department, Royal Brisbane Hospital, Herston 4029, QLD, Australia.

Stephens, S. D. G. (1980). Evaluating the problems of the hearing impaired. *Audiology, 19,* 205–220.

Stephens, D., & Zhao, F. (1996). Hearing impairment: Special needs of the elderly. *Folia Phoniatrica et Logopaedica, 48,* 137–142.

Stumer, J., Hickson, L., & Worrall, L. (1996). Hearing impairment, disability and handicap in elderly people living in residential care and in the community. *Disability and Rehabilitation, 18*(2), 76–82.

Terrell, B., & Ripich, D. N. (1989). Discourse competence as a variable in intervention. *Seminars in Speech and Language Disorders, 10,* 282–297.

Ventry, I. M., & Weinstein, B. E. (1982). The Hearing Handicap Inventory for the Elderly: A new tool. *Ear & Hearing, 3,* 128–134.

Ventry, I. M., & Weinstein, B. E. (1983). Identification of elderly people with hearing problems. *American Speech, Language, and Hearing Association, 25,* 37–42.

Ward, E. C., & Conroy, A-L. (1999). Validity, reliability and responsivity of the Royal Brisbane Hospital Outcome Measure for Swallowing. *Asia Pacific Journal of Speech, Language and Hearing, 4,* 109–129.

World Health Organization. (2001). *International classification of functioning, disability and health.* Geneva: Author.

Worrall, L. (1999). *Functional communication therapy planner.* Oxon, UK: Winslow Press.

Worrall, L. E., & Egan, J. (in press). The use of outcome measures by Australian speech pathologists. *Asia Pacific Journal of Speech-Language and Hearing.*

Yorkston, K. M., Beukelman, D. R., Strand, E. A., Bell, K. R., & Hustad, K. C. (1999). Optimizing communicative effectiveness: Bringing it together. In K. M. Yorkston, D. R. Beukelman, E. A. Strand, & K. R. Bell (Eds.), *Management of motor speech disorders in children and adults* (pp.483–541). Austin, TX: Pro-Ed.

Yorkston, K. M., & Beukelman, D. R. (1984). *Assessment of intelligibility of dysarthric speech.* Pro-Ed: Austin, TX.

Chapter 6

Participation and Quality of Life

M easuring participation and quality of life is an emerging area of
practice for speech-language pathologists and audiologists working with older people with communication disabilities. This chapter
first defines participation and quality of life and relates the WHO component of participation to the concept of quality of life. Assessments
of participation and quality of life are reviewed. Many of the measures
are as yet unfamiliar to audiologists and speech-language pathologists,
and reviewing them helps to clarify the concepts of participation
and quality of life. Finally, in this chapter, healthy older people's
descriptions of their quality of life are presented, followed by specific
findings about how people with communication disability describe
their quality of life.

In the last two chapters, the communication-related impairments and the communicative
activity limitations that occur in older people with and without a specific communication
disability were described. In addition, assessments for communication impairments and
activities were discussed. Speech-language pathology and audiology practice has traditionally been limited to these two domains. Moving along the continuum of functioning
and disability, this chapter focuses on the broader concepts of participation and quality of
life. These concepts have not previously been the focus of assessment and intervention for
audiologists and speech-language pathologists, but they are rapidly emerging areas, particularly for clinicians adopting a social model of practice (see Chapter 3).

The chapter begins by describing what is meant by the terms *participation* and *quality of life*. Following this description, a range of assessments is described that could be used by speech-language pathologists and audiologists, and results are presented from studies that have employed these assessments to date. Such studies indicate the adverse effects that communication disability can have on an older person's participation in life and on quality of life.

Participation in the WHO Model

In Chapter 2, the WHO framework of functioning, disability, and health was described in detail. In the WHO model, participation was defined as "involvement in a life situation" (WHO, 2001, p. 10). The participation domains in the WHO model are the same as those in the activities list provided in Chapter 5.

1. Learning and Applying Knowledge
2. General Tasks and Demands
3. Communication
4. Mobility
5. Self-Care
6. Domestic Life
7. Interpersonal Interactions and Relationships
8. Major Life Areas
9. Community, Social, and Civic Life

It is evident that communication would have a major impact on an older person's ability to participate in all of these areas. The importance of communication is obvious for participating in interpersonal interactions and relationships, but it would also be important for other areas such as participating in self-care and mobility. For example, an older person with communication disability such as severe dysarthria living in a residential care environment may not be able to participate in decisions about which clothes to wear and whether they want assistance to walk.

Assessment of Participation

No standardized measures of communication participation are currently available. The most effective way to assess participation is through an interview asking the older person about his or her level of involvement and degree of satisfaction with participation in the WHO domains listed in the previous section. Hickson and Worrall (2001) suggested the following interview questions for older people with hearing impairment, but they could equally be applied to other impairments.

- What were you involved in 2 years ago?
- What are you doing now?
- Why the change?
- What is stopping you from participating now?
- What can be done so that you can return to things you used to like to do?

The areas identified by the individual as being things that he or she would like to return to (e.g., going to the movies, attending church meetings) subsequently become the goals of rehabilitation. It may also be useful to interview significant others about their perceptions of the older person's participation, what stops the person from doing what he or she wants, and what helps.

Using the WHO model, barriers (i.e., things that prohibit participation) and facilitators (i.e., things that assist participation) can be environmental or personal. Environmental barriers for older people with hearing impairment may include poor acoustic conditions, no loop system, not being given enough time to respond, lack of support, or attitudes of others. Personal barriers may include poor coping strategies, denial of their own difficulties, resistance to new technologies, and lack of assertiveness. Once the barriers have been identified, appropriate action can be taken at the personal and/or societal level to facilitate participation.

Parr, Byng, and Gilpin (1997) conducted in-depth interviews with 50 people with aphasia about their experiences. Parr and Byng (2000) summarized the disabling barriers that emerged from the interviews as

- environmental barriers (e.g., background noise, people talking all at once)
- attitudinal barriers (e.g., hostile and discriminatory reactions)
- structural barriers (e.g., restricted access to support and services)
- informational barriers (e.g., not being given information relevant to their concerns in an appropriate form).

Simmons-Mackie and Damico (1996) also recommend in-depth interviews as a first step for people with aphasia. The other steps include observation of the person in real life and a conversational analysis from a video recording of the person with aphasia. This process of determining barriers to participation can help to direct future rehabilitation. As discussed previously in Chapter 5 in relation to the assessment of activities, real-life observation can be extremely informative. It is understood that this is frequently not possible for the audiologist or speech-language pathologist who is clinic bound, but there are occasions when visits beyond the therapy setting do occur (e.g., a visit to a frail older person in a residential care facility). Clinicians should take such opportunities to carefully examine the barriers and facilitators to their older client's participation.

Another potentially useful method of determining the extent of participation, particularly in the area of social participation, is the Social Activities Survey (SOCACT; Cruice, 2001, see Chapter 6 Appendix A). The SOCACT was based on research within the stroke and gerontology literature (Bowling, Farquhar, Grundy, & Formby, 1993; Cummins, 1995; Labi, Phillips, & Gresham, 1980; Niemi, Laaksonen, & Kotila, 1988; Reitzes, Mutran, & Verrill, 1995). Twenty leisure, informal, and formal social activities are checked for frequency of participation. The same social activities are then marked for the most frequent social activity partner, that is, the person is asked *With whom do you usually do these activities?* Thus, the SOCACT yields data on the number of social activities, frequency, and partners. Some older people are found to have low levels of social participation and are socially isolated. The person should then be asked if he or she is satisfied with this (remembering that, for some people, solitude is a choice) and, if not, then barriers and facilitators to participation can be identified. The speech-language pathologist or audiologist can then assist in overcoming environmental or personal barriers that exist and can work with other professionals and family members to enhance the participation of the individual.

In summary, an older person's participation is assessed most frequently by means of an interview that identifies areas of participation, as well as barriers that restrict participation, and facilitators that enhance it. Assessment information can also be obtained from interviewing significant others and from observation. The clinician must work collaboratively with the client and other stakeholders (e.g., family, caregivers) to develop an appropriate rehabilitation plan based on these assessment results. Examples of interventions that focus on participation for older people in the community, hospital, and residential care facility for the aged are included in Chapters 7, 8, and 9 in the following section of this book. This chapter focuses on assessment only.

Quality of Life

Quality of life is a concept that has received far greater attention in the health and aged care sectors than participation. Whereas participation assessments are rare, there is a plethora of assessments that measure various aspects of quality of life. The reason for this most probably is because the two concepts are similar. In addition, the term quality of life has been used to encompass participation. For example, Hirsch and Holland (2000) stated that participation and quality of life are too similar to differentiate. In essence, when most people are asked about their quality of life, they will often refer to their participation in life situations as a contributing factor to the quality of their lives. When people are asked about their participation in life situations, they will consider it within the context of their overall quality of life.

It is important, however, from a theoretical perspective, to point out that the two concepts do emanate from two different areas. The WHO term participation is from the health area, and quality of life concepts have been widely used across a range of disciplines (e.g., health, social welfare, psychology, economics) and have not been traditionally linked to the WHO model. Cruice, Worrall, and Hickson (2000b) conceptualized the dimensions of the WHO model and quality of life as separate yet related entities (see Figure 2–4, in Chapter 2), and that is the approach adopted in the text. Participation and quality of life are related but not the same.

To date, audiologists and speech-language pathologists have not incorporated quality of life measures into routine clinical practice (Hesketh & Hopcutt, 1997; Steering Committee of the Quality Improvement Study Section of ASHA Special Interest Division 11, 1996; Worrall & Egan, 2001). Most clinicians, however, would argue that effective communication is integral to a good quality of life. Most would agree that enhanced quality of life is the ultimate aim of intervention. Many believe that quality of life is compromised following a communication disability. How much evidence is there for these statements? Is communication as important to quality of life as clinicians think? How can communication specialists place greater emphasis on quality of life issues in the management of communication disability in older clients? The first step to answering these questions is to find out more about the concept of quality of life, how it is affected by health conditions, and how it can be measured.

One of the best ways to understand the concept of quality of life is to reflect on one's own quality of life. How would you rate your quality of life? Why do you say that? (Farquhar, 1995). Farquhar found that most healthy people reflect on the strength of family relationships (e.g., *My quality of life is good because I have a loving family*) or their economic status (e.g., *My quality of life is good because I earn a good salary*). Some place more emphasis on their emotional health (e.g., *I am generally happy*) or their physical health (e.g., *I am fit and healthy*). This is particularly the case if the person has some experience of mental health or physical health problems. Certainly, it is easy to see why some people who are depressed, socially isolated, poor, or chronically ill might rate their quality of life as poor. However, it is not always possible to predict quality of life. It is an individual concept. It is important to recognize that people's perception of their quality of life varies according to the values they hold and the experiences they have.

For example, some people who have aphasia following a stroke have described their lives as being better than before. One man found his aphasia to be a good excuse to finish a job that he did not like and escape to his shed to pursue his hobby away from his very talkative wife. Another claimed that his life was too hectic before and that his strokes have made him appreciate the simple things in life. In contrast, some people with very mild communication disabilities consider the quality of their lives to have changed dramatically. People who have little experience of health problems often take their health for granted and do not see it as a priority for quality of life. The same might be said for communication problems.

The term, quality of life, has become part of modern everyday vocabulary. It has also been overused within the health sector. Definitions vary; however, the World Health Organization's definition is considered to be the foremost authority. Quality of life is defined as "an individual's perception of their position in life in the context of the culture and value systems in which they live and in relation to their goals, expectations, standards and concerns" (World Health Organization Quality of Life Assessment Group, 1993, p. 5).

Older people have described quality of life to be based on happy marriages, contentment, social relations, income, standards of living, and possession of goods (Seed & Lloyd, 1997). They have also described it as an understanding of self, an ability to adapt to changing situations, staying afloat, enjoying life through losses and problems, and dependent on the extent to which older people can find value and meaning in their lives (Lundh & Nolan, 1996).

Assessment of Quality of Life

Numerous measures of quality of life exist. Development of a range of measures has largely been driven by the agenda of governments and payers to measure the outcomes of health care services. Quality of life measures are used for the development and evaluation of health care policies, allocation of resources, planning of future health care needs, implementation of nationwide health-related surveys, and evaluation of the efficacy of clinical treatments and research trials (Berkman, Chauncey, & Holmes, 1999; McCallum, 1995; McHorney, Kosinski, & Ware, 1994). The increase in emphasis on quality of life measures is due to (a) an increasing recognition of quality of life as a crucial outcome, (b) a shift in focus from life prolongation to quality of life in health care settings, (c) the possibility of health status comparisons across different conditions or target populations using general health status measures, and (d) a general agreement about the importance of the "centrality" of the patient's self-perceptions of health (Bruley, 1999; McCallum, 1995; Ware & Sherbourne, 1992; Ware, Snow, Kosinski, & Gander, 1993).

For speech-language pathologists and audiologists, incorporating an assessment of quality of life into a test battery allows the clinician to access a global perspective of the client. It can help to establish long-term goals and measure success in achieving them. It enhances the clinician's accountability by determining whether the intervention makes a difference to quality of life. It may ultimately improve practice by determining which interventions most benefit quality of life. Finally, it is potentially important for clinicians to talk about quality of life outcomes when seeking funding for services from administrators and payers. Such people may not necessarily understand the outcomes of speech, language, or hearing assessments, but may be impressed by a discussion of intervention affecting quality of life for older people.

There are three main types of quality of life measures that are potentially useful for speech-language pathology and audiology practice. These are (a) health-related quality of life measures, (b) nonhealth-related quality of life measures, and (c) communication-related quality of life measures. Figure 6–1 is a list of quality of life measures that have been cited in the literature about communicatively disabled populations. Each of the three different types of measures have been used in various studies.

The following sections of this chapter contain a description of health-related, nonhealth-related, and communication-related quality of life measures. A number of frequently used measures are reviewed, and many partial or whole measures are included in the Appendixes. The reader is also directed to reviews of communication-related quality of life assessment in Hirsch and Holland (2000) and Frattali (1998). For more generic measures, readers are referred to the text *Measuring health: A guide to rating scales and questionnaires* (McDowell & Newell, 1996). This text provides full descriptions, including copies of instruments, of over 80 measurement methods in the areas of physical disability and handicap, social health, psychological well-being, depression, mental status testing, pain measurements, general health status, and quality of life.

HEALTH-RELATED QUALITY OF LIFE MEASURES

Heath-related quality of life can be measured in a number of ways. First, a person's overall health can be evaluated using a generic multidimensional measure. Such a measure attempts to paint an overall picture of health-related quality of life through measuring each of the domains or dimensions that are thought to make up quality of life. Second, overall health can be broken down into the common domains of physical, emotional, social, and mental health, and one of these domains can be specifically examined. These are called domain-specific measures of quality of life. Third, there are also measures that evaluate subcomponents of each of the domains. These can be called factor-specific measures of quality of life. For example, social health has the subcomponents of social integration, social networks, social adjustment, relationships, interaction, or social support, and there are measures that evaluate each of these constructs specifically. All three levels of measurement may have application to speech-language pathology and audiology for older people, depending on the reason for the assessment. For example, the clinician may want to determine the overall quality of life of an older client, or may be specifically focused on social health, or even more specifically, social support.

GENERIC MULTIDIMENSIONAL MEASURES

There are many generic measures of quality of life including the SF-36 (Ware & Sherbourne, 1992), the Sickness Impact Profile (Bergner et al., 1981), the Nottingham

Instruments previously used with the general aging population

Schedule for Evaluation of Individual Quality of Life (SEIQoL) (Browne et al., 1994)

Short Form 36 (SF-36) (Ware & Sherbourne, 1992)

Sickness Impact Profile (SIP) (Bergner, Bobbit, Carter, & Gibson, 1981)

Nottingham Health Profile (NHP) (Hunt, McKenna, Williams, & Papp, 1981)

Quality of Well-Being Scale (QWB Scale) (Anderson, Kaplan, Berry, Bush, & Rumbaut

Euroqol (The Euroqol Group, 1990)

Life Satisfaction Index (LSI) (Neugarten, Havighurst, & Tobin, 1961)

Affect Balance Scale (ABS) (Bradburn, 1969)

Philadelphia Geriatric Morale Scale (PGMS) (Lawton, 1972)

Reintegration to Normal Living (RNL) (Wood-Dauphinee, Opzoomer, Williams, Marchand, & Spitzer, 1988)

Instruments previously used with people with stroke

Sickness Impact Profile (SIP) (Bergner et al., 1981)

Ferrans and Powers Quality of Life Index—Stroke Version (Ferrans & Powers, 1985)

Reintegration to Normal Living (RNL) (Wood-Dauphinee et al., 1988)

Instruments previously used with people with aphasia

How I Feel About Myself—modification of the Ryff Psychological Well-being Scale (Thelander, Hoen, & Worsley, 1994)

Geriatric Evaluation of Relative's Rating Instrument (GERRI) (Schwartz, 1983)

Functional Life Scale (FLS) (Sarno, Sarno, & Levita, 1973)

Caregiver Burden Interview (Zarit, Reever, & Bach-Peterson, 1980)

Psychosocial Wellbeing Index (PWI) (Lyon et al., 1997)

Affect Balance Scale (ABS) (Bradburn, 1969)

Short Form 36 (SF-36) (Ware & Sherbourne, 1992)

FIGURE 6–1. Quality of life instruments. Reprinted with permission from Cruice, M., Worrall, L., and Hickson, L., (2000b). Quality-of-life measurement in speech pathology and audiology. *Asia Pacific Journal of Speech, Language and Hearing, 5*(1), 1–20.

Instruments previously used with people with laryngectomy, glossectomy, or oesophageal carcinoma

Short Form 36 (SF-36) (Ware & Sherbourne, 1992)

General Health Questionnaire (12 item version) (Goldberg & Hillier, 1979)

Psychosocial Adjustment to Illness Scale (PAIS) (Derogatis, 1986)

Performance Status Scale for Head and Neck Cancer Patients (PSS-HN) (List, Ritter-Sterr, & Lansky, 1990)

Functional Assessment of Cancer Therapy—General and Head and Neck (Cella et al., 1993)

Rotterdam Symptom Checklist (De Haes, van Knippenberg, & Neijt, 1990)

Voice Handicap Index (VHI) (Jacobson et al., 1997)

Instruments previously used with people with hearing impairment

Hearing Handicap Inventory for the Elderly (HHIE) (Ventry & Weinstein, 1982)

Short Portable Mental Status Questionnaire (Pfeiffer, 1975)

Geriatric Depression Scale (GDS) (Brink et al., 1982)

Self Evaluation of Life Function (SELF) (Linn & Linn, 1984)

Beck's Depression Inventory (Beck, Ward, Mendelson, Mock, & Erbaugh, 1961)

Mental Status Questionnaire (Kahn et al., 1960)

Life Satisfaction Index Z (Neugarten et al., 1961)

Short Form 36 (SF-36) (Ware & Sherbourne, 1992)

Instruments previously used with people with other audiological disabilities (cochlear implants, acoustic neuroma, otitis media)

Otitis Media-6 Survey (OM-6) (Rosenfeld, Goldsmith, Tetlus, & Balzano, 1997)

Performance Inventory for Profound Hearing Loss Answer Form (Owens & Raggio, 1988)

Center for Epidemiologic Studies—Depression Scale (CES-D) (National Institute of Mental Health, 1972) (cited in Radloff, 1977)

Quality of Well-Being Scale (QWB) (Anderson et al., 1989)

Patient Quality of Life Form (Wexler Miller, Berliner, & Crary, 1982)

Index Relative Questionnaire Form (Wexler et al., 1982)

FIGURE 6–1. Continued.

Health Profile (Hunt et al., 1981), the Euroqol (Euroqol Group, 1990), the General Health Questionnaire (Goldberg & Hillier, 1979), and the Dartmouth COOP Charts (Nelson et al., 1987). Two specific measures are reviewed in detail here. The SF-36 (Ware & Sherbourne, 1992) is a common tool and is used in many health settings. It has also been used to measure the health of large populations such as those of a state or a nation. The measure has a heavy emphasis on the physical domain and does not appear to capture the effects of a communication disability particularly well. However, because norms are available on many populations, it is a useful comparative tool. The other measure reviewed in this section is the COOP Charts. It was chosen because it has been found to be the most aphasia-friendly generic tool in a comparison study of quality of life measures for people with aphasia (Cruice, Hirsch, Worrall, Holland, & Hickson, 2000a).

SF-36 The Medical Outcome Study Short Form-36 (SF-36) is a general survey of health status (see Chapter 6 Appendix B). The SF-36 is a well-recognized, frequently used, and psychometrically sound measure of health status. An online literature search conducted in various health sciences databases produced a list of more than 1,400 published studies related to the SF-36. The assessment can be administered by telephone, by written questionnaire, or by interview. The results are analyzed in terms of a set of subscales rather than a total score. Hence, there are scores for eight subscales of physical functioning, role-physical, bodily pain, general health, vitality, social functioning, role-emotional, and mental health. Readers can measure their own health status by completing the SF-36 online at www.sf-36.com. There are shorter versions of the measure (SF-12 and SF-6), and norms are available for many populations on all versions.

There are, however, documented limitations to using this measure with older people. Brazier, Walters, Nicholl, and Kohler (1996) and Jenkinson, Wright, and Coulter (1994) reported that high levels of missing data often occur in older age groups. Concerns have emerged about the use of the SF-36 in the self-completion format by older people (Brazier et al., 1992; Dyer & Sinclair, 1998). Unsatisfactory response rates and a high number of missing or incompleted items have been found particularly problematic among older postal respondents (Hayes, Morris, & Wolfe, 1995; Mallinson, 1998). Researchers have also questioned the use of the SF-36 with specific groups, such as those with dementia, severe hearing or visual loss, stroke, or those who live in nursing homes (Hayes et al., 1995; Lyons, Perry, & Littlepage, 1994; O'Mahony, Rodgers, Thomson, Dobson, & James, 1998; Weinberger et al., 1991). Although telephone and postal survey collection methods are endorsed as being more cost-effective than direct interviews, and may be the only feasible method for large population surveys, it is still unclear how aging and its affiliated communication changes affect the quality of the responses obtained. The concern for audiologists and speech-language pathologists is that health care planning is often based on these large-scale surveys, and the needs of older people with communication difficulties may be overlooked through such measures.

COOP Charts The Dartmouth COOP Charts (Nelson et al., 1987) were originally developed as a quick and easy tool to measure patient's health status in physicians' offices. The charts consist of nine items and cover physical fitness, feelings, daily activities, social activities, pain, overall health, change in health, social support, and quality of life. The participants record their responses to each item on a vertical 5-point scale that has words, pictures, and numbers as categories of response. More information about the COOP project is available at www.dartmouth.edu/~coopproj/index.html.

In a study of the usability of a variety of quality of life measures for people with aphasia, Cruice et al. (2000a) found that the COOP Charts were rated the most usable standardized quality of life measure for people with aphasia. The measure received the highest rating for length (mean length 8–12 minutes), wording of instructions, understanding instructions, and overall appropriateness. The SF-36 and the Sickness Impact Profile (SIP; Bergner et al., 1981) received the lowest ratings and are not recommended for use with people with aphasia. A global rating of quality of life received a very high rating. In this simple measure, which can be used as a screening tool, participants were asked to rate their quality of life as *very poor, poor, average, good,* or *very good.*

DOMAIN-SPECIFIC MEASURES

As noted earlier, health-related quality of life can be divided into domains such as physical health, social health, emotional health, and mental health. Whereas generic multidimensional measures take some or all of these domains into account, another approach is to focus on the measurement of a single domain. The domain of social health is particularly relevant to speech-language pathologists and audiologists because of the ramifications of a communication disability on social factors. Effective communication is essential for socialization and maintaining social networks.

McDowell and Newell (1996) describe three different ways of defining social health: in terms of adjustment, social support, and the ability to perform normal roles in society. There are a number of scales that seek to measure aspects of social health, but none that encompass all aspects. The Rand Social Health Battery (Donald & Ware, 1982) was an attempt to measure social functioning, defined as "the ability to develop, maintain and nurture major social relationships" (Sherbourne, 1992, p. 173) (see Chapter 6 Appendix C). This measure, however, does not determine the level of support received from these relationships. The Medical Outcomes Study Social Support Survey (Sherbourne & Stewart, 1991) (see Chapter 6 Appendix D) was developed to fill this need. Rather than asking about the frequency of social activities as in the Rand Social Health Battery, this measure asks the person how often he or she receives support (e.g., from someone the person can confide in, or from someone to help with daily chores if the person is sick). While there are a number of scales of social health, none have been applied to a population with communication disability. More recently, another aspect of social health, social network analysis, has been gaining popularity.

FACTOR-SPECIFIC MEASURES

Social network analysis is a factor-specific level of the broader concept of social health. Social network analysis is a widely used method to describe the manner in which people are linked with others in their social environment. Antonucci and Akiyama (1987) devised a method based on face-to-face interviews in which the composition and size of an individual's social network may be described. Figure 6–2 provides an example. This social network method identifies each person with whom the individual comes into contact during the course of routine activities and classifies the contact by its importance (immediacy or closeness), frequency of contact, and the relationship between the people involved.

If a social network analysis is conducted with a client with a communication disability, what is the average social network size for older people? Several studies throughout the world have found that older people's social network size is between 7 and 10 people (Antonucci & Akiyama, 1987; Mugford & Kendig, 1987; Phillipson, Bernard, Phillips, & Ogg, 1998; Smith & Baltes, 1998). Mugford and Kendig (1987) developed a social network typology and investigated the influence of disability on network size and *multiplexity* (the number of different types of contacts). Networks were classified as *attenuated* (small numbers, few types), *intense* (small numbers, many types), *diffuse* (large numbers, few types), *complex* (large numbers, many types), or *balanced* (medium numbers, medium types). The authors report that the presence of a (nonspecified) disability was found to influence social network structure by modestly increasing the number of kin, especially more distant relatives, while decreasing the number of contacts with friends. The implications that this finding has for speech-language pathologists and audiologists are that there are likely to be a larger number of family members involved with older clients and that many clients may want to renew contact with friends.

Non-Health-Related Quality of Life or Well-Being Measures

Non-health-related quality of life measures typically assess psychological well-being and life satisfaction. Some indicators of well-being and life satisfaction are morale, affect, coping ability, and self-esteem. An example of such a measure is the Short-Form Ryff Scales of Psychological Well-Being (Ryff, 1989). This scale is an 84-item measure of well-being that incorporates the domains of self-acceptance, positive relations with others, autonomy, environmental mastery, purpose in life, and personal growth. Administration time with people with no communication disability is between 15 and 30 minutes.

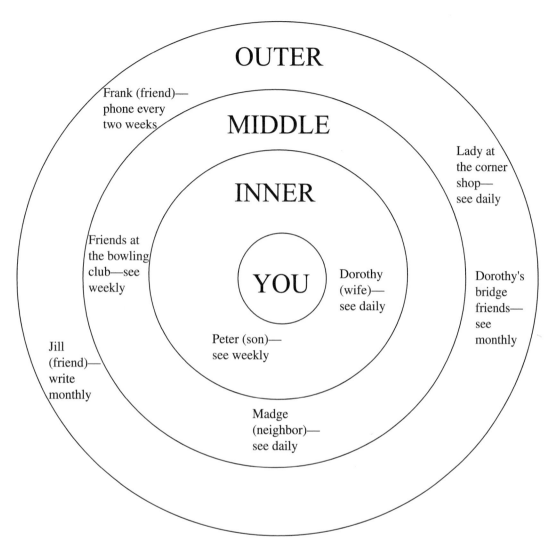

FIGURE 6–2. Example of a social network.

There is a shorter 24-item version devised for people with aphasia (Hoen, Thelander, & Worsely, 1997) (see Chapter 6 Appendix E) that was used to document change in a pretest/posttest evaluation of an aphasia program at the York-Durham Aphasia Center, Ontario, Canada. The 24 items for this version were chosen from the original 84 items by selecting the items that people with aphasia best understood. Although there is no available data on the psychometrics of this condensed scale, this scale is certainly suitable for people with a communication disability.

Communication-Related Quality of Life Measures

Communication-related quality of life measures include measures with a focus on the quality of life of people with specific communication impairments (e.g., Voice Handicap Index: Jacobson et al., 1997; Hearing Handicap Inventory for the Elderly: Ventry & Weinstein, 1982), or existing measures of quality of life that are suitable for people with communication disability (e.g., the COOP Charts: Nelson et al., 1987), or have been adapted for people with aphasia (e.g., Aachen Quality of Life Inventory: Engell, Huber, & Huetter, 1998), or measures that seek to encapsulate the effect of a communication disability on quality of life (e.g., the Quality of Communicative Life Scales: Paul-Brown, Frattali, Holland, Thomson, & Caperton, 2001). There are few quality of life measures with a specific focus on communication. Some of the measures potentially most useful for the assessment of older people's quality of life are described below.

QUALITY OF COMMUNICATIVE LIFE SCALES

The Quality of Communicative Life Scales (Paul-Brown et al, 2001) is still in development and at the time of publication was not available for purchase. However, a research edition has been demonstrated in conference presentations and has been available for field testing over the past few years. This measure was developed by ASHA and is seen as an extension to the work on the ASHA FACS (Frattali, Thompson, Holland, Wohl, & Ferketic, 1995). It has been specifically developed for people who have neurogenic communication disorders. The research edition of the measure contains 18 items such as *I like to talk with people, My role in the family is the same, I stay in touch with family and friends, I make my own decisions,* and *In general, my quality of life is good.* Each item is on a separate page, and the participant responds directly on the same page using a vertical visual analogue scale. The Quality of Communicative Life Scales has the potential to be a useful tool for many speech-language pathologists and audiologists.

VISUAL ANALOG SCALES FOR SELF-ESTEEM

The Visual Analog Scales for Self-Esteem (VASES; Brumfitt & Sheeran, 1999) is a simple 10-item measure of self-esteem designed for people with aphasia, but it could also be used with other populations. With only 10 items, the VASES is quick to administer, taking only 2 or 3 minutes. The examiner needs no special training, and the process of administering the measure is easy to understand. For example, examiners would be confident that most people with aphasia could understand the process of rating responses. There is also a balance of positive and negative concepts so that the focus is not entirely on negative self-esteem. Self-esteem is defined as "part of the self-concept that has to do with how the person evaluates their group memberships, physical attributes and typical thoughts and feelings" or "as the way people judge themselves in positive or negative terms" (Brumfitt & Sheeran, 1999, p. 2).

The VASES has one practice item and then 10 items. These include items relating to being understood, confident, cheerful, outgoing, mixed up, intelligent, angry, trapped, optimistic, and frustrated. The two anchors for the visual analogue scale for each item are illustrated (e.g., not confident plus/minus confident). The respondents are asked to choose one of the pictures that best represents them. They are then asked to look at a rating scale below the picture and grade the degree of their response (e.g., ++, +, or 0). Scores from 10 to 50 can then be calculated for the measure. The interpretation of the results is left to the clinician, with an argument being provided that normative data are not necessary and that any negative scores should be interpreted as indicative of low self-esteem. However, the authors do caution that very high positive scores can be indicative of lack of insight or defensiveness.

CODE MULLER PROTOCOL

The Code Muller Protocol (Muller, Code, & Mugford, 1983) is a well-established scale of psychosocial adjustment developed specifically for people with aphasia. It was designed to measure differences between levels of optimism between the speech-language pathologist and the significant other of the person with aphasia. Ten items (e.g., *Do you think the ability to work will . . .*) are rated on a 5-point scale from *get much worse* to *improve a lot*. Other items refer to getting more speech therapy, independence from others, ability to meet friends, cope with depression, follow interests and hobbies, speak to strangers, cope with frustration, make new personal relationships, and cope with embarrassment.

HEARING HANDICAP INVENTORY FOR THE ELDERLY

The HHIE (Ventry & Weinstein, 1982) was discussed in Chapter 5 because it includes a number of items concerning activity limitations relevant to older people with hearing impairment. In addition, the HHIE includes items about participation, for example, *Does a hearing problem cause you to visit friends, relatives, or neighbors less often than you would like?* This assessment measure has also been described as a health-related quality of life measure because it includes a number of items about the social and emotional impact of hearing impairment on the lives of older adults, for example, *Does a hearing problem cause you to feel depressed?* Other self-report hearing disability and handicap assessments include items about aspects of quality of life; however, the HHIE has the greatest number of items about quality of life and has been most widely used in audiology practice with older people.

Quality of Life of Older People

The measures just described have gone some way toward describing the concept of quality of life. In studies that examined quality of life in older people, what has been found? In contrast to agist assumptions that older people have a poor quality of life, Browne et al. (1994)

found that older people reported significantly higher levels of quality of life than younger people reported on The Schedule for the Evaluation of Individual Quality of Life (SEIQoL) (Browne et al., 1994). This report confirms the results of other studies that have found higher levels of life satisfaction, psychological well-being and subjective well-being in older people compared to their younger counterparts. Browne et al. suggested that the higher levels of quality of life reported by older people in the study is a result of the lack of sensitivity of traditional measures of quality of life to older people's concerns. The SEIQoL allowed older people to select their own domains and weight the importance of each one. Health was not a major domain of the older people in this study.

Farquhar (1995) conducted interviews about quality of life with 210 older participants from an urban and a rural region of England. Each participant was asked a series of questions.

- How would you describe the quality of your life? Why do you say that?
- What things give your life quality?
- What things take the quality away from your life?
- What would make the quality of your life better?
- What would make the quality of your life worse?

Responses were written verbatim and coded. Coded responses from the whole interview were categorized from very positive to very negative. Sixty-one percent described the quality of their lives positively, and the reasons provided included that, compared to others, they had a good quality of life, they had social contacts such as their families, they had their health, they had enough money, and they were still engaged in activities. Sixteen percent described their quality of life negatively. The reasons included helplessness, disability or ill health, unhappiness, old age and the desire to be young, reduced social contacts (often due to the death of friends or family members), and material circumstances. There were more people who described the quality of life negatively in the over-85-year age group and in the urban region compared to the rural region. When asked what gave their life quality, many mentioned family (children), activities, other social contacts, health and material circumstances, whereas reduced social contacts, ill health, and disability figured prominently in the responses about what takes quality away from their life. These themes were repeated throughout the interviews.

These interviews indicate that older people value social health as well as physical health. The importance of social contacts, especially with family, is a particular theme throughout the interviews. There is no mention of communication specifically; however, older people clearly value communication with family, friends, and others. The ability to communicate combined with the opportunity to communicate is implicit in the domain of social health. Opportunity, rather than ability to communicate, is viewed as the key feature of quality of life. However, what happens when the ability to communicate is also affected? How does this affect quality of life?

Quality of Life of Older People With a Communication Disability

Quality of life research in populations with communication disabilities is limited, and quality of life instruments are used infrequently in clinical practice (Hesketh & Hopcutt, 1997; Steering Committee of the Quality Improvement Study Section of ASHA Special Interest Division 11, 1996). There are two main reasons why quality of life is difficult to measure in people with communication disabilities. The first is that most measures use self-report, and this format causes difficulty for people with a communication disability, particularly those with a language impairment such as aphasia, or the cognitive-communication disorders associated with dementia or head injury. The second issue relates to the strong emphasis on the physical dimension in many health-related quality of life measures. Communication is rarely mentioned in quality of life definitions and often is not considered in measurement tools (e.g., SF-36, Chapter 6 Appendix B). Hence, many available measures fail to capture the effect that a communication disability has on quality of life. Nevertheless, interest in measuring quality of life in communicatively disordered populations is growing.

Studies of adult speech-language pathology populations that have included quality of life measurement include studies of head and neck surgical procedures for cancer of the larynx (Clements, Rassekh, Seikaly, Hokanson, & Calhoun, 1997; DeSanto, Olsen, Perry, Rohe, & Keith, 1995; Morton, 1997; Stewart, Chen, & Stach, 1998), oesophagus (O'Hanlon et al., 1995), and tongue (Ruhl, Gleich, & Gluckman, 1997), and studies of aphasia (Records & Baldwin, 1996; Sarno, 1997) and TBI (Webb, Wringley, Yoels, & Fine, 1995). Quality of life research into aphasia has been initiated under the labels of psychosocial well-being (Lyon et al., 1997) and life satisfaction (Hinckley, 1998). In audiology, there are studies that include quality of life measurement in age-related hearing loss (Bess, Lichtenstein, Logan, Burger, & Nelson, 1989; Magilvy, 1985; Morgan, Hickson, & Worrall, 2002; Mulrow et al., 1990; Stephens & Hétu, 1991), cochlear implants (Harris, Anderson, & Novak, 1995; Maillet, Tyler, & Jordan, 1995), otitis media (Rosenfeld et al., 1997), and acoustic neuroma (Parving, Tos, Thomsen, Moller, & Buchwald, 1992). The two communication disabilities that have been most investigated in terms of quality of life are people with aphasia and older people with hearing impairment. These are reviewed in more detail in the following sections.

Quality of Life in Aphasia

Le Dorze and Brassard (1995) interviewed 18 people with aphasia and their relatives and/or friends about their perceptions of the consequences of aphasia. A standardized assessment tool was not used. People with aphasia reported changes in

- communication situations (e.g., effort on communication, fatigue in keeping up the conversation, irritation with not finding the right word)
- interpersonal relationships (e.g., disruption of family relations, friction with spouse, loss of friends)
- loss of autonomy (e.g., loss of employment, physical dependency, reduced recreational activities)
- stigmatization (e.g., aphasia being associated with mental illness, dementia or drunkenness, change in self-image, embarrassment about speaking and walking).

  The family and friends reported changes in

- situations of communication (e.g., stress in realizing that what the person with aphasia says is not always what he or she thinks, irritation at not being able to guess what the person with aphasia means)
- interpersonal relationships (e.g., changed perception of person with aphasia, change in intimate relationships)
- heightened responsibilities (e.g., reading for the person with aphasia, worrying about the person with aphasia's health and safety)
- consequences arising from behavioral changes of the person with aphasia (e.g., difficulty in adapting to these changes, difficulty in accepting some of the person with aphasia's emotional reactions)
- restricted activities (e.g., giving up shared common leisure activities, abandoning plans for a vacation)
- stigmatization (e.g., uneasiness when others address the relative or friend instead of the person with aphasia).

Despite these negative consequences, people with aphasia rate the quality of their lives as *average* to *good* on a range of measures (Cruice et al., 2000a; Cruice, Worrall, & Hickson, 2000c). Proxies typically rate the quality of life of the person with aphasia as between *poor* and *average*, that is, one scale point lower (Cruice et al., 2000c). Healthy older people typically rate the quality of their lives as between *good* and *very good* (Cruice et al., 2000c).

La Pointe (1999) stressed that social isolation and exclusion have a particular impact on the quality of life of people with aphasia and their relatives. Sarno (1992, 1997) found that improved perception of quality of life was related to the intensity and length of reha-bilitation services during the first year. Hoen et al. (1997) found improved well-being for their clients who had attended group treatment programs at the York-Durham Aphasia Center. Both these studies suggest that inclusion through rehabilitation and aphasia centers is an important factor in improving the quality of lives of people with aphasia and their relatives.

Quality of Life of Older People With Hearing Impairment

Both disease-specific and generic health-related quality of life measures have been used to investigate the far-reaching effects of hearing impairment on the lives of older people and to investigate change in quality of life subsequent to aural rehabilitation (for a review, see Bess, 2000). Generic measures that have been used with the older population with hearing impairment are listed in Figure 6–1.

Bess et al. (1989) conducted a comprehensive study of 153 older people using the Sickness Impact Profile (SIP; Bergner et al., 1981), a 135-item health-related quality of life measure. Multivariate analysis was used to adjust for the following possible confounding variables: age, race, gender, education level, number of illnesses, presence of diabetes and ischemic heart disease, number of medications, near visual acuity, and mental status. A 10-dB increase in hearing impairment was found to result in a 2.8 increase in SIP scores on the physical scale and a 2.0 increase in scores on the psychosocial scale. Thus, hearing impair-ment was associated with higher SIP scores and increased dysfunction in the elderly. Bess et al. then went on to compare the mean SIP score of their subjects with hearing impair-ment with those of other published reports of SIP results. In comparison to the mean SIP score of 13.4 for subjects with hearing impairment, the mean for the unimpaired adult pop-ulation is 2–3; the mean for heart transplant recipients after one year is 9–10; and the mean for people with chronic obstructive airways disease is 24–25 (Hart & Evans, 1987; McSweeney, Grant, Heaton, Adams, & Timms, 1982). Thus, hearing impairment was associated with adverse quality of life changes somewhere between those experienced by heart transplant recipients and people with chronic obstructive airway disease.

Morgan et al. (2002) examined the relationship between the responses of older people with and without hearing impairment using the disease-specific HHIE (Ventry & Weinstein, 1982) and the generic health-related quality of life measure, the SF-36. A significant rela-tionship was found between hearing impairment and the mental health subscale of the SF-36. Significant relationships were also found between the HHIE and the mental health, bodily pain, and physical functioning subscales of the SF-36. These relationships existed inde-pendently of age. The significant relationship between hearing impairment and mental health confirms the results of other studies that have found an association between depression and hearing loss (Carabellese et al., 1993; Garland, 1978; Herbst & Humphrey, 1980; Jones, Victor,

& Vetter, 1984; Thara, 1993; Vesterager, Salomon, & Jagd, 1988). This study confirmed that disease-specific measures are more sensitive to hearing impairment in older people. On the other hand, the study showed the importance of assessing the broader field of quality of life. The impact of hearing loss on mental health is only shown when using generic quality of life measures, and the likely presence of mental health problems in older people with hearing impairment is an important implication for audiologists.

Some researchers have used generic quality of life measures to investigate the impact of hearing aid fitting on quality of life. Overall, the research in this area has shown that current health-related quality of life measures are not sufficiently sensitive to pick up changes to quality of life evident with the disease-specific measures (Bess, 2000). This is because such measures have an emphasis on physical health and do not contain many, or indeed any, items related to communication health. The development of a communication-sensitive generic quality of life measure should be a priority for future research.

This chapter has highlighted an emerging area of practice for gerontological audiology and speech-language pathology, the measurement of participation, and quality of life. Some of the key measures appropriate to older people with communication disabilities have been reviewed and are provided in the Appendixes. Asking older clients about their participation and quality of life will provide the clinician with the client's own perspective of what matters. It will, therefore, guide the overall direction of intervention and may serve to measure the outcome of intervention. It is for these reasons that it is becoming increasingly important to measure older people's participation and quality of life.

Interventions that target participation and quality of life issues are beginning to emerge in clinical practice and in the literature. In Chapter 3, interventions that focus on these dimensions were considered to be using a social approach. Some examples of social approaches to intervention used in the community, hospital, and residential care facility for the aged are described in Chapters 7, 8, and 9, respectively.

 KEY POINTS

- Participation is one of the dimensions of the WHO's International Classification of Functioning and Disability (2001).
- Participation is about an individual's involvement in life situations such as mobility and social relationships.

- Participation can be assessed through open-ended questions such as *What were you involved in two years ago? What are you doing now?*

- Asking about clients' involvement in a range of social activities is relevant to the participation of older people with a communication disability.

- Participation can also be assessed by interviewing significant others and by direct observation in the real world.

- Quality of life measurement is becoming increasingly prevalent in population surveys and in health care settings.

- Speech-language pathologists and audiologists do not routinely measure quality of life, although it is an emerging area of interest.

- Quality of life emanates from the unique perspective of each individual and is sometimes difficult to predict.

- There are three main types of quality of life measures relevant to speech-language pathology and audiology: health-related, non-health-related, and communication-related quality of life measures.

- There are several levels of health-related quality of life measures from the generic to the specific.

- There are many measures of quality of life that have been used with communicatively disabled populations, and these are listed in Figure 6–1.

- Measures such as the SF-36, COOP Charts, Rand Social Health Battery, Social Support Survey, social network analysis, Ryff Scales of Psychological Well-Being, Quality of Communicative Life, Visual Analog Scales for Self-Esteem, Code-Muller Protocols, and the Hearing Handicap Inventory for the Elderly are described, and many are provided in the Appendixes.

- Older people rate their quality of life significantly higher than younger people rate theirs.

- Social health (e.g., relationship with family) is an important consideration for older people when they describe the quality of their lives.

- People with aphasia continue to rate the quality of their life as *average* to *good*, compared to healthy older people who rate it between *good* and *very good*.

- Older people with hearing impairment have significantly poorer quality of life than healthy older people with normal hearing.

CLASS ACTIVITIES

1. Divide the students into pairs and have each student ask his or her partner these questions.
   - How would you describe the quality of your life? Why do you say that?
   - What things give your life quality?
   - What things take the quality away from your life?
   - What would make the quality of your life better?
   - What would make the quality of your life worse?

   Students should compare their answers and discuss the similarities and differences.

2. Ask students to measure their own health-related quality of life by logging on to www.sf-36.com and completing the SF-36 online. In class, students should compare their results with others and discuss the differences. Other discussion questions for the class are: What are the advantages and disadvantages of this tool? What problems might arise when assessing older people with communication difficulties using the SF-36?

3. Ask students to complete their own social network using Figure 6–2 as an example. They should then compare the network to the average networks for older people described in this chapter and discuss reasons why social networks may decrease with age.

RECOMMENDED READING

Bess, F. H. (2000). The role of generic health-related quality of life measures in establishing audiological rehabilitation outcomes. *Ear and Hearing, 21*(4), 74S–79S.

Cruice, M., Worrall, L., & Hickson, L. (2000a). Quality-of-life measurement in speech pathology and audiology. *Asia Pacific Journal of Speech, Language and Hearing, 5*(1), 1–20.

Cruice, M., Hirsch, F., Worrall, L., Holland, A., & Hickson, L. (2000b). Quality of life for people with aphasia: Performance on and usability of quality of life assessment. *Asia Pacific Journal of Speech, Language and Hearing, 5*, 85–91.

Frattali, C. M. (Ed.). (1998). Measuring modality-specific behaviors, functional abilities, and quality of life. In C. M. Frattali (Ed.), *Measuring outcomes in speech-language pathology* (pp. 55–88). New York: Thieme.

Hirsch, F. M., & Holland, A.L. (2000). Beyond activity: Measuring participation in society and quality of life. In L. E. Worrall & C. M. Frattali (Eds.), *Neurogenic communication disorders: A functional approach* (pp. 35–54). New York: Thieme.

McDowell, I., & Newell, C. (1996). *Measuring health: A guide to rating scales and questionnaires* (2nd ed.). New York: Oxford University Press.

Morgan, A., Hickson, L., & Worrall, L. (in press). Quality of life of older people with hearing impairment. *Asia Pacific Journal of Speech, Language and Hearing.*

Parr, S., Byng, S., & Gilpin, S. (1997). *Talking about aphasia*. Buckingham, UK: Open University Press.

Parr, S. P., & Byng, S. C. (2000). Perspectives and priorities: Accessing user views in functional communication assessment. In L. E. Worrall & C. M. Frattali (Eds.), *Neurogenic communication disorders: A functional approach* (pp. 55–66). New York: Thieme.

REFERENCES

Anderson, J. P., Kaplan, R. M., Berry, C. C., Bush, J. W., & Rumbaut, R. G. (1989). Interday reliability of function assessment for a health status measure: The quality of well being scale. *Medical Care, 27,* 1076–1083.

Antonucci, T. C., & Akiyama, H. (1987). Social networks in adult life and a preliminary examination of the Convoy Model. *Journal of Gerontology, 42,* 519–527.

Beck, A. T., Ward, C. H., Mendelson, M., Mock, J., & Erbaugh, J. (1961). An inventory for measuring depression. *Archives of General Psychiatry, 4,* 561–571.

Bergner, M., Bobbitt, R. A., Carter, W. B., & Gilson, B. S. (1981). The Sickness Impact Profile: Development and final revision of a health status measure. *Medical Care, 19,* 787–805.

Berkman, B., Chauncey, S., & Holmes, W. (1999). Standardized screening of elderly patients' needs for social work assessment in primary care: Use of the SF-36. *Health and Social Work, 24*(1), 9–16.

Bess, F. H. (2000). The role of generic health-related quality of life measures in establishing audiological rehabilitation outcomes. *Ear and Hearing, 21*(4), 74S–79S.

Bess, F. H., Lichtenstein, M. J., Logan, S. A., Burger, M. C., & Nelson, E. (1989). Hearing impairment as a determinant of function in the elderly. *Journal of the American Geriatric Society, 37,* 123–128.

Bowling, A., Farquhar, M., Grundy, E., & Formby, J. (1993). Changes in life satisfaction over a two and a half year period among very elderly people living in London. *Social Science and Medicine, 36*(5), 641–655.

Bradburn, N. M. (1969). *The structure of psychological well-being.* Chicago: Aldine.

Brazier, J. E., Harper, R., Jones, N. M., O'Cathain, A., Thomas, K. J., Usherwood, T., & Westlake, L. (1992). Validating the SF-36 health survey questionnaire: A new outcome measure for primary care. *British Medical Journal, 305*(6846), 160–164.

Brazier, J. E., Walters, S. J., Nicholl, J. P., & Kohler, B. (1996). Using the SF-36 and Euroqol on an elderly population. *Quality of Life Research, 5*(2), 195–204.

Brink, T. L., Yesavage, J. A., Lum, O., Heerseman, P. H., Adey, M., & Rose, T. L. (1982). Screening tests for geriatric depression. *Clinical Gerontologist, 1,* 37–43.

Browne, J., O'Boyle, C., McGee, H., Joyce, C., McDonald, N., O'Malley, K., & Hiltbrunner, B. (1994). Individual quality of life in the healthy elderly. *Quality of Life Research, 3,* 235–244.

Bruley, D. K. (1999). Beyond reliability and validity: Analysis of selected quality-of-life instruments for use in palliative care. *Journal of Palliative Medicine, 2*(3), 299–309.

Brumfitt, S., & Sheeran P. (1999). *Vases: Visual Analog Self-Esteem Scale.* Bicester, UK: Winslow Press.

Carabellese, C., Appollonio, I., Rozzini, R., Bianchetti, A., Frisoni, G., Frattola, L., & Trabucchi, M. (1993). Sensory impairment and quality of life in a community elderly population. *Journal of American Geriatrics Society, 4,* 401–407.

Cella, D. F., Tulsky, D. S., Gray, G., Sarafian, B., Linn, E., Bonomi, A., Silberman, M., Yellen, S. B., Winicour, P., Brannon, J., (1993). The Functional Assessment of Cancer Therapy Scale: Development and validation of the general measure. *Journal of Clinical Oncology, 11*(3), 570–579.

Clements, K. S., Rassekh, C. H., Seikaly, H., Hokanson, J., & Calhoun, K. (1997). Communication after laryngectomy. *Archives of Otolaryngological Head and Neck Surgery, 123,* 493–496.

Cummins, D. R. A. (1995, May). *The Comprehensive Quality of Life Scale: theory and development.* Paper presented at the Health Outcomes and Quality of Life Measurement Conference, Canberra, Australia.

Cruice, M. (2001) *Communication and quality of life in older adults with aphasia and healthy older adults.* Unpublished doctoral thesis, The University of Queensland, Brisbane Australia.

Cruice, M., Hirsch, F., Worrall, L., Holland, A., & Hickson, L. (2000a). Quality of life for people with aphasia: Performance on and usability of quality of life assessments. *Asia Pacific Journal of Speech, Language and Hearing, 5,* 85–91.

Cruice, M., Worrall, L., & Hickson, L. (2000b). Quality-of-life measurement in speech pathology and audiology. *Asia Pacific Journal of Speech, Language and Hearing, 5*(1), 1–20.

Cruice, M., Worrall, L., & Hickson, L. (2000c, May). The well-being and quality of life of older people with aphasia: What they and their significant others have to say. Paper presented at the Speech Pathology Australia National Conference, Adelaide.

De Haes, J. C. J. M., van Knippenberg, F. C. E., & Neijt, J. P. (1990). Measuring psychological and physical distress in cancer patients: Structure and application of the Rotterdam Symptom Checklist. *British Journal of Cancer, 62,* 1034–1038.

Derogatis, L. R. (1986). The Psychosocial Adjustment to Illness Scale (PAIS). *Journal of Psychosomatic Research, 30,* 77–91.

DeSanto, L. W., Olsen, K. D., Perry, W. C., Rohe, D. E., & Keith, R. L. (1995). Quality of life after surgical treatment of cancer of the larynx. *Annals of Otology, Rhinology and Laryngology, 104,* 763–769.

Donald, C. A., & Ware, J. E. (1982). *The quantification of social contacts and resources.* Santa Monica, CA: Rand Corporation.

Dyer, C., & Sinclair, A. (1998). The use of Short-Form (SF)-36 questionnaire for older adults. *Age and Ageing, 27*(6), 756.

Engell, B., Huber, W., & Huetter, B. O. (1998, August). *Quality of life measurement in aphasic patients.* Proceedings of the 24th International Association of Logopedics and Phoniatrics Congress, Amsterdam, Netherlands.

Farquhar, M. (1995). Elderly people's definitions of quality of life. *Social Science and Medicine, 41*(10), 1439–1446.

Ferrans, C., & Powers, M. (1985). Quality of life index: Development and psychometric properties. *Advances in Nursing Science, 8,* 15–24.

Frattali, C. M. (Ed). (1998). Measuring modality-specific behaviors, functional abilities, and quality of life. In C. M. Frattali (Ed.), *Measuring outcomes in speech-language pathology* (pp. 55–88). New York: Thieme.

Frattali, C. M., Thompson, C. M., Holland, A. L., Wohl, C. B., & Ferketic, M. M. (1995). *American Speech-Language-Hearing Association: Functional assessment of communication skills for adults (ASHA-FACS).* Rockville, MD: American Speech-Language-Hearing Association.

Garland, M. H. (1978). Problems in the elderly: Depression and dementia. *Hospital Update, 4,* 313–319.

Goldberg, D., & Hillier, V. (1979). A scaled version of the General Health Questionnaire. *Psychological Medicine, 9,* 139–145.

Harris, J. P., Anderson, J. P., & Novak, R. (1995). An outcomes study of cochlear implants in deaf patients. *Archives of Otolaryngological Head and Neck Surgery, 121,* 398–404.

Hart, L. G., & Evans, R. W. (1987). The functional status of ESRD patients as measured by the Sickness Impact Profile. *Journal of Chronic Diseases, 40,* 117s–130s.

Hayes, V., Morris, J., & Wolfe, C. (1995). The SF-36 health survey questionnaire: Is it suitable for use with older adults? *Age and Ageing, 24,* 120–125.

Herbst, K. G., & Humphrey, C. (1980). Hearing impairment and mental state in the elderly living at home. *British Medical Journal, 281,* 903–905.

Hesketh, A., & Hopcutt, B. (1997). Outcome measures for aphasia therapy: It's not what you do, it's the way that you measure it [special issue]. *European Journal of Disorders of Communication, 32,* 189–202.

Hickson, L., & Worrall, L. (2001). Older people with hearing impairment: Application of the new World Health Organization International Classification of Functioning and Disability. *Asia Pacific Journal of Speech, Language, and Hearing, 6,* 129–133.

Hinckley, J. (1998). Investigating the predictors of lifestyle satisfaction among younger adults with chronic aphasia. *Aphasiology, 12*(7/8), 509–518.

Hirsch, F. M., & Holland, A. L. (2000). Beyond activity: Measuring participation in society and quality of life. In L. E. Worrall & C. M. Frattali (Eds.), *Neurogenic communication disorders: A functional approach* (pp. 35–54). New York: Thieme.

Hoen, B., Thelander, M., & Worsely, J. (1997). Improvement in psychological well-being of people with aphasia and their families: Evaluation of a community-based program. *Aphasiology, 11*(7), 681–691.

Hunt, S. M., McKenna, S. P., McEwen, J., Williams, J., & Papp, E. (1981). The Nottingham Health Profile: Subjective health status and medical consultations. *Social Science and Medicine, 15a,* 221–229.

Jacobson, B., Johnson, A., Grywalski, C., Silbergleit, A., Jacobson, G., Benninger, M., & Newman, C. (1997). The Voice Handicap Index (VHI): Development and validation. *American Journal of Speech-Language Pathology, 6*(3), 66–70.

Jenkinson, C., Wright, L., & Coulter, A. (1994). Criterion validity and reliability of the SF-36 in a population sample. *Quality of Life Research, 3,* 7–12.

Jones, D. A., Victor, C. R., & Vetter, N. J. (1984). Hearing difficulty and its psychological implications for the elderly. *Journal of Epidemiology and Community Health, 38,* 75–78.

Kahn, R. L., Goldfarb, A. I., Pollock, M. & Gerber, I. E. (1960). Brief objective measure for the determination of mental status in the aged. *American Journal of Psychiatry, 117,* 326–328.

Labi, M., Phillips, T., & Gresham, G. (1980). Psychosocial disability in physically restored long-term stroke survivors. *Archives of Physical and Medical Rehabilitation, 61,* 561–565.

LaPointe, L. (1999). Quality of life with aphasia. *Seminars in Speech and Language, 20*(1), 5–17.

Lawton, M. P. (1972). The dimension of morale. In D. P. Kent, R. Kastenbaum, & S. Sherwood (Eds.), *Research planning and action for the elderly: The power and potential of social science* (pp. 144–165). New York: Behavioral Publications.

Le Dorze, G., & Brassard, C. (1995). A description of the consequences of aphasia on aphasic persons and their relatives and friends, based on the WHO model of chronic diseases. *Aphasiology, 9*(3), 239–255.

Linn, M. W., & Linn, B. S. (1984). Self-Evaluation of Life Function (SELF) Scale: A short comprehensive self-report of health for elderly adults. *Journal of Gerontology, 39,* 603–612.

List, M., Ritter-Sterr, C., & Lansky, S. B. (1990). A performance status for head and neck cancer patients. *Cancer, 66,* 564–569.

Lundh, U., & Nolan, M. (1996). Ageing and quality of life 1: Towards a better understanding. *British Journal of Nursing, 5*(20), 1248–1251.

Lyon, J. G., Cariski, D., Keisler, L., Rosenbek, J., Levine, R., Kumpala, J., Ryff, C., Coyne, S., & Blanc, M. (1997). Communication partners: Enhancing participation in life and communication for adults with aphasia in natural settings. *Aphasiology, 11*(7), 693–708.

Lyons, R., Perry, H., & Littlepage, B. (1994). Evidence for the validity of the Short Form 36 questionnaire (SF-36) in an elderly population. *Age and Aging, 23,* 182-184.

Magilvy, J. K. (1985). Quality of life in hearing-impaired older women. *Nursing Research, 34*(3), 140–144.

Maillet, C. J., Tyler, R. S., & Jordan, H. N. (1995). Change in the quality of life of adult cochlear implant patients. *Annals of Otology, Rhinology, and Laryngology,* Suppl. 165, 31–48.

Mallinson, S. (1998). The Short-Form 36 and older people: Some problems encountered when using postal administration. *Journal-of-Epidemiology-and-Community-Health, 52*(5), 324–328.

McSweeney, A., Grant, I., Heaton, R. K., Adams, K. M., & Timms, R. M. (1982). Life quality of patients with chronic obstructive pulmonary disease. *Archives of Internal Medicine, 142,* 473–478.

McCallum, J. (1995). The SF 36 in an Australian sample: Validating a new, generic health status measure. *Australian Journal of Public Health, 19*(2), 160–166.

McDowell, I., & Newell, C. (1996). *Measuring health: A guide to rating scales and questionnaires* (2nd ed.). New York: Oxford University Press.

McHorney, C. A., Kosinski, M., & Ware, J. E. (1994). Comparisons of the costs and quality of norms for the SF-36 Health Survey collected by mail versus telephone interview: Results from a national survey. *Medical Care, 32*(6), 551–567.

Morgan, A., Hickson, L., & Worrall, L. (2002). Quality of life of older people with hearing impairment. *Asia Pacific Journal of Speech, Language and Hearing, 7 (1), 39–53.*

Morton, R. P. (1997). Laryngeal cancer: Quality of life and cost effectiveness. *Head and Neck, 19,* 243–250.

Mugford, S., & Kendig, H. (1987). Social relations: Networks and ties. In H. L. Kendig (Ed.), *Aging and families: A social network perspective* (pp. 38–59). Sydney: Allen & Unwin.

Muller, D. J., Code, C., & Mugford, J. (1983). Predicting psychological adjustment to aphasia. *British Journal of Disorders of Communication, 18,* 23–29.

Mulrow, C. D., Aguilar, C., Endicott, J. E., Tuley, M. R., Velez, R., Charlip, W. S., Rhodes, M.C., Hill, J. A., & DeNino, L. A. (1990). Quality-of-life changes and hearing impairment: A randomized trial. *Annals of Internal Medicine, 113,* 188–194.

Nelson E., Wasson, J., Kirk, J., Keller, A., Clark, D., Dietrich, A., Stewart, A., & Zubkoff, M. (1987). Assessment of function in routine clinical practice: Description of the COOP Chart method and preliminary findings. *Journal of Chronic Diseases, 40*(1), 55S–63S.

Neugarten, B. L., Havighurst, R. J., & Tobin, S. S. (1961). The measurement of life satisfaction. *Journal of Gerontology, 16,* 134–143.

Niemi, M., Laaksonen, R., & Kotila, M. (1988). Quality of life 4 years after stroke. *Stroke, 19,* 1101–1107.

O'Hanlon, D. M., Harkin, M., Karat, D., Sergeant, T., Hayes, N., & Griffin, S. M. (1995). Quality of life assessment in patients undergoing treatment for esophageal carcinoma. *British Journal of Surgery, 82,* 1682–1685.

O'Mahony, P. G., Rodgers, H., Thomson, R. G., Dobson, R., & James, O. F. (1998). Is the SF-36 suitable for assessing health status of older stroke patients? *Age and Aging, 27,* 19–22.

Owens, E., & Raggio, M. (1988). Performance inventory for profound and severe hearing loss. *Journal of Speech and Hearing Disorders, 53,* 42–57.

Parr, S., Byng, S., & Gilpin, S. (1997). *Talking about aphasia.* Buckingham, UK: Open University Press.

Parr, S. P., & Byng, S. C. (2000). Perspectives and priorities: Accessing user views in functional communication assessment. In L. E. Worrall & C. M. Frattali (Eds.), *Neurogenic communication disorders: A functional approach* (pp. 55–66). New York: Thieme.

Parving, A., Tos, M., Thomsen, J., Moller, H., & Buchwald, C. (1992). Some aspects of life quality after surgery for acoustic neuroma. *Archives of Otolaryngological Head and Neck Surgery, 118,* 1061–1064.

Paul-Brown, D., Frattali, C. M., Holland, A. L., Thompson, C. K., & Caperton, C. J. (2001). *Quality of Communication Life Scale. Field test version.* Unpublished manuscript. Available from the American Speech-Language-Hearing Association, 10801 Rockville Pike, Rockville, MD 20852.

Pfeiffer, E. (1975). A short portable mental status questionnaire for the assessment of organic brain deficit in elderly patient. *Journal of American Geriatrics Society, 23,* 433–441.

Phillipson, C., Bernard, M., Phillips, J., & Ogg, J. (1998). The family and community life of older people: Household composition and social networks in three suburban areas. *Age and Aging, 18,* 259–288.

Radloff, L. S. (1977). The CES-D Scale: A self-report depression scale for research in the general population. *Applied Psychological Measurement, 1,* 385–401.

Records, N. L., & Baldwin, K. (1996, November). *A tool to measure "quality of life" of aphasic individuals.* Paper presented at the ASHA Annual Convention, Seattle, WA.

Reitzes, D., Mutran, E., & Verrill, L. (1995). Activities and self-esteem: Continuing the development of activity theory. *Research on Aging, 17*(3), 260–277.

Rosenfeld, R., Goldsmith, A. J., Tetlus, K., & Balzano, A. (1997). Quality of life for children with otitis media. *Archives of Otolaryngological Head and Neck Surgery, 123,* 1049–1054.

Ruhl, C. M., Gleich, L. L., & Gluckman, J. L. (1997). Survival, function and quality of life after total glossectomy. *The Laryngoscope, 107,* 1316–1321.

Ryff, C. D. (1989). Happiness is everything, or is it? Explorations on the meaning of psychological well-being. *Journal of Personality and Social Psychology, 57*(6), 1069–1081.

Sarno, M. (1992). Preliminary findings in a study of age, linguistic evolution, and quality of life in recovery from aphasia. *Scandinavian Journal of Rehabilitation Medicine Supplement, 26,* 43–59.

Sarno, M. (1997). Quality of life in aphasia in the first post-stroke year. *Aphasiology, 11*(7), 665–679.

Sarno, J. E., Sarno, M. T., & Levita, E. (1973). The functional life scale. *Archives of Physical Medicine and Rehabilitation, 54,* 214–220.

Schwartz, G. (1983). Development and validation of the Geriatric Evaluation by Relative's Rating Instrument (GERRI). *Psychological Reports, 53,* 479–488.

Seed, P., & Lloyd, G. (1997). *Quality of life.* London: Jessica Kingsley Publishers Ltd.

Sherbourne, C. D. (1992). Social functioning: Social activity limitations measure. In A. L. Stewart, & J. E. Ware Jr., (Eds.), *Measuring functioning and well-being: The Medical Outcomes Study approach* (pp. 173–181). Durham, NC: Duke University Press.

Sherbourne, C. D., & Stewart, A. L. (1991). The MOS Social Support Survey. *Social Science and Medicine, 32,* 705–714.

Simmons-Mackie, N., & Damico, J. (1996) Accounting for handicaps in aphasia: Communicative assessment from an authentic social perspective. *Disability and Rehabilitation, 18,* 540–549.

Smith, J., & Baltes, M. M. (1998). The role of gender in very old age: Profiles of functioning and everyday life patterns. *Psychology and Aging, 13,* 676–695.

Steering Committee of the Quality Improvement Study Section of ASHA Special Interest Division 11. (1996). Clinical use of Outcome Measures: Results of a survey. *ASHA Special Interest Division 11 Newsletter, 6*(3), 2–8.

Stephens, D., & Hétu, R. (1991). Impairment, disability and handicap in audiology: Towards a consensus. *Audiology, 30,* 185–200.

Stewart, M. G., Chen, A. Y., & Stach, C. B. (1998). Outcomes analysis of voice and quality of life in patients with laryngeal cancer. *Archives of Otolaryngology, Head and Neck Surgery, 124,* 143–148.

Thara, K. (1993) Depressive states and their correlates in elderly people in rural community. *Nippon-Koshu-Eisei-Zasshi, 40,* 85–94.

The Euroqol Group. (1990). Euroqol: A new facility for the measurement of health related quality of life. *Health Policy, 19,* 199–208.

Thelander, M. J., Hoen, B., & Worsley, J. (1994). *York-Durham Aphasia Center: Report on the evaluation of effectiveness of a community program for aphasic adults.* Ontario, Canada: York-Durham Aphasia Center.

Ventry, I., & Weinstein, B. E. (1982). The Hearing Handicap Inventory for the Elderly: A new tool. *Ear and Hearing, 3,* 128–134.

Vesterager, V., Salomon, G., & Jagd, M. (1988). Age related hearing difficulties: Psychological and sociological consequences of hearing problems. *Audiology, 27,* 179–192.

Ware, J., & Sherbourne, C. (1992). The MOS 36-Item Short Form Health Survey (SF-36). *Medical Care, 30,* 473–483.

Ware, J. E., Snow, K. K., Kosinski, M., & Gander, B. (1993). SF-36 health survey manual and interpretation guide. Boston: Nimrod Press.

Webb, C. R., Wrigley, M., Yoels, W., & Fine, P. R. (1995). Explaining quality of life for persons with traumatic brain injuries 2 years after injury. *Archives of Physical Medicine and Rehabilitation, 76,* 1113–1119.

Weinberger, M., Samsa, G. P., Hanlon, J. T., Schmader, K., Doyle, M. E., Cowper, P. A., Uttech, K. M., Cohen, H. J., & Feussner, J. R. (1991). An evaluation of a brief health status measure in elderly veterans. Journal of American Geriatrics Society, 39, 691–694.

Wexler, M., Miller, L. W., Berliner, K. I., & Crary, W. G. (1982). Psychological effects of cochlear implant: Patient and "index relative" perceptions. *Annals of Otology, Rhinology and Laryngology, 91*(Suppl.), 59–61.

Wood-Dauphinee, S. L., Opzoomer, A., Williams, J. I., Marchand, B., & Spitzer, W. O. (1988). Assessment of global function: The reintegration to normal living index. *Archives of Physical Medicine and Rehabilitation, 69,* 583–590.

World Health Organization Quality of Life Assessment Group. (1993). Study protocol for the World Health Organization project to develop a quality of life assessment instrument (WHOQOL). *Quality of Life Research, 2,* 153–159.

World Health Organization. (2001). *International classification of functioning, disability and health*. Geneva: Author.

Worrall, L. E., & Egan, J. (2001). A survey of outcome measures used by Australian speech pathologists. *Asia Pacific Journal of Speech, Language, and Hearing, 6*(3), 149–162.

Zarit, S. H., Reever, K. E., & Bach-Peterson, J. (1980). Relatives of the impaired elderly: Correlates of feeling of burden. *Gerontologist, 20,* 649–655.

Practice in Different Gerontological Settings

In the previous section, the nature and assessment of older people's communication and swallowing impairments, activity limitations and participation restrictions, and their overall effect on quality of life were described. In this section, the emphasis is on intervention. Continuing with the theme of the WHO's model (WHO, 2001) in which environmental factors are important, this section describes prevention and intervention strategies for older people in three different environments. Chapter 7 describes approaches appropriate for both healthy older people and older people with communication disability living in the community. Chapter 8 focuses on older people in the hospital environment, and Chapter 9 addresses the complex issue of audiology and speech-language pathology intervention for older people living in residential care facilities for the aged. Interventions are discussed using the WHO framework and there is an emphasis on enhancing activity, participation, and quality of life, rather than more traditional impairment-based treatments.

Chapter 7

The Community Environment

Despite agist stereotypes of older people living in nursing homes, the fact is that the vast majority of older people (>90%) live in the community. A major aim of health care programs and policies around the world is to ensure that older people continue to live independent lives in the community for as long as possible. Speech-language pathologists and audiologists have traditionally not been part of this healthy aging movement that focuses on prevention rather than traditional intervention. This chapter argues that students and clinicians need to be better prepared to face the challenge of preventing communication disability.

A communication education program, developed by the authors, which aims to maintain communication skills with age is described, and the results of evaluations of the program are presented. The chapter also discusses the role of audiologists and speech-language pathologists who provide a service to older people with known communication disability in the community. This service is known as home health care in North America, domiciliary care in the United Kingdom, and generically community health services in Australia. Group programs developed for people with hearing impairment and aphasia are described. Finally, options for individual intervention in the community are outlined.

The role of speech-language pathologists and audiologists with older people in the community is less well defined than their role in organizational settings such as hospitals and extended care facilities. The focus of this chapter is on working with community-based older people along the health-disease continuum, as discussed in Chapter 2. Audiologists and speech-language pathologists have a role with the following three groups of older people living in the community: (a) those who do not have a communication disability but who want to plan for the future and prevent disability from occurring, (b) those with unidentified communication disabilities that are posing a risk for the maintenance of their independence, and (c) those with known communication disabilities who need assistance to function in the community. Hence, communication professionals' roles with these client groups encompass both prevention and intervention.

Healthy Aging: Prevention of Communication Disability

Although working with healthy older people has not been a primary activity of audiologists and speech-language pathologists in the past, the indications are that this approach has great potential for improving the communication and, therefore, the quality of life of older people in the long term. Work in this area comes under the auspices of health promotion, which is defined by The Ottawa Charter for Health Promotion as a process for enabling people to increase control over and improve their own health (WHO, 1986). A great deal of emphasis has been placed by governments on health promotion for older people, but unfortunately programs have generally been limited to the maintenance and improvement of physical health. An exception to this is Canada Health's Communicating with Seniors (www.hc-sc.gc.ca/seniors-aines), an approach that takes a broad perspective on communication and contains information about age-friendly communication from a number of disciplines.

It is important that audiologists and speech-language pathologists become involved in health promotion and that they access some of the funding being allocated by governments for this purpose. In the United States, for example, the primary driving force in health promotion is Healthy People 2010 (www.health.gov/healthy people). ASHA defines the role of speech-language pathologists and audiologists in Healthy People 2010 on its website (www.professional.asha.org/resources/factsheets/2010_fact_sheet.cfm). As part of this Healthy People 2010 initiative, The Office of Disease Prevention and Health Promotion advertises funding opportunities on its website (http://odphp.osophs.dhhs.gov). In May, 2002, for example, community implementation microgrants were being advertised. Certainly, funding for health promotion activities may not be reimbursable through normal channels, but it appears there is an increasing amount of funding becoming available for these important activities.

The *Keep on Talking* Program

To promote the communication health of older people, the *Keep on Talking* program was developed (Hickson, Worrall, Yiu, & Barnett, 1996). A summary of the key features of this communication education program is contained in Figure 7–1. The program was developed by an interdisciplinary team of three speech-language pathologists, an audiologist, and an optometrist who worked in consultation with older people as well as their health providers. This section begins with a description of the development of the program. This description is included so that other clinicians can replicate the team's procedures and design a program specific to the needs of their local populations. A detailed description of *Keep on Talking* is then provided, followed by the results of the program evaluation (Worrall, Hickson, Barnett, & Yiu, 1998).

PROGRAM DEVELOPMENT

To plan an appropriate communication education program for older people, the project team needed to know what communication difficulties older people commonly experience in everyday life and what they want to learn more about. This approach is in line with the views of other researchers who consider it essential to consult with older consumers and their service providers for the appropriate planning of health promotion programs (e.g., Carson & Pichora-Fuller, 1997; Marginson, 1991). In the development phase, nine group

---

- Designed for healthy older people living in the community
- Developed in consultation with older people and health care workers (Hickson et al., 1996)
- Five weekly group sessions on different topics
- Each session lasts 2 hours
- Recommended group size is six to eight participants
- Participants may or may not have communication problems
- Groups are facilitated by a volunteer group leader
- A detailed manual is provided, with "script" and handout materials
- Each session is a mix of reflection, information, discussion, and planning for action

FIGURE 7–1. Features of the *Keep on Talking* program.

consultation meetings were held, consisting of seven groups of older people ($N = 36$) and two groups of health professionals ($N = 10$) who worked regularly with older people living in the community.

The technique employed for the consultation process is known as the Nominal Group Technique (NGT) and was described by Delbecq, Van de Ven, and Gustafson (1975) as a strategy for generating ideas and solving problems in planning situations. Standard survey techniques were considered to be too limiting and would not allow people to state their opinions in their own words. The NGT involves the generation of ideas by individual group members initially, followed by group discussion of ideas, and finally the independent rating of ideas by individual group members. This rating process results in a final set of prioritized ideas for the group. Because individual members are called upon to generate ideas, and then to rate the ideas independently, the NGT allows all group members to contribute without the risk of a few group members dominating the process.

The questions asked at each meeting and the NGT process are summarized in Figure 7–2. The most common oral communication problems reported by the older participants were hearing, memory, and word-finding difficulties. In terms of reading and writing, the most common problems cited were those to do with vision, motivation, and physical difficulties with writing. The results obtained for the health professional groups were similar for the written communication question but were quite different for the oral communication question. Although the health professionals agreed that hearing loss was a major difficulty, they also reported that lack of appropriate conversational skills (e.g., manner of questioning, inappropriate topics) and personality factors (e.g., attitude, egocentricity, denial) were major difficulties. The differences between responses obtained from older people and responses from health professionals who work with older people may have been because the health professionals spent most of their time working with older people in the community who needed support, that is, those with disability, rather than the healthy elderly. Differences may have also occurred because the health professionals were describing what they saw as general problems of the older population based on their professional experience, and their responses may reflect the agist perceptions of the population as a whole.

Because different responses were obtained from older people and from health professionals highlights the need for speech-language pathologists and audiologists to actively consult with their older clients when developing communication programs. Clinicians' views may be biased, and it is important not to assume what people need. As older people (and not health professionals) were the target group for the program, the final program development was based on the findings from the consultations with the older participants, rather than those obtained from health professionals.

Questions:

1. What problems do you have in talking, hearing, understanding, or just generally getting your message across?

2. What problems do you have in reading or writing?

3. We are devising an educational program about maintaining communication in old age. What would you like to see included?

Procedure:

1. Silent generation of ideas.

2. Presentation of an idea by each group member in turn and recording of each idea on a board in front of the group.

3. Discussion, clarification, and grouping of ideas.

4. Individual ranking of ideas. Each group member is given three post-it stickers with the numbers 1, 2, and 3 on them and asked to place the numbers next to his or her top three priority items in order. The results for all members are then collated, and the group's priorities are established.

FIGURE 7–2. Summary of the consultation process for development of the *Keep on Talking* program: Questions put to the groups and the Nominal Group Technique process.

The older participants identified a number of topics for inclusion in the final *Keep on Talking* program. The major topic areas, in order of priority, were

1. Motivational (i.e., how to maintain and improve communication skills, social networks, and self-confidence)
2. Conversational skills practice
3. Information about hearing loss, hearing aids, and services for those with hearing impairment
4. General education about communication.

THE PROGRAM

In line with the expressed desire of older people for the *Keep on Talking* program to be motivational, the program concentrated on challenging participants to consider what they would do if they experienced any communication difficulties in the future, or if they were having problems now, what they should do to maintain their communication skills. Thus, the aims of the program were to

1. Increase participants' understanding about communication changes that are likely to occur with age
2. Provide information (techniques and services) necessary to maintain or improve communication skills
3. Encourage participants to consider how best to go about improving or maintaining their communication skills.

The *Keep on Talking* program consisted of five group sessions (approximately 2 hours each) on the following topics:

1. Communication and well-being
2. Coping with hearing loss
3. Services for people with hearing loss
4. Maintaining literacy skills and memory
5. Summary and planning for the future

The program was led by a volunteer who had the experience of being a *Keep on Talking* group member and was, therefore, an older adult. The advantages of such volunteers are (a) that they generally have empathy with group members and can relate to the needs of the group, and (b) their involvement substantially reduces the costs of running the program.

The manual for the program included a script for the volunteer to follow, references to additional sources to assist the volunteer to learn about the topic, as well as handout materials to be photocopied for group members. Sessions contained a mixture of reflection, information, discussion, and planning for action. An example of a reflective activity, which was part of the first session on Communication and Well-Being, is shown in Chapter 7 Appendix A. Information was provided in each session about communication and about changes to communication. Participants were told that changes occur with age for both internal reasons (i.e., changes to the human body) and external reasons (i.e., lifestyle changes). An example of a handout providing information about reading and writing is shown in Chapter 7 Appendix B. Planning for action was an important component of each session, and participants were asked to respond to a number of "what if" questions. In the final session, these responses were summarized for future reference (see Chapter 7 Appendix C). In addition, in the final session, participants were asked to undertake an annual review of their social and communication activities (see Chapter 7 Appendix D). This review was designed to raise their awareness about possible changes to communication and to help generate possible solutions. Chapter 7 Appendix E contains an example of a completed review.

PROGRAM EVALUATION

Two hundred and fifty participants aged 56 to 93 years took part in the program evaluation. All participants were volunteers recruited by advertising in newspapers, in community newsletters, on notice boards at seniors' groups, and on television. The majority of the participants was female (70%), and all were community-based (i.e., not living in residential care): 79% lived in his or her own home, 16% lived in a retirement village, and the remainder lived in the homes of others. A controlled-comparison quasiexperimental research approach (Green & Kreuter, 1991) was used to evaluate the intervention. In this approach, a control group similar to the experimental group is used for comparison purposes. This control group does not receive the intervention. The research is quasiexperimental because participants are not randomly allocated to either a control or experimental group, as they would be in a strict experimental approach.

All 250 participants were initially assessed on a range of communication impairment, activity limitation, and participation restriction screening tasks. The impairment level tests were pure-tone audiometry, near and distance visual acuity tests, forward and backward digit span, and a confrontation naming test. Communication activity limitations were assessed through interview via self-report. Participation restrictions were evaluated by interviewing participants about their social networks and decision-making abilities. All participants were provided with the results of their assessment, and any questions about difficulties were discussed or necessary advice was given. For example, if a hearing impairment was found and the participant asked about possible treatment, he or she was given information about rehabilitation services. Articles by Cruice, Worrall, and Hickson (2000); Hickson et al. (1999); Hickson, Worrall, Barnett, and Yiu (1995); and Worrall, Yiu, Hickson, and Barnett (1995) contain details about the assessment results for all participants.

Following the initial assessment, participants were allocated to the experimental group ($n = 120$) if they were interested in attending the 5-week *Keep on Talking* program and were available at the session times. The control group consisted of 130 participants.

The program was evaluated in three ways, and a summary of the major findings of the study is contained in Table 7–1. First, the experimental group completed a questionnaire at the beginning and at the end of the *Keep on Talking* program. The questionnaire included 10 items that tested participants' knowledge base (e.g., *Hearing deteriorates with age, and I am aware of some strategies to maintain my communication skills into old age*) as well as five items that were attitudinal (e.g., *I believe hearing is an important part of communication*). Significant improvements were found for many of the knowledge-based items, with participants increasing their knowledge about communication changes with age and about strategies to maintain communication skills.

Second, participants who undertook the *Keep on Talking* program were asked for feedback about the program immediately after they had completed it. Participants were asked

TABLE 7-1

SUMMARY OF FINDINGS FROM THE *KEEP ON TALKING* PROGRAM EVALUATION

Comparison of pre- and postprogram questionnaires	Increased awareness of strategies to maintain communication skills, hearing, memory, and word recall into old age Increased knowledge about memory and word recall changes that can occur with age Increased awareness of the importance of eyesight to communication
Examples of participants' qualitative feedback postprogram	Gave me a better understanding of the problem and know where to go for help Learned about aging and strategies Very informative, gave insight into the future Discovered my contemporaries have similar problems My hearing problem is worse than I realized New ways of coping with my disabilities Lots of learning from others' experiences
Satisfaction ratings postprogram	51.9% very satisfied; 28.3% satisfied
Group comparison 1 year after initial assessment	45% of experimental group and 10% of control group had taken some action
Examples of actions taken by experimental group participants	Memorized numbers using association of ideas Applied for a hearing aid More involvement in local groups Reflected on my social interactions Have endeavored to keep my mind alert (e.g., crosswords) Ask husband to repeat/speak up Have been more conscious of needing to be more outgoing

to rate their level of satisfaction with the program and were asked for general qualitative impressions about the program. Overall, positive results were obtained (see Table 7–1).

The third means of program evaluation was an interview of both control and experimental participants 1 year after their initial communication assessment. A total of 117 participants were reviewed, and 45% of the experimental group compared to 10% of the control group reported taking some action in the past year as a result of their involvement with the study. Some examples of actions taken are presented in Table 7–1.

In summary, the program evaluation indicated that *Keep on Talking* was an enjoyable and valuable experience for healthy older people. The older participants developed strategies to maintain their communication skills and were motivated to take some action to maintain or improve their communication. This result is important because such preventative action may mean fewer older people experience communication disability in the long term. Audiologists and speech-language pathologists should become more involved in health promotion in the community and should promote strategies for enhancing communication and quality of life to policy makers and funding bodies. A volunteer-run program such as the one described here is one cost-effective way of doing this. The *Keep on Talking* program was developed in consultation with healthy older Australians living in an urban setting and as such may not meet the needs of healthy older people in other settings. The development, implementation, and evaluation of the program have been detailed so that others can use it as a template.

Other Group Programs for Healthy Older People

The focus of the *Keep on Talking* program is the maintenance of communication skills with age. Rose and Wotton (1992) pointed out that this is just one type of group that can be run for older people. They list a number of other group activities that could benefit older people (Table 7–2). It is hoped their ideas may be useful for audiologists and speech-language pathologists devising group programs for older people. Such ideas might be useful across a range of settings (e.g., community, clinics, extended care facilities), and may benefit healthy older people and people with known communication disability.

Of the groups listed in Table 7-2, those most applicable to healthy older people and the prevention of communication disability are social groups and groups that focus on strengths, in particular, reminiscence. A social group should not be seen merely as a venue to share a cup of tea or coffee. Such groups are extremely valuable for interaction. People listen, talk, laugh, meet new people, and can be motivated to maintain their communication. Similarly, reminiscence is an important communication activity. Bevan and Jeeawody (1998) define reminiscence as "a process involving people recollecting, reflecting on and recreating events, feelings, incidents, and happenings, either individually or collectively" (p.20). It has been found to be a significant factor in successful aging and in the enhancement of quality of life in older people.

TABLE 7–2

EXAMPLES OF GROUP ACTIVITIES FOR OLDER PEOPLE

Type of Group	Aims	Examples of Activities
Social	To decrease feelings of isolation To promote self-esteem To foster relationships between group members	Discuss members' interests, hobbies, and so forth Looking at the day's newspapers and discussing current events Celebrations such as birthdays, anniversaries
Assessment	To conduct a functional assessment of members' skills in particular areas by observing their performance in the group	Shopping Cooking
Skills teaching	Focus on particular skill development	Listening skills Appropriate use of eye contact Starting a conversation Taking turns in conversation
Focusing on strengths	To focus on the maintained skill of long-term memory To increase members' self-esteem and confidence	Reminiscence of members' past achievements Discussion of old photographs, newspapers Listening to music from the past
Psychotherapy groups	To allow members to express their feeling of loss To provide support to group members	Discussion of loss and grief Drawing lines on papers marking significant life events
Reality orientation	To allow members to keep in touch with the world	Discuss newspapers and current events Discuss familiar objects Discuss photographs of location

Note: Adapted from Rose and Wotton (1992).

Intervention for Older People With Communication Disability Living in the Community

Intervention for people with communication disability living in the community may take the form of group sessions, individual sessions, or a combination of the two. A number of group programs have been devised for older people with hearing impairment and for those with aphasia, and some examples of these are described in this section. Group or individual sessions may take place in the clinic situation or in the community (e.g., in a person's home, in a center for older people), and the agent of intervention may be a speech-language pathologist, an audiologist, or a volunteer.

Group Programs

OUTREACH TO OLDER PEOPLE WHO ARE HARD OF HEARING

Many older people with hearing impairment living in the community access conventional clinic-based audiological services. It is well known, however, that there are many who do not. Hickson et al. (1999) found that 57% of a sample of 240 community-based older people had some degree of hearing impairment; however, only 15% of the sample reported that they owned or used hearing aids. Some of the reasons why older people are not accessing audiological services are that they are concerned about the cost of hearing aids, their cosmetic appearance, the comfort of wearing hearing aids, hearing annoying noises, and the hearing aid calling attention to their disability (Franks & Beckman, 1985; Kricos, Lesner, & Sandridge, 1991).

Hoek, Paccioretti, Pichora-Fuller, McDonald, and Shyng (1997) describe a two-tiered program, Outreach to Hard-of-Hearing Seniors, for community-based older people with hearing impairment who were unable or unwilling to access traditional clinic-based services. The program was developed as a community partnership between older people's groups, a health center, and a university. Most important, "it was the seniors who were responsible for creating the partnership involving groups that had not previously collaborated in this fashion" (Hoek et al., 1997, p. 199). Level 1 of the program consisted of education and hearing screening and was designed for older people living independently in the community who attended community centers or lived in designated housing for older people. Level 2 consisted of education, hearing screening, diagnostic assessment, and rehabilitation, and was designed for older people who attended adult day care centers or lived in personal care housing. This type of housing means that people live in their own apartments, but come together for some activities and for meals in a central dining area. Nursing support is available if requested.

Steps in running the Level 1 service are shown in Table 7–3. The services are provided by audiometric technicians under the supervision of audiologists. This service is an excellent example of a program aimed at raising healthy older people's awareness about hearing impairment, its effects on everyday life, and possible intervention options. The program is user-friendly because it is conducted in the community setting, in a familiar environment for the older people. Another important feature of the program is the use of the Hearing Handicap Inventory for the Elderly—Screening Version (Ventry & Weinstein, 1983) as the primary tool on which recommendations are based. This focuses the intervention on the everyday activity limitations and participation restrictions important to the clients. Of the 141 older people assessed in the Level 1 service, 34% were referred to a physician, 28% to a hearing aid dispenser, and 27% to an audiologist. No further action was indicated for only 23% of the sample. Thus, many of these older people needed help and were willing to accept referral for further assistance, but they had not accessed conventional clinic-based audiological services.

The Level 2 program is similar to Level 1, with the major differences being that the program had more audiological input and that staff education was included. Increased audiological input was provided by audiologists being available on-site for consultation, rather than being accessed by referral as they were in the Level 1 program. In terms of staff education, the audiologists provided inservices to nurses who worked at the day care centers or personal care housing centers. Topics covered in staff education were communication strategies, hearing aid use, room acoustics, and assistive listening devices. Of the 122 older people seen in the Level 2 service, 44% were seen by the on-site audiologist, 25% were referred to a physician, 10% to a hearing aid dispenser, 13% to an audiologist, and 17% required no further action.

In summary, community programs such as those described by Hoek et al. (1997) can be employed to reach older people with hearing impairment who are not seen at traditional audiology clinics. Many of the clients seen in such programs are describing communication difficulties and require assistance to maintain their communication abilities. Perhaps they do not knock at the audiology clinic door because they are not aware that a hearing impairment is the source of their communication problems, or perhaps it is just too daunting to arrange the appointment. Whatever the reason, the needs of these older people are not being met by existing services, and audiologists should be innovative and broaden services to meet the needs of the community-based population.

HEARING AID ORIENTATION

Another type of group program that has been devised for older people who have accessed traditional audiological services and obtained a hearing aid is the Hearing Aid

TABLE 7-3

OUTLINE OF LEVEL 1, OUTREACH FOR OLDER PEOPLE WHO ARE HARD-OF-HEARING.

Preparation: Site visit to community center or housing complex	Program explained to staff Advertising posters displayed Determine best locations for group and individual sessions
Education: Group presentation on hearing	A talk on hearing loss, communication strategies, hearing aids, and assistive listening devices Group size limited to 10 Assistive listening devices provided to older people who need them to hear the talk
Individual consultations provided on request	Further discussion of material covered in the talk Any questions related to individual concerns are answered Written material provided on various topics that the individual is interested in (e.g., assistive listening devices, tinnitus) Some hearing aids and assistive listening devices are displayed Otoscopic examination Brief case history about ear pain, discharge, tinnitus, dizziness, onset of loss Administration of the HHIE-S (Ventry & Weinstein, 1983) Pure-tone air conduction screening provided if requested by client or if the client cannot be assessed with the HHIE-S (e.g., non-English speaker)
Individual recommendation if indicated after consultation	Referral to a physician *if* cerumen blocking, ear pain, discharge, continuous or annoying tinnitus, unexplained dizziness, or sudden hearing loss Referral to hearing aid dispenser *if* client has a hearing aid that is broken, HHIE-S score > 12 *and* has hearing aid, needs batteries for hearing aid, or needs new mold Referral to audiologist *if* HHIE-S score > 1 *and* wants help, HHIE-S score unreliable *and* failed pure-tone screening, unusual findings, hearing aid is broken and dispenser is unknown Referral for telephone or television device *if* client only has trouble with telephone or television No further action *if* client has no desire for further consultation or help, HHIE-S score < 10 with hearing aids, HHIE-S score unreliable but passed pure-tone screening

Note: Adapted from Hoek et al. (1997).

Orientation program (e.g., Lesner, 1995). These programs generally consist of four or five didactic sessions that focus on education about hearing, hearing aids, and hearing in difficult listening situations. In terms of the WHO model (2001), such programs focus on the level of body (impairment), rather than on the everyday effects of the impairment. Although somewhat limited in scope, the programs can be very useful for clients who are struggling to manage with the new technology they have obtained. A number of audiologists have pointed out that such programs can also be beneficial to the clinician because there will be fewer hearing aid returns, fewer follow-up visits to the audiologist, and happier and more loyal customers (Madell & Montano, 2000; Ross, 1997).

COMMUNICATION PROGRAMS FOR PEOPLE WITH HEARING IMPAIRMENT

A number of audiologists have advocated that rehabilitation programs must extend beyond hearing aids and should focus on the effects of hearing impairment on communication in everyday life (e.g., Beynon, Thornton, & Poole, 1997; Montgomery & Houston, 2000). Thus, in WHO terminology, the aim of such programs is to decrease the activity limitations and participation restrictions associated with hearing impairment. In this section, some examples of communication courses designed for people fitted with hearing aids and for people with hearing impairment (with and without hearing aids) are described. Common features of these programs are that they are for small groups (up to 10 participants), that significant others are included, that each session lasts for approximately 2 hours, and that the sessions are run by audiologists. Lesner (1995) provides excellent practical guidelines for clinicians running such group programs for older adults.

Beynon et al. (1997) described a 4-week communication course for first-time hearing aid users, which covers the following topics:

1. Anatomy and physiology of the ear, the nature of hearing impairment, and the effects of hearing impairment in different situations.
2. Benefits and disadvantages of hearing aids, hearing aid maintenance, adjusting the hearing aid in different listening environments, the nature of speech, the effects of hearing impairment on speech perception, and elements of lip-reading.
3. Coping strategies for better communication and solutions to communication problems.
4. Lip-reading, hearing tactics, stress and anxiety associated with communication, and use of relaxation techniques.

Beynon et al. evaluated the efficacy of this communication course by comparing pre- and postrehabilitation scores on the Quantified Denver Scale of Communication Function (Schow & Nerbonne, 1980) for a control group ($n = 27$), who received hearing aid fitting only, and an experimental group ($n = 26$), who received hearing aid fitting and the communication course. The average age for both groups of participants was 68 years. The experimental group showed a significantly greater improvement in communication than the control group.

Another example is the 6-session course described by Montgomery and Houston (2000), which is presented in Chapter 7 Appendix F. This program includes didactic information, discussion, problem solving, written handout material, and homework between sessions. Although Montgomery and Houston do not present any quantitative evidence to support their program, they do list a number of benefits for their group members:

- improving speech-reading and auditory-visual speech recognition
- sharing of feelings with the group
- receiving support from the group
- gaining perspective on their situation
- meeting role models for effective communication
- admitting their hearing problems in the safe group
- practicing strategies in the group situation that they can apply in the real world
- having regular contact with an audiologist in the early days of adjusting to hearing aids.

The programs described thus far are designed for people with hearing impairment who have been fitted with hearing aids. However, as stated earlier, there are many older people with hearing impairment who choose not to use hearing aids and not to access conventional rehabilitation services that focus on hearing aids. In view of this, the authors developed, in collaboration with another colleague (Christopher Lind), a communication program for older people with hearing impairment that is appropriate whether or not the participants are hearing aid users. This program is called *Active Communication Education.*

The program consists of a series of modules about everyday communication activities that have been found to be problematic for older people with hearing impairment, for example, using the telephone, listening to television, going to a restaurant, and conversing at the dinner table. The particular modules undertaken by each group depend on the communication needs identified in the first session by the group members (see Chapter 7 Appendix G). In this way, the program is less prescriptive than previous communication courses in that the content varies depending on the communication difficulties described by the participants. Within each module, there is a detailed discussion of the communication activity itself, the sources of difficulty in the activity, possible solutions, and practical exercises. In the period between each session, participants are encouraged to use the newly learned strategies in their daily communication. An example module on the topic of conversation in noise is shown in Chapter 7 Appendix H.

Another difference between the *Active Communication Education* program and other communication courses for people with hearing impairment is that the focus is firmly on communication activity limitations and participation restrictions, and issues of impairment rarely arise. Participants have been responsive to this approach and are happy to discuss their everyday communication difficulties rather than hearing loss or hearing aid use. Of course, such issues are not ignored if they come up in group discussion. The *Active Communication Education* program represents a social model approach to intervention as discussed in Chapter 3. The major features of this approach are that the client's difficulties are not viewed in isolation, but are considered in the context of the society in which he or she lives, and that decision making is shared between client and clinician. It is envisaged that the benefits of the *Active Communication Education* program will not only be measurable as improvement in communication but also as improvement in quality of life. Program evaluation is to be undertaken within the next few years.

CONSUMER GROUPS FOR PEOPLE WITH HEARING IMPAIRMENT

In addition to the group programs described thus far that are, in the main, run by audiologists, there are numerous programs offered by consumer groups for people with hearing impairment. Examples of such consumer groups are the Canadian Hard of Hearing Association (http://www.chha.ca), Better Hearing Australia (www.betterhearing.org.au), Hearing Concern in the United Kingdom (www.hearingconcern.com), and Self Help for Hard of Hearing People (www.shhh.org) and the League for the Hard of Hearing (www.lhh.org) in the United States. The services offered by these groups vary depending on resources, but typically they provide information, counseling, and peer support to people with hearing impairment either individually or in a group format. They are also important in terms of advocacy for the needs of the group members. It is essential that audiologists are aware of the consumer organizations in their area and work collaboratively with them so that duplication of programs does not occur and so that optimal services can be developed. Consumer groups are aware of the needs and concerns of their members and can relay this important information to the health professional. Likewise, the audiologist can inform the consumer groups about new issues in rehabilitation that would be of interest to the members.

APHASIA GROUPS AND CENTERS

In the public arena, aphasia is not a well-known disorder (Code, Simmons-Mackie, Armstrong, & Armstrong, 2000). It is for this reason that people with aphasia and their families respond well to meeting other people and families with aphasia. They can share common concerns, learn from each other's successes and disappointments, and join forces to advocate for better services for people with aphasia. The benefits of group therapy for people with aphasia are well articulated in texts such as those by Elman (1999) and Marshall (1999). Roger Ross, a person with aphasia, stated that he did not feel that he began to recover until he joined a group (Holland & Ross, 1999). He maintains that joining a group can be the most important action a stroke survivor can take. In the same article, Audrey Holland, an aphasiologist with immense experience with people with aphasia, states that she once thought that individual therapy should be supplemented by group therapy, but now maintains that group therapy should be the main intervention in chronic aphasia; individual therapy should be an adjunct (Holland & Ross, 1999).

The concept of aphasia centers has taken the notion of group therapy an extra step. Support organizations for people with hearing impairment, such as those described previously, have been established for many years. Aphasia centers, on the other hand, are a relatively new concept. At present, there are approximately five aphasia centers operating worldwide. There are also several university-based aphasia programs with similar aims at The University of Arizona and The University of Queensland, for example; however, these programs operate differently from the independent aphasia centers. The first and best known is The Aphasia Institute in North York, Ontario, Canada (www.aphasia.on.ca/index.shtml; Kagan & Cohen-Schneider, 1999; Kagan & Gailey, 1993). This center, which is one of several throughout Canada, was founded by Pat Arato in 1979 as a self-help group for seven people with aphasia.

Each week over 100 people with aphasia and their families come to the center in Toronto. Some come just once, whereas others attend on multiple occasions. They come for a range of activities. For example, there is a 12-week introductory course that uses Supported Conversation (Kagan, 1998) to discuss aphasia and its consequences with participants, some of whom are discovering what aphasia is all about for the first time. Volunteers, who meet regularly with the speech-language pathologists and social workers at the center, facilitate the introductory course. People with aphasia and their families may then attend conversational groups or various classes, such as art therapy or public speaking. The professional staff conduct home assessments to establish the applicants' suitability for the Aphasia Institute. The center has a base level of funding from the Provincial Ministry of Health but relies on bequests, grants, membership fees, charitable donations, and fundraising events to provide other services that are considered essential to the success of the program.

Connect is an aphasia center recently established in London in the United Kingdom (www.ukconnect.org/). Funded by a large charitable donation, Connect is situated on the south bank of the Thames River in London. While the eventual aims are to expand the service to a range of communication disabilities, and to establish a regional network of such centers throughout the United Kingdom, the first step is to consolidate the operation of Connect in London. The Connect project grew out of the City University's aphasia groups.

The Aphasia Center of California is funded by program fees, in-kind services, individual and organizational contributions, and grants (http://www.employees.org/~accadmin/). This aphasia center began in 1996 and is housed within a center for older people in Oakland, California. The program includes communication treatment groups, reading and writing groups, individual speech-language pathology sessions, and a caregiver's group. Speech-language pathologists facilitate all these groups. There are also recreational classes (fitness/relaxation and art classes) facilitated by adult education instructors.

Although these aphasia centers have some differences, the commonalities are

- a focus on enabling people to live well with chronic aphasia (i.e., a social model approach)
- an independent existence outside institutions such as universities or hospitals
- a predominantly charitable funding base
- a collaboration between consumers and speech-language pathologists.

DEVELOPING A COMMUNITY GROUP

Community organizations for older people with communication disabilities provide a valuable service to older people, their families, and the community at large. How can audiologists and speech-language pathologists provide a similar level of service to people with chronic communication disability in their local community when such an organization is not available? Establishing smaller groups for people with specific communication disabilities (e.g., aphasia, hearing impairment, dysarthria) is a good starting point. The steps in beginning a group program for people with communication disability in the community are

1. Determine whether there are other community-based groups in the area for people with similar communication disabilities and find out whether there is a need for another group.
2. Seek approval from the organization to establish the group, if needed.
3. Recruit four to six people with similar communication disabilities to the group. Include the families, caregivers, and friends if possible.
4. Conduct an NGT (see Figure 7–2) with the group to determine what they want to get out of the group sessions. The lead question that might be asked is "What would you like to achieve by attending this group?"
5. The WHO model could be used to classify individual goals into body, activity, or participation levels. For example, goals might be to communicate with families better (activity level), to return to work (participation level), or to just speak better

(impairment level). The final set of goals may need to be negotiated with the group. These goals will direct the content of therapy in the group.

6. Take baseline measures. Outcome measures such as Goal Attainment Scaling; the Therapy Outcome Measures (Enderby & Johns, 1997); the Client Oriented Scale of Improvement (Dillon, James, & Ginis, 1997); or specific measures at the body, activity, or participation levels could be used to measure success in the goals before and after the group program (see Frattali, 1999; Hesketh & Sage, 1999; Worrall, 2000; Worrall & Egan, 2001, for more details on these measures).

7. Work on the specific goals of the group as a whole and also on the specific goals of individuals within the group. This work can be done through practice, practice, practice or through discussion and compensation. For example, if the spouses in the group whose partners are aphasic feel they cannot leave their partner because of safety issues, then practicing tasks like getting help in an emergency are excellent group activities. Hopper and Holland (1998) provided details and evaluation on this type of situation-specific therapy. A common goal of the group may be to answer the telephone effectively. One member of the group may have found an answering machine a useful way around this problem. The machine screens the messages and then the person with a communication disability can call back if and when he or she chooses. Other members of the group may decide to try this easy solution.

8. Gather resources, act as a consultant, facilitate the group, and learn from the group about what all participants want. Use this knowledge to develop another group. Share the knowledge and resources with professional colleagues so that others can begin to learn about the power of groups for people with communication disabilities.

Individual Programs

In many situations, group programs are not available or clients do not want to participate in them; therefore, speech-language pathologists and audiologists need to provide individual programs to assist older people with a known communication disability to function in the community. What are the roles of the clinician in such individual programs?

In community settings, the health professional is not confined to the medical model described in Chapter 3. The rehabilitation and social models are more relevant to community settings because the focus is on integration with the community and everyday life goals. This section, therefore, describes two programs, one that is based on a rehabilitation model and another based on a rehabilitation-social model. Both are designed for people with aphasia, but the principles are directly transferable to any communication disability.

INTERVENTION BASED ON THE REHABILITATION MODEL

The rehabilitation model has a focus on activity level communication. It does not use a shared decision-making approach but instead uses an approach where the clinician seeks the input of the client, but ultimately the decision rests with the clinician (see Chapter 3). Older people are sometimes more comfortable with the clinician making the final decision because this way has been their experience of health care over the years. The following section describes an intervention program for aphasia that focuses on activity level communication.

The *Speaking Out* program described by Worrall and Yiu (2000) consists of 10 modules that address some everyday communication activities with which people with aphasia struggle. These include using the telephone, buying a gift, repairing communication breakdowns, and financial management. The *Speaking Out* program used some adult learning principles. Each module begins with a trigger. This trigger may simply be a discussion of how aphasia has affected a person's ability in a topic such as managing finances. This is followed by some aphasia-friendly information (with written handouts), and then the participant sets some goals and practices them throughout the intervening week. The 10-week program emphasizes that the person with aphasia and his or her family take primary responsibility for finding solutions to problems. There is also an emphasis on creating awareness that there are potential solutions or helpful strategies in overcoming some of the person's everyday communicative problems. In the evaluation of the program (Worrall & Yiu, 2000), a trained volunteer was used to implement the program in the person's home; however, the program could also be administered by a speech-language pathologist. In addition, in the evaluation, two groups of participants received the program at different times.

The program had variable and complex effects across all three WHO dimensions and was more effective with some participants than others. Overall there was significant improvement on the impairment measure (the WAB; Kertesz, 1982), and improvements for some participants on the activity level measure (the ASHA FACS; Frattali, Thompson, Holland, Wohl, & Ferketic, 1995) and on the health-related quality of life measure (the Short Form-36 health survey; Ware & Sherbourne, 1992). It was concluded that long-standing speakers who were aphasic might benefit from a 10-week functional communication therapy program delivered by trained volunteers.

In summary, the *Speaking Out* program is a good example of an intervention program that targets the activity level of the WHO model. It seeks the input of the client because the client can choose which modules are relevant; however, there is a fixed menu of intervention options.

INTERVENTION BASED ON THE REHABILITATION-SOCIAL MODEL

The Functional Communication Therapy Planner (FCTP: Worrall, 1995, 1999, 2000) describes a step-by-step process for establishing, treating, and evaluating intervention goals with individuals who have communication disability. The everyday communication activities targeted in the intervention are those undertaken by people living in their homes in the community. The FCTP can, therefore, be used for readying people for discharge to the community from a hospital or providing relevant functional therapy for people with communication disability who have returned to their homes. In the next section, the application of the FCTP to older people who are receiving services from a speech-language pathologist or an audiologist is described.

Step 1: Collaborative Goal Setting Autonomy, or the right of self-determination, is a key concept in intervention for older adults. Sometimes clinicians assume clients want independence. In fact, they want to be free to make their own decisions about how to function in the community (Jordan & Kaiser, 1996; Marks, 1997). The decision may be to function independently or the decision may be to be dependent on others. Of course, the needs and wishes of the significant others should be taken into account. For example, a person with a severe hearing impairment or aphasia may be perfectly happy not using the telephone, and the person's spouse may be happy to make and accept calls on the partner's behalf. On the other hand, the person with communication disability may want to use the telephone and may resent someone taking over. Thus, it is essential that the communication needs of the client are individually determined.

The principles of shared decision making (Coulter, 1997) are used in this goal-setting process. This approach means that the therapist does not make the decisions for the client, nor does the therapist assume that he or she knows what is best for the client. Additionally, the client does not dictate the type of service that will be provided. It is a negotiation between equal partners in the interaction about what the goals of therapy should be. The FCTP uses a structured interview to determine the everyday communicative needs that are important to the client (see Chapter 7 Appendix I for an example of some of the everyday communicative activities discussed in the interview).

Step 2: Preservice Evaluation Before intervention begins, the performance of the client in his or her specific goals is assessed. For example, if a client wants to purchase tickets for a football match as a surprise for his or her family, the clinician may ask the client to attempt a simulation of this task. In the Functional Communication Therapy Planner, performance is rated on a 7-point multidimensional rating scale of communicative effectiveness. It rates parameters of adequacy, independence, efficiency, and appropriateness of the communication attempts. Another way to establish a baseline is through the use of Goal Attainment Scaling (GAS) (see Worrall, 2000). In this system, the client and the clinician determine what would be an achievable level of performance for a particular goal, as well as establishing outcomes that would be better than expected and poorer than expected. For example, a realistic outcome for the football match scenario may be that the client can telephone the ticket outlet and give credit card details if a friend or the therapist writes out the script beforehand and waits in the background while the transaction is taking place. A better-than-expected outcome may be that the client is now able to complete the transaction alone, modifying the generic script, and feeling confident enough to make the call without a friend providing backup. The negotiated outcomes are given numerical values (e.g., $+2, +1, 0, -1, -2$) and these then form the basis of a quantifiable measure of outcome.

Step 3: Service Provision Actual service provision will depend on the goals set by the client and the clinician. When working with people in the community, it is most likely that the clinician's role will be somewhat different from the traditional clinical role. For example, it is more likely the clinician will act as a consultant, advising clients about community support services available to them. The importance of this role cannot be underestimated. In a social model approach, the clinician often helps the client to find the resources he or she needs. The audiologist or speech-language pathologist may also become involved in advocacy for their clients in the community. For example, it may be necessary for an audiologist to approach a local club about purchasing a loop system for the auditorium. Another important aspect of working with older people with communication disability in the community is the use of the strength's perspective (Saleeby, 1997), an approach where the therapist focuses on the client's strengths and uses these to achieve goals. Examples of this approach include using strong family ties to enhance the communication between the individual with communication disability and the family, or using the artistic talents of an individual to help the individual deal with the grief of losing language, speech, or hearing abilities.

Step 4: Postservice Evaluation It is important to review progress and outcomes regularly and to change clients' goals during the course of providing service. The goals of clients with chronic disabilities change as the course of the disability progresses. For example, the goals of clients immediately after a hearing aid fitting are likely to concern management of the hearing aid. Goals may change as hearing aid management is mastered and are more likely to focus on maximizing communication in specific situations. In aphasia, the goals of clients change as they adjust to the idea of living with aphasia for some time. Goal changing occurs with many chronic disabilities.

In addition to providing an effective consumer-oriented service by monitoring goals, it is important to review and measure outcomes from the perspective of increasing accountability within a health system. Modern health systems must account for where the money is spent. Health care payers and consumers are, therefore, rightly asking for evidence that worthwhile outcomes are achieved. It is, therefore, important that audiologists and speech-language pathologists measure the effect of their interventions and convey this information in a meaningful way to their employers and to their clients. For further information on how increased accountability is affecting speech-language pathologists, see Frattali (1999). In the Functional

Communication Therapy Planner, outcomes are measured simply by repeating the baseline measure. The Goal Attainment Scaling process described earlier can also be used.

Similarly, outcomes measurement is important in audiology, and audiologists have begun to use an approach that is similar to, but not quite the same as, the FCTP described previously. The approach involves the use of the Client Oriented Scale of Improvement (COSI: Dillon et al., 1997). With the COSI, rehabilitation begins with the client and audiologist collaboratively setting goals. These goals become the focus of subsequent rehabilitation. Unlike the FCTP, there is no preservice evaluation and no determination of expected outcomes. There is, however, measurement of outcome, with the client asked to rate his or her final ability and degree of change for each goal at the end of rehabilitation.

CASE STUDIES OF COMMUNITY-BASED INTERVENTIONS

Two case studies are provided that demonstrate effective community-based services. One of the cases has aphasia and the other has a hearing impairment.

This chapter has described numerous communication intervention programs for older people who are living in the community. With such a large proportion of healthy or "at-risk"

Case Study: Mr. Pollock

Mr. Pollock developed aphasia following a stroke six months ago. He has been discharged from therapy at the hospital and has sought the help of the speech-language pathologist at the local community health center. The speech-language pathologist interviewed Mr. Pollock and his wife about what they wanted from speech therapy. They talked about the social isolation they were feeling now that many of their friends no longer visited. They also described the difficulties they were having getting access to services in the community and finding a new purpose in life despite the presence of aphasia. Mr. Pollock also expressed frustration about not being able to use money anymore or to pay the bills. His wife is also afraid of leaving him alone because he cannot use the telephone.

To reduce their social isolation and address some of the other goals, the speech-language pathologist refers Mr. Pollock and his wife to an aphasia group at the local university. To tackle Mr. Pollock's frustration with finances and the need for Mr. Pollock to use the telephone, the *Speaking Out* program would also be appropriate. Through the volunteer network at the local health center, the speech-language pathologist seeks a volunteer for Mr. Pollock and trains him or her on the use of the *Speaking Out* program. The speech-language pathologist monitors Mr. Pollock's progress on the program. Mr. and Mrs. Pollock, therefore, are receiving the services that they require, with the speech-language pathologist acting primarily as a consultant.

Case Study: Mrs. Moore

Mrs. Moore has a moderate bilateral sensorineural hearing loss and has worn in-the-ear hearing aids for 18 months. She was initially satisfied with the hearing aids and happy with her improved ability to communicate with her family and to hear the television, which were her original goals on the COSI (Dillon et al., 1997). Mrs. Moore returns to the audiology clinic to complain about the performance of the hearing aids. In her consultation with the audiologist, it becomes clear that the hearing aids are working well, that they are providing appropriate amplification, and that their performance has not changed since she first obtained them. Mrs. Moore's hearing impairment has not changed. What has happened is that she has started to notice other communication difficulties that she would like to do something about. She has joined a group of older people in her area and the group arranges a number of outings (e.g., bus trips, walking tours) and activities (e.g., guest speakers, discussion sessions, musical mornings). Mrs. Moore has found it difficult to join in a number of these activities and has become embarrassed about her hearing problems. The first goal that Mrs. Moore and her clinician decide to address is that of Mrs. Moore's difficulties with guest speakers. A number of possible strategies are discussed, and it is agreed that (a) Mrs. Moore will position herself closer to the guest speakers, (b) Mrs. Moore will confide in her closest friend at the group that she is having difficulties and ask her friend to help her by writing notes during the talk, (c) Mrs. Moore will contact the local support organization for people with hearing impairment and inquire about speech reading classes they offer, and (d) the audiologist will contact the group's convener and find out about the acoustics in the group meeting room and if a loop system or other group amplification is available. A follow-up appointment is arranged at which the outcomes of the intervention will be evaluated and Mrs. Moore's other goals addressed.

older people living in the community, a preventative or health promotion approach is appropriate. For those older people with a known communication disability who are receiving home health care services, a range of communication interventions that focus on functioning in the community have been described. If aged care services continue to place emphasis on community-based interventions, speech-language pathologists and audiologists need to expand their services into this important domain.

 KEY POINTS

- Speech-language pathologists and audiologists have both prevention and intervention roles with older people living in the community.
- Group programs are particularly appropriate and useful for community-based work.

- *Keep on Talking* is a group education program designed to maintain and improve the communication skills of community-based older people. It consists of five weekly 2-hour sessions run by volunteers.

- The Nominal Group Technique (NGT) was used for consultation with key stakeholders in the development of the *Keep on Talking* program. It is a useful technique for identifying and prioritizing goals when working with older people.

- The program evaluation of *Keep on Talking* showed that older people learned strategies to maintain their communication and were motivated to take some action to maintain or improve their communication.

- There are a number of group programs designed for older people living in the community with the specific communication disabilities of hearing impairment and aphasia. For people with hearing impairment, there are outreach programs, hearing aid orientation courses, communication programs, and consumer support programs. For people with aphasia, a number of specialized aphasia centers have been developed.

- The rehabilitation and social models of practice are more relevant to community settings than the medical model.

- The *Speaking Out* program is an individual program designed for people with aphasia living in the community. The focus of the program is on activity-level communication.

- The steps in the *Functional Communication Therapy Planner* can be applied to individual service provision for older people with communication disability living in the community. The steps are collaborative goal setting, determination of expected outcomes, service provision, and postservice evaluation of outcomes.

CLASS ACTIVITIES

1. Divide the class into small groups of five to six students. Each group has been asked to run a *Keep on Talking* program in their local community. Develop an implementation plan that answers these questions: How and where will the program be run? How will it be advertised? What marketing is necessary? How will participants be recruited to attend?

2. The *Keep on Talking* program is one way that audiologists and speech-language pathologists can become involved in health promotion for older people. Use the Nominal Group Technique with the class to develop a prioritized list of other health

promotion activities that speech-language pathologists and audiologists could undertake for older people.

3. Interview a client about what he or she wants from your intervention (either speech-language pathology or audiology). Did the client say what you thought he or she would say? Do you think the client should have a say in what services are provided? As a class, talk about your beliefs about the shared decision-making model.

4. What resources are available for older clients in your area? How do you access this information?

RECOMMENDED READING

Beynon, G. J., Thornton, F. L., & Poole, C. (1997). A randomized, controlled trial of the efficacy of a communication course for first time hearing aid users. *British Journal of Audiology, 31,* 345–351.

Hickson, L., Worrall, L., Yiu, E., & Barnett, H. (1996). Planning a communication education program for older people. *Educational Gerontology, 22,* 257–269.

Hoek, D., Paccioretti, D., Pichora-Fuller, K., McDonald, M., & Shyng, G. (1997). Outreach to hard-of-hearing seniors. *Journal of Speech-Language Pathology and Audiology, 21*(3), 199–208.

Montgomery, A. A., & Houston, K. T. (2000). The hearing-impaired adult: Management of communication deficits and tinnitus. In J. G. Alpiner & P. A. McCarthy (Eds.), *Rehabilitative audiology: Children and adults,* (3rd ed.), (pp. 377–401). Baltimore: Lippincott Williams & Wilkins.

Worrall, L. E. (1999). *Functional communication therapy planner.* Oxon, UK: Winslow Press.

Worrall, L., Hickson, L., Barnett, H., & Yiu, E. (1998). An evaluation of the Keep on Talking program for maintaining communication skills into old age. *Educational Gerontology, 22,* 257–269.

REFERENCES

Bevan, C., & Jeeawody, B. (1998). *Successful aging: Perspectives on health and social construction.* Sydney: Mosby.

Beynon, G. J., Thornton, F. L., & Poole, C. (1997). A randomized, controlled trial of the efficacy of a communication course for first time hearing aid users. *British Journal of Audiology, 31,* 345–351.

Carson, A. J., & Pichora-Fuller, M. K. (1997). Health promotion and audiology: The community-clinic link. *Journal of Academy of Rehabilitative Audiology, 30,* 29–51.

Code, C., Simmons-Mackie, N., Armstrong, J., & Armstrong, E. (2000, August). *Public awareness of aphasia.* Paper presented at the 9th International Aphasia Rehabilitation Conference, Rotterdam, The Netherlands.

Coulter, A. (1997). Partnerships with patients: The pros and cons of shared decision-making. *Journal of Health Services Research and Policy, 2,* 112–121.

Cruice, M. N., Worrall, L. E., & Hickson, L. M. H. (2000). Boston Naming Test results for healthy older Australians: A longitudinal and cross-sectional study. *Aphasiology, 14* (2), 143–155.

Delbecq, A. L., Van de Ven, A. H., & Gustafson, D. H. (1975). *Group techniques for program planning.* Glenview, IL: Scott, Foresman.

Dillon, H., James, A., & Ginis, J. (1997). Client Oriented Scale of Improvement (COSI) and its relationship to several other measures of benefit and satisfaction provided by hearing aids. *Journal of the American Academy of Audiology, 8*(1), 27–43.

Elman, R. (Ed.). (1999). *Group treatment of neurogenic communication disorders: The expert clinician's approach.* Boston: Butterworth-Heinman.

Enderby, P., & Johns, A. (1997). *Therapy outcome measures (speech and language therapy).* Clifton Park, NY: Delmar Learning.

Erber, N. (1996). *Communication therapy for adults with sensory loss.* Melbourne: Clavis Publishing.

Franks, J. R. & Beckman, N. J. (1985). Rejection of hearing aids: Attitudes of a geriatric sample. *Ear & Hearing, 6*(3), 161–166.

Frattali, C. M. (1999). *Measuring outcomes in speech-language pathology.* New York: Thieme.

Frattali, C. M., Thompson, C. M., Holland, A. L., Wohl, C. B., & Ferketic, M. M. (1995). *ASHA Functional Assessment of Communication Skills for Adults (FACS).* Rockville, MD: American Speech-Language-Hearing Association.

Green, L. W., & Kreuter, M. W. (1991). *Health promotion planning: An educational and environmental approach.* Toronto: Mayfield Publishing Company.

Hesketh, A., & Sage, K. (1999). For better for worse: Outcome measurement in speech and language therapy. *Advances in Speech-Language Pathology, 1*(1), 37–45.

Hickson, L., Worrall, L., Barnett, H., & Yiu, E. (1995). The relationship between communication skills, social networks and decision-making strategies: An exploratory study. *Australian Journal on Ageing, 14,* 89–94.

Hickson, L., Lind, C., Worrall, L., Lovie-Kitchin, J., Yiu, E., & Barnett, H. (1999). Hearing and vision in healthy older Australians: Objective and self-report measures. *Advances in Speech Language Pathology, 1*(2), 95–105.

Hickson, L., Worrall, L., Yiu, E., & Barnett, H. (1996). Planning a communication education program for older people. *Educational Gerontology, 22*, 257–269.

Hoek, D., Paccioretti, D., Pichora-Fuller, K., McDonald, M., & Shyng, G. (1997). Outreach to hard-of-hearing seniors. *Journal of Speech-Language Pathology and Audiology, 21*(3), 199–208.

Holland, A. L., & Ross, R. (1999). The power of aphasia groups. In R. Elman (Ed.), *Group treatment of neurogenic communication disorders: The expert clinician's approach* (pp. 15–17). Boston: Butterworth-Heinman.

Hopper, T., & Holland, A. (1998). Situation-specific training for adults with aphasia: An example. *Aphasiology, 12*, 933–944.

Jordan, L., & Kaiser, W. (1996). *Aphasia: A social approach.* London: Chapman & Hall.

Kagan, A. (1998). Supported conversation for adults with aphasia: Methods and resources for training conversation partners. *Aphasiology, 12*(9), 816–830.

Kagan, A., & Cohen-Schneider, R. (1999). Groups in the "Introductory Program" at the Pat Arato Aphasia Center. In R. J. Elman (Ed.), *Group treatment of neurogenic communication disorders: The expert clinician's approach* (pp. 97–106). Boston: Butterworth-Heinemann.

Kagan, A., & Gailey, G. F. (1993). Functional is not enough: Training conversation partners for aphasic adults. In A. L. Holland & M. M. Forbes (Eds.), *Aphasia treatment: World perspectives* (pp. 199–225). Clifton Park, NY: Delmar Learning.

Kaplan, H., Garretson, C., & Bally, S. J. (1995). *Speechreading: A way to improve understanding* (2nd ed.). Washington, DC: Gallaudet University Press.

Kertesz, A. (1982). *Western Aphasia Battery.* New York: Grune & Stratton.

Kricos, P. B., Lesner, S. A., & Sandridge, S. A. (1991). Expectations of older adults regarding the use of hearing aids. *Journal of the American Academy of Audiology, 2*, 129–133.

Lesner, S. A. (1995). Group hearing care for older adults. In P. B. Kricos & S. A. Lesner (Eds.), *Hearing care for the older adult: Audiologic rehabilitation* (pp. 203–225). Boston: Butterworth-Heinemann.

Madell, J. R., & Montano, J. (2000). Audiologic rehabilitation in different employment settings. In J. G. Alpiner & P. A. McCarthy (Eds.), *Rehabilitative audiology: Children and adults* (3rd ed., pp. 60–79). Baltimore: Lippincott Williams & Wilkins.

Marginson, B. (1991). Needs of older people: Do education programs meet the challenge? *Australian Journal on Aging, 10*(2), 8–11.

Marks, D. (1997). Models of disability. *Disability and Rehabilitation, 193*, 85–91.

Marshall, R. C. (1999). *Introduction to group treatment for aphasia: Design and management.* Boston: Butterworth-Heinemann.

Montgomery, A. A., & Houston, K. T. (2000). The hearing-impaired adult: Management of communication deficits and tinnitus. In J. G. Alpiner & P. A. McCarthy (Eds.),

Rehabilitative audiology: Children and adults (3rd ed., pp. 377–401). Baltimore: Lippincott Williams & Wilkins.

Rose, G., & Wotton, G. (1992). Group work with the elderly. In M. Fawcus (Ed.), *Group encounters in speech and language therapy* (pp. 125–140). Kibworth, UK: Far Communications.

Ross, M. (1997). A retrospective look at the future of aural rehabilitation. *Journal of the Academy of Rehabilitative Audiology, 30,* 11–28.

Saleeby, D. (Ed.). (1997). *The strengths perspective in social work practice* (2nd ed.). New York: Longman.

Schow, R. L., & Nerbonne, M. A. (1980). Hearing handicap and Denver scales: Applications, categories and interpretation. *Journal of the Academy of Rehabilitative Audiology, 13,* 66–77.

Ventry, I. M., & Weinstein, B. E. (1982). The Hearing Handicap Inventory for the Elderly: A new tool. *Ear & Hearing, 3,* 128–134.

Ventry, I. M., & Weinstein, B. E. (1983). Identification of elderly people with hearing problems. *American Speech, Language, and Hearing Association, 25*(7), 37–42.

Ware, J. E., & Sherbourne, C. D. (1992). The MOS 36-item Short-Form Health Survey (SF-36). I. Conceptual framework and item selection. *Medical Care, 30,* 473–483.

Wilson, J., Hickson, L., & Worrall, L. (1998). Use of communication strategies by adults with hearing impairment. *Asia Pacific Journal of Speech, Language and Hearing, 3,* 29–41.

World Health Organization. (1986). *Targets for health for all.* Geneva: World Health Organization Regional Office for Europe.

World Health Organization. (2001). *International classification of functioning and disability.* Geneva: Author.

Worrall, L. E. (1995). The functional communication perspective. In D. Muller & C. Code (Eds.), *Treatment of aphasia* (pp. 47–69). London: Whurr Publishers.

Worrall, L. E. (1999). *Functional communication therapy planner.* Oxon, UK: Winslow Press.

Worrall, L. E. (2000). The influence of professional values on the functional communication approach in aphasia. In L. E. Worrall & C. M. Frattali (Eds.), *Neurogenic communication disorders: A functional approach* (pp. 191–205). New York: Thieme.

Worrall, L. E., & Egan, J. (2001). A survey of outcome measures used by Australian speech pathologists. *Asia Pacific Journal of Speech, Language, and Hearing, 6*(3), 149–162.

Worrall, L., Hickson, L., Barnett, H., & Yiu, E. (1998). An evaluation of the Keep on Talking program for maintaining communication skills into old age. *Educational Gerontology, 24*(2), 129–140.

Worrall, L., & Yiu, E. (2000). Effectiveness of functional communication therapy by volunteers for people with aphasia following stroke. *Aphasiology, 14*(9), 911–924.

Worrall, L. E., Yiu, E. M-L., Hickson, L. M. H., & Barnett, H. (1995). Normative data for the Boston Naming Test for Australian Elderly. *Aphasiology, 9*(6), 541–551.

Chapter 8

The Hospital Setting

This chapter describes interventions suitable for older people who are patients in a hospital. Speech-language pathology and audiology services provided to this population generally take a more medical model approach than services in the community or in the residential care environment. However, with the increasing emphasis on consumer-focused care and measurable functional outcomes, it is argued that a rehabilitation and social model approach is also needed. This approach is necessary in both the inpatient and outpatient hospital settings.

This chapter begins with a case study of an older person with a communication disability in a hospital. The case study serves to illustrate the importance of the context of hospital care. A description of the hospital communicative environment follows. The process of speech-language pathology in acute stroke is described, and the role of the hospital audiologist is also discussed. Some of the issues associated with acute care are highlighted, and a summary of outpatient services is provided.

Older people are disproportionate consumers of health care. In the United States, they account for 38% of all discharges from short-stay non-federal hospitals, even though they constitute 13% of the population (National Center for Health Statistics, 1999). They also stay in the hospital for longer periods of time (6.5 days compared to 5.2 days). Hence, speech-language pathologists and audiologists who work in medical settings such as hospitals are likely to encounter many older people in their caseloads.

It is currently estimated that in the United States 19% of the overall speech-language pathology caseload and 33% of the overall audiology caseload are older people (Shadden & Toner, 1997). By 2050, these numbers are expected to increase to 39% and 59%, respectively. What special considerations are needed for older people in hospital settings? What are the features of these environments that are problematical for older people? How can speech, language, and hearing interventions be sensitive to the needs of older people in modern-day health care settings?

This chapter focuses on the hospital setting but is equally valid for other medical centers such as rehabilitation units, community health centers, and clinics. Within the continuum of health care, definitions vary worldwide about the nature of acute, subacute, outpatient, and rehabilitation services. As it is almost impossible to define these concepts within each country, let alone across the many countries of the world, this chapter will use a simple dichotomy of inpatient and outpatient services. *Inpatient* refers to those who are in the hospital full time, and *outpatient* refers to those who have been discharged, yet still return to the hospital to participate in intervention.

Hospitals, rehabilitation units, community health centers, and clinics are common working environments for audiologists and speech-language pathologists. These settings are where many interventions for voice, speech, language, swallowing, and hearing impairment occur. What else can be said in this chapter that has not been written about in other standard texts on aphasia treatment or treatment of motor speech, voice, swallowing, or hearing disorders? First, this text has a focus on aging; hence, this chapter specifically focuses on older people with these disorders. Second, this text has a focus on prevention to intervention, and within this chapter a new approach to prevention of communication disability in hospitals is described that is based on the social model of accessibility. Finally, Chapter 2 described the principles on which this text is based: the health-disease continuum, the WHO model, healthy aging construct, and Communication Accommodation Theory. These principles suggest approaches to rehabilitation that are different from the more medical model approach described in some audiology and speech-language pathology texts. To illustrate the reason for this different perspective, the chapter begins with a description of a typical case of an older person with communication disabilities in a hospital.

Mrs. Simon: Inpatient Services

The case study stems from an often cited and powerful story titled "My name is Mrs. Simon" (Elliot, 1984). This was a true story written by the daughter of Mrs. Simon, who died in a large, university-affiliated hospital known throughout the United States for its outstanding research record. Mrs. Simon was an active and well groomed 85-year-old woman who, prior to hospital admission for some routine tests, managed her large home independently, worked as a volunteer for a number of organizations, read books, and listened to classical music. During Mrs. Simon's 2 weeks in the hospital, her daughter described a systematic and gradual stripping of her mother's individuality and dignity. On visiting her mother for the first time, her daughter was appalled. Her mother was unkempt, her dentures had been removed, she was in a hospital gown, and her glasses were nowhere to be found. The staff were labeling her as senile, and according to staff, it appeared as if the daughter had caught the disease of senility when she questioned the ultimate benefit of painful procedures, such as a spinal tap, in an 85-year-old woman. The final event began when Mrs. Simon started having difficulty breathing. The resident ordered yet another X ray and when Mrs. Simon refused to get onto the gurney that was brought for her, the orderly said "Now don't you be difficult, Dolly." She announced firmly and with dignity, "My name is Mrs. Simon" and died as she got to the elevator. This story is a poignant reminder to all hospital staff who work with older people in a hospital.

Mr. Worthington: Inpatient Services

The next case study again seeks to bring the patient's perspective of a hospital admission to the attention of health professionals. This case is a patient with a communication disability. The first perspective is that of the speech-language pathologist and the audiologist. The second perspective is the patient's view of the same event.

The Speech-Language Pathology and Audiology Perspective

The hospital speech-language pathologist receives a referral for a stroke patient, 78-year-old Mr. Douglas Worthington. This is the third referral of the day, so the speech-language pathologist visits Mr. Worthington at 3:30 p.m. The medical chart states he was admitted the day before with a left hemisphere stroke caused by middle cerebral artery infarct. Mr. Worthington is in bed asleep when the speech-language pathologist arrives, but the nurse wakes him so that she can take his temperature. The speech-language pathologist notices that Mr. Worthington continues to be drowsy, is drooling from the left side of his mouth, and does not respond well to the nurse's commands. A brief clinical bedside examination for swallowing is conducted and

continues

it is evident that Mr. Worthington cannot manage any fluid or food orally at the present time. The speech-language pathologist recommends nil by mouth, writes this directive in the medical chart, and informs the nurse in charge.

Next day, Mr. Worthington is a little brighter and his wife is by his bed when the speech-language pathologist visits. As the speech-language pathologist begins to talk to Mrs. Worthington, Mr. Worthington attempts to communicate but becomes quite distressed at his inability to talk. Mrs. Worthington tells him to rest and asks the speech-language pathologist for information about his condition. It is explained that Mr. Worthington has some swallowing difficulties, and it has been recommended that he not eat or drink anything until his swallow improves. The speech-language pathologist also explains that she has not had a chance to assess Mr. Worthington further, and asks for 15–30 minutes now so that she can assess him. The speech-language pathologist conducts the hospital's informal aphasia screening test and determines that Mr. Worthington has moderate comprehension difficulties and severe expressive problems. He was able to say some automatic speech (e.g., days of the week) with substantial prompting and help. There was considerable oral dyspraxia, and the speech-language pathologist considers that a verbal dyspraxia is contributing significantly to Mr. Worthington's communication difficulties. The speech-language pathologist also notices that Mr. Worthington is cupping his ear with his hand and asking for repeats, hence she refers him for an audiological assessment. His swallow has improved and he now tolerates thickened fluids and a pureed diet. There is still drooling, of which Mr. Worthington is not aware. Mrs. Worthington is told that her husband will now be fed thickened fluid and pureed food, and aphasia is verbally explained to her. She seems pleased that Mr. Worthington will now be able to eat and drink and goes to explain this to her husband.

The speech-language pathologist continues to visit the Worthingtons daily to check on their progress. Within 7 days, Mr. Worthington is eating a normal diet but is still drinking thickened fluids. He is becoming more frustrated with his speech and with the hospital staff generally each day. Mrs. Worthington is upset by his anger and confides to the speech-language pathologist that even she cannot always understand what he wants and that the staff are not always helpful. He often does not have his glasses on when she arrives to visit him, and he is distressed because he cannot get help to go the toilet and is often incontinent. Mrs. Worthington implies that the nurses ignore her husband's requests for help, and the doctor is not able to stay long to respond to their questions. She asks whether Mr. Worthington will ever get his speech back. The speech-language pathologist tries to reassure Mrs. Worthington that everything will be done to help her husband get his speech back, but it is probably too early to tell how much progress he will make. The speech-language pathologist undertakes to advocate to the nursing and medical staffs on the Worthingtons' behalf.

The audiological assessment is arranged for Mr. Worthington and he is taken in a wheelchair to the hospital audiology clinic. Mrs. Worthington attends the appointment with him. The audiologist takes case history information from Mrs. Worthington about her husband. Mr.

Worthington has had hearing difficulties for some time. He had been fit with a hearing aid approximately 5 years previously, but had not found it particularly helpful and had not continued to use it. Mr. Worthington is able to complete pure-tone audiometry, responding consistently by nodding in response to sound. Speech audiometry is attempted unsuccessfully. Mr. Worthington is not capable of word repetition and becomes upset when presented with a closed-set word-pointing task. Therefore, his aphasic expression and comprehension problems prohibit this form of assessment. Immittance audiometry is performed. The test results indicate a moderate sensorineural hearing impairment, and the results are explained to Mr. and Mrs. Worthington. The possibility of hearing aid fitting is discussed, but they do not want to proceed with the fitting at the present time, as Mrs. Worthington thinks it would be too much for her husband to cope with. The audiologist provides the couple with information about how to obtain a hearing aid should they reconsider at a later date. In the meantime, Mr. Worthington is provided with a personal amplification assistive listening device (see Chapter 9, Figure 9–3) to help him with one-on-one conversation. The audiologist includes a report in the medical chart and advises the speech-language pathologist of the outcome of the assessment. It is agreed that Mr. Worthington's hearing impairment could be contributing to his comprehension difficulties and that amplification will be beneficial for him.

The speech-language pathologist develops a communication chart with the help of Mr. and Mrs. Worthington and the hospital staff who routinely work with Mr. Worthington. The small book has a page of photographs of Mr. Worthington's family and some drawings of things Mr. Worthington might need. There is also a page of photographs of the hospital staff, with their professions written underneath. There are some common topics listed on another page (e.g., home, the stroke, money), and everyone involved has participated in selecting them. There are also aphasia-friendly explanations of stroke and aphasia inserted into the book. Aphasia-friendly materials are specially adapted written materials designed to suit the reading comprehension skills of people with aphasia. They often include pictures or icons to assist with comprehension, and the language is often simplified. Mrs. Worthington borrows the speech-language pathologist's easy-to-read book about stroke and aphasia from the National Stroke Foundation. Mr. Worthington and the hospital staff use the communication book whenever they get stuck, but this is happening less often because the speech-language pathologist's instructions to the staff about accommodating to Mr. Worthington's speech and hearing difficulties have helped. One nurse in particular has been good at communicating with him. Mr. Worthington's frequent outbursts have eased somewhat now that he is able to get his message across more readily and he believes his needs are being heard. Mrs. Worthington has also learned to accommodate to her husband's communication a little more successfully through a process of conversational coaching. Mr. Worthington is now on a normal diet and is keen to attend speech therapy. He is also attending daily physical therapy and occupational therapy sessions, and the speech-language pathologist and audiologist have discussed Mr. Worthington's communication needs with these other staff members in order to optimize the communication process for both Mr. Worthington and his therapists.

continues

At the weekly case conference, it is decided that Mr. Worthington will go home as soon as he is able to walk up stairs with a cane. His wife expresses concern about her husband going home, as she is 77 years of age and has arthritis that limits her mobility. In addition, she gave up driving some years ago and asks about her husband's ability to drive. The Worthington's have no family living nearby, and their friends and neighbors are also mostly older people. The speech-language pathologist asks to accompany the occupational therapist on a home visit. During the home visit, the speech-language pathologist determines that Mrs. Worthington thinks she will not be able to leave her husband alone in the house to go shopping or attend her own medical appointments. The speech-language pathologist's priority in therapy is to ensure that Mr. Worthington can get help if he needs it while his wife is away. With Mrs. Worthington looking on, dialing the telephone in an emergency is rehearsed, as well as answering the telephone and the door. Mrs. Worthington agrees to rehearse these tasks at home when her husband is discharged. A few weeks after discharge, Mrs. Worthington puts the emergency contact telephone numbers in the telephone's memory function so that Mr. Worthington needs only to press one button. She also installs an answering machine for the telephone, and her son is able to arrange for a personal alarm system to be installed in his parents' house. Mrs. Worthington now takes short trips out of the house. Mr. Worthington starts to attend outpatient therapy once a week. The continued program of intervention for Mr. Worthington is described later in this chapter.

THE PATIENT AND FAMILY'S PERSPECTIVE

This is the same case study of Mr. Doug Worthington, but this time seen through the eyes of the patient, Doug, and his wife, Beryl. Doug was mowing the lawn and called to his wife just before he collapsed. Beryl thought he had a heart attack and had to dial the emergency number three times because she was so panicked. The ambulance came quickly and although the emergency medical technicians reassured her he would be all right, she feared the worst. She had been preparing herself for this day for years. The young physician at the hospital was not in any hurry to see her husband, and Beryl had to ask the nurses twice about when the physician would see him. Doug was unconscious. He was taken away for a while, Beryl cannot remember where to, and then she was asked to follow him to his hospital bed. The staff were friendly but they were all busy. A nurse explained that Mr. Worthington had a stroke and that the physician would see him when he did his rounds next morning. When Beryl got home, she rang her son who lived in another city. He offered to come home, but she said to wait to hear what the physician said the following day.

Beryl talked to the physician the next day, and he said that Doug had experienced a stroke and that he would need to remain in the hospital for a while longer. Doug woke up but did not seem to understand where he was or what had happened. He tried to get out of bed to go to the toilet but he fell. The nurse actually scolded him for "being so silly." Doug's reaction to this was to shout in garbled words and curse the nurses, a reaction that Beryl had never seen in her husband. Beryl became upset when she spoke to her son on the telephone that night. He decided to come home as soon as he could but advised that he would only be able to stay a few days.

When Doug's son, Frank, arrived at the hospital, Doug cried. He knew it must be serious if his son had come home. Doug had been in a prisoner-of-war camp in Poland during World War II, and he was reminded of how frightened he had been then. He felt like a 2-year-old again. He could not walk, could not talk, and no one was telling him anything. Frank was also distressed to see his father cry and vent his frustration.

As the days went by, Doug found that Lucy, one of the nurses, seemed to understand what he was saying and took special care of him. The fog in his head began to clear, and he was beginning to understand what was required of him each day. He was having daily physical therapy, occupational therapy, and speech therapy, and he found the personal amplifier that the audiologist had provided helped him to understand what people were saying. Other staff talked to Doug, but he could not remember who they all were. He desperately wanted to go home because he knew everything would be all right once he got home.

Beryl was anxious about Doug coming home. She was relieved when the occupational therapist and speech-language pathologist came home with her and gave her some practical help about how to manage. Doug was eventually discharged home and began outpatient therapy. The story is continued later in the chapter.

Communication Difficulties in the Hospital

Hospitals are unique environments. Anyone who has been a patient in a hospital will agree that it is a foreign environment. It is not a homelike place: hospital beds, furnishings, and different food create a hard and clinical ambience. There are often many staff to meet, which is done when the patient is in crisis, dependent for all care, or is ill or in pain. This section describes the features of the environment that contribute to communication difficulties in hospitals. McCooey, Toffolo, and Code (2000) described these as features concerned with the communication impairments of the patients, the communication difficulties of hospital staff, and the communication-related environment barriers in hospitals. The environmental barriers include the administrative culture of the organization and the economic realities of the system.

In the Worthington case study, it is evident that going into the hospital with a life-threatening illness is a traumatic event for all the family. It is also evident that the hospital did not always respond well to Mr. and Mrs. Worthington's needs. What is it about hospitals that make them so different from people's everyday experiences? What do hospital workers need to know about how to respond to patients' individual needs? What roles do the speech-language pathologists and audiologists have in creating a positive hospital experience for all patients?

These questions can be answered by examining the sources of communication problems in hospitals: the patients, the staff, and the environment.

THE PATIENTS

Chapter 4 summarized many of the voice, speech, language, sensory, and other communication-related associated impairments associated with normal and pathological aging. The traditional older adult speech-language pathology caseload in hospitals consists of people with dysphagia and communication disabilities caused by diseases such as aphasia, dysarthria, or dyspraxia or caused by injury. However, as noted in earlier chapters, one of the distinguishing features of older people is the multitude of impairments that occur. Therefore, as in Mr. Worthington's case, not only did he have acute aphasia but he also had dysphagia, dyspraxia, facial paresis, and a hearing and visual impairment.

The typical older adult inpatient caseload for audiologists is made up of those who are in the hospital primarily for treatment related to hearing (e.g., surgery for otosclerosis, acoustic neuroma) and those who are in the hospital for other treatment (e.g., related to a stroke or a fall at home) and who are identified as having hearing difficulties. This latter group is far more common than the former in most hospital settings. The prevalence of hearing impairment among older people in hospitals is high. Poltl and Hickson (1990) found that 80% of older inpatients had a hearing impairment. Subsequent medical referral was necessary in approximately 40% of cases in the study because of excessive wax and/or middle ear dysfunction. These prevalence figures are similar to those obtained in nursing homes (see Chapters 4 and 9).

In addition to barriers caused by patients' communication impairments, there are barriers associated with the older person's reluctance to ask for information while in the hospital. He or she may develop a passive or dependent role in the hospital, may feel the need to show deference to staff, and may not want to bother busy and overworked staff (Field, 1992). Hence, older patients in hospitals are often not able communicators. This situation, combined with the emotional stress of a hospital admission, means that older patients need special attention for their communication while in the hospital.

THE STAFF

There is a range of professional and support staff working in hospitals. Although nurses have the most contact with patients, there are many others who communicate with patients (e.g., cleaners, radiographers, and receptionists). In addition, there are different workers in each shift. Consequently, there are potentially many different people with whom the older person needs to communicate in the hospital.

Staff need to have both the skills and attitude to communicate well with patients. Research into nurse-patient communication in hospitals has concluded that most communication is automatic, routine, and focused on physical care (see Jarrett & Payne, 1995, and Llenore & Ogle, 1999, for reviews). It has also been found that the time spent in communication is proportional to the communicative ability of the patient. If a patient is having difficulty communicating, then the staff will spend less time talking to the person. Nursing staff require special communication skills to interact with those who do not respond or who have difficulty understanding instructions or expressing their needs. They also require excellent communication skills to elicit the worries and concerns of patients.

Staff attitudes toward older people may also be a barrier to effective communication in the hospital environment. Stereotypical views of older people can lead to patronizing talk (see Chapters 2 and 9). The frail, ill, passive, and depersonalized role of older people when they are in the hospital contributes to staff's agist attitudes that manifest themselves in patronizing talk.

To create a positive communication environment (see Lubinski, 1995), all hospital staff need to be skilled communicators and need to learn to treat each older person as an individual. It is important that the hospital values the communication skill of the people it employs and is prepared to support training for staff about effective communication.

THE ENVIRONMENT

Environmental factors may include the physical environment as well as the policy and legislative environment (WHO, 2001). This section describes the barriers to communication that the physical environment of the hospital creates. It also sets the hospital environment into policy and legislative contexts.

The physical environmental barriers to communication in hospitals include excessive noise and access to the nurse call button (McCooey et al., 2000). Hospitals are noisy places. There is often a lack of privacy, and the acoustic environment produces significant reverberation and background noise. The most basic communication channel in the hospital, the nurse call button, may also be a problem for older people in the hospital. Call buttons can be difficult to see, recognize, reach, and operate for some patients.

The policy and legislative environment includes the laws, regulations, and policies that govern a context. The accessibility of institutions such as hospitals to people with disabilities has become a significant policy issue. Most countries have antidiscrimination legislation that binds public institutions to nondiscriminatory practices. In the United States, the Self Help for Hard of Hearing (SHHH) group has developed a program to assist hospitals to provide services for people with hearing loss and to comply with the Americans with Disabilities Act (www.shhh.org). Individuals with disabilities who perceive they have been discriminated against have been testing the antidiscrimination laws. Many hospitals are, therefore, conducting audits of their practices to ensure that people with disabilities receive fair treatment. Forster, Towers, and Buttner (1999) conducted one such audit at a hospital in Australia and reported that people who were hearing impaired or deaf found it difficult to make appointments or inquire about inpatients through the hospital's telephone service, and had difficulty using the public or bedside telephones. Other hearing access difficulties included hospital televisions, education videos, religious services, and public seminars at the hospital. Similar audits for patients with other communication disabilities need to be undertaken.

At the institutional level, it is important that hospitals value and reward good communication. Referring to institutions for people with TBI, Ylvisaker, Feeney, and Urbanczyk (1993) stated that an institution that values effective communication would express this principle through its mission statement and annual reports. It would commit resources to enhance communication in the hospital and identify barriers and facilitators for communication throughout the hospital. Most hospitals do not value communication, and an attitudinal barrier exists that prizes physical and medical care over all else.

In summary, many older people have multiple preexisting or new communication difficulties when admitted to the hospital. The multitude of staff involved in hospital services do not necessarily have the skills or nonagist attitudes to communicate well with those who have a communication disability, and the physical and policy environments of hospitals do not necessarily create a positive communication environment. Just as Lubinski (1995), Ylvisaker et al. (1993), and others have described modifying the communication environment for residents in care facilities for the aged and TBI facilities, McCooey et al. (2000) have described this approach in the hospital setting. This social model approach focuses on creating a positive communication environment within the hospital.

McCooey et al. (2000) described a process that begins with identifying patients who are experiencing communication difficulties in hospital situations such as "telling about pain and discomfort" and "indicating when he or she does not understand." Speech-language pathologists can identify patients with communication difficulties using a screening tool called the Inpatient Functional Communication Interview (IFCI). The specific problems of each patient are then addressed through education of staff and family, modifying the physical environment if possible, and working with management to facilitate policy changes if needed (e.g., valuing communication in the mission statement of the facility, ensuring that good communication skills are valued in recruitment of staff). The IFCI and interventions arising from it are described in more detail later in this chapter.

The social model approach described previously is a new model of service that has not been fully evaluated and may require a paradigm shift for those embracing the medical model. More important, in some health care funding systems, this type of approach may not be approved for reimbursement. However, the social model approach to service delivery may be a useful adjunct to more traditional services and has the potential to make a difference to many hospital patients.

Speech-Language Pathology Intervention

Although there are many texts that describe the management of communication disability, there are few that describe the acute management stage, that is, the case management in the first few weeks following admission to a hospital. The next section describes the steps involved in managing cases in the acute stages.

Stroke is the most frequent reason why older people are referred to hospital-based speech-language pathology. Other less common medical admissions are as a result of cancers of the larynx, pharynx, or tongue; TBI; spinal injury; neurosurgical problems; or neurological disorders such as Guillain-Barré syndrome. Preexisting disorders such as Parkinson's disease or ALS may also occur in patients who are admitted to a hospital for reasons such as a fall, an operation, or some other medical need. However, because stroke is the most common referral, the process of acute care will focus on this type of case, although there are certainly similar processes involved in managing patients with the other disorders.

The process for acute care patients with stroke typically begins when the speech-language pathologist receives the referral and pays an initial visit to the patient. As seen in the case study of Mr. Worthington described earlier in this chapter, the first step is usually some bedside screening process during which the speech-language pathologist aims to provide a general indication about the communication and/or swallowing status of the patient to the staff, the patient, and the family. The medical status of the patient often takes priority at this stage. If a communication disability is present, the next step is to establish some form of communication among the patient, staff, and family. Monitoring the status of the disorder, and communicating the results of these assessments to staff, as well as to the patient and family, are important parts of the process. Patient and family education and counseling are ongoing during the whole stay in the hospital, and discharge planning occurs when a likely destination becomes evident. Beginning impairment-based language treatment in these early stages is a much-debated topic, and the debate is summarized in the following sections. Johnson, Valachovic, and George (1998), however, describe a useful consultative approach that concludes that the role of the acute care speech-language pathologist is to prepare for rehabilitation activities that will follow discharge. This assumes a short length of stay typical of most modern-day hospitals. Each step of acute speech-language pathology intervention is discussed in detail in the following sections.

STEP 1: SCREENING ASSESSMENT AND DIAGNOSIS

Screening assessment in an acute care setting is a delicate balance between obtaining sufficient valid information and being as least intrusive as possible. The context is a busy hospital and a nonalert or fatiguing patient whose medical status is rapidly changing and who is still coming to terms with the hospital admission, the stroke, and the foreign environment in the hospital.

Bedside screening assessments are ideal for this situation. In patients with stroke, the first urgent concern is often swallowing status. Identifying the presence or absence of other speech, language, and hearing impairments is a second priority at this stage. The management of dysphagia has become the major role for speech-language pathologists in acute care settings. Accurate assessment of dysphagia has been identified as a major contributor to positive medical outcomes, especially in neurological cases. In older people in particular, the identification of dysphagia is important in the prevention of aspiration pneumonia, an all-too-frequent cause of death in frail older people (Palmer & Hunter, 1998). Dysphagia management is also important for adequate nutrition, another issue of concern for older people admitted to a hospital.

The medical chart is a source of much information and must be consulted prior to seeing the patient. In a bedside clinical examination of swallowing, typically the overall status of the patient's medical and cognitive situations is observed first, and an examination of the processes involved in swallowing follow. If it is perceived to be safe to do so, the clinician will often perform some trial swallows to determine the success of the swallow. The presence of silent aspiration is always a possibility; hence, some facilities routinely provide nonoral feeding in the first few days poststroke, whereas others rely on modified barium swallows or videofluoroscopy to confirm the presence of aspiration. See, for example, Logemann (1998) and Musson (1998) for a detailed description of these procedures. Outcome measures such as the Checklist for Daily Monitoring of Patients With Communication or Swallowing Disorder (Johnson et al., 1998) or the Royal Brisbane Hospital's Outcome Measure for Swallowing (1998) (see Chapter 5, Table 5–8) are useful for tracking the progress of the patient through the stages of swallowing rehabilitation. Intervention techniques predominantly involve a modified diet (i.e., thickening fluids and pureeing solids); supervision and monitoring of aspiration symptoms (e.g., wetness of vocal quality, choking); and techniques such as supraglottic swallows, chin tucks, and altered head positioning that all modify the pathways for the food, to minimize aspiration. Indirect therapy, such as oromotor exercise, is also an option.

Once the condition of dysphagia has been established and management initiated, the presence of an accompanying speech or language impairment is the next focus. As Johnson et al. (1998) noted, informal testing is frequently used in the acute care setting due to poor patient tolerance of testing and the inability to accurately administer a standardized test at bedside. In addition, they noted that even the most experienced and organized speech-language pathologist must rely on flexible online decision making to complete an assessment of an acute stroke patient. Many hospitals and clinicians have developed their own informal screening tests or they will sometimes use subtests of larger standardized tests with different patients. The speech-language pathologist takes a portfolio of brief assessment materials to the bedside and uses whatever is appropriate for the patient at the time of the evaluation.

If dysarthria is present, it is likely to be evident when the patient speaks. Slurred speech accompanied by some loss of intelligibility is the key feature of a dysarthria. The presence of oral and verbal groping behaviors and articulatory errors may lead the clinician to suspect dyspraxia. Although the clinician may be able to observe the groping articulatory movements during speech or hear the poor sequencing of phonemes, it is often necessary to conduct further testing to confirm the presence of an accompanying dyspraxia. Another contributing factor to a tentative diagnosis of verbal dyspraxia would be the presence of an oral or limb dyspraxia. Tests such as the Apraxia Battery for Adults (Dabul, 1979) may be used to further test for the presence of a subtle verbal dyspraxia. The presence of aphasia may be immediately evident when the patient attempts to communicate, but a screening test such as the BNT (Kaplan, Goodglass, & Weintraub, 1983) is often used to differentially diagnose aphasia from a cognitive-communication disorder caused by dementia or TBI. It may also be necessary to test for aphasia when the patient is nonresponsive. In this case, the clinician is determining whether the reason for a lack of response is aphasia or another cause such as decreased levels of alertness or confusion or a combination of these.

There is a range of formal aphasia screening measures available, and these are described in Table 8–1. There are differences in the use of tests worldwide, and the comments on the frequency of use of these tests in each region have been drawn from Katz et al. (2000). For full reviews of these tests, see Beech, Harding, and Hilton-Jones (1993), Kersner (1992), or Peterson and Marquardt (1994). For a description of assessments not designed specifically for screening but that may also be usefully applied in the hospital setting, see Chapter 4.

STEP 2: COMMUNICATING WHILE IN THE HOSPITAL

Once a diagnosis becomes clearer, there is first a need to communicate diagnostic information to other staff involved in the care of the patient. There may also be a need to provide information about how to communicate effectively with the patient if significant communication impairment is apparent. The IFCI (McCooey, 2001; see Figure 8–1 for a list of items from the IFCI) is a way of initiating this process. The items on the IFCI were generated by observing the communication between staff and patients and through staff and patient interviews. The assessment is conducted like an interview and is as naturalistic as possible as the patient is interviewed many times in the hospital. Sometimes the interview simulates natural situations; for example, an instruction relevant to the context is given for Item 7, "The patient's ability to ask you questions about his or her care." For this item, the speech-language pathologist asks "I will be talking with the doctors and nurses later. Do you have any questions for the doctors and nurses? Would you like me to find anything out

TABLE 8–1

FORMAL LANGUAGE SCREENING TESTS.

Test, Author, Publisher	Description
Aphasia Screening Test–2. (Whurr, 1996, Whurr Publishers, U.K.)	A language-screening test for moderately to severely impaired brain-damaged patients. Administration time 30–60 minutes. Popular measure in the United Kingdom and Australia.
Aphasia Language Performance Scales (Keenan & Brassel, 1975, Pinnacle Press, U.S.A.)	Screening test for aphasia using four scales (Listening, Talking, Reading, Writing), each with 10 items. Administration time 20–35 minutes. More popular in the United States, particularly the VA hospitals.
Frenchay Aphasia Screening Test (Enderby, Wood, & Wade, 1987; NFER-Nelson, U.K.)	Designed to be used by all health professionals, not just speech-language pathologists, to detect the presence of aphasia. Administration time 3–10 minutes. Developed in the United Kingdom, not used frequently by speech-language pathologists.
Bedside Evaluation Screening Test II (West, Sands, & Ross-Swain, 1998)	Assesses auditory comprehension, speaking, and reading. Does not assess writing. Administration time 20–30 minutes. Predominantly used in the United States.
Boston Naming Test (Kaplan, Goodglass, & Weintraub, 1983; Lea & Febiger, U.S.A)	A popular 60-item confrontation naming test to detect anomia. See Chapter 4 for a full description.
Sklar Aphasia Scale (Sklar, 1983; Western Psychological Services, U.S.A)	Administration time 30–60 minutes. Often used in the United States.

for you? Would you like me to find out about . . . (e.g., when you are going home or any issues raised earlier)?" The ability of the patient is rated for each item, and communicative strategies that help the patient are noted. Communicative strategies used during the interview may have included verbal prompting, additional time, use of a communication book, asking the patient to write the message down, or writing key words for the patient. The IFCI provides a baseline measure for how well the patient is communicating in the hospital and also provides information about how best to communicate with the patient.

The IFCI may also point to the need for intervention in a variety of areas. It may alert the speech-language pathologist or audiologist to the need for environmental changes (e.g.,

1. The patient's ability to understand descriptions about what is happening or going to happen or has happened as it relates to hospital procedures

2. The patient's ability to understand information about his or her current medical condition

3. The patient's ability to follow instructions

4. The patient's ability to tell you if he or she has any pain or discomfort

5. The patient's ability to tell you about his or her medical condition at present

6. The patient's ability to express feelings

7. The patient's ability to ask you questions about his or her care

8. The patient's ability to call for a nurse

9. The patient's ability to ask for something he or she needs

10. The patient's ability to tell you what has happened to bring him or her into hospital

11. The patient's ability to tell you what he or she likes or does not like

12. Gaining the patient's attention

FIGURE 8–1. Items from the Inpatient Functional Communication Interview (reprinted with permission from McCooey, R. (2001). *Communication in the acute hospital setting.* Unpublished Masters thesis.)

better acoustic conditions, need for binaural listeners to be available for clients who are hearing impaired), changes to staff communication (e.g., training for nurses about hearing aids, use of elderspeak), or changes to the family's communication (e.g., communication training for family members, increasing knowledge about communication disability).

There is sometimes a need for an alternative or augmentative communication system for patients in acute care. These systems are often communication charts or communication books and range from a copied one-page piece of cardboard or paper with standard pictures or drawings (e.g., toilet, doctor, nurse) to books with photos of family members, staff, and common objects. The communication aid can serve several purposes. The first is to assist the patient to successfully transmit important messages such as "I want to see the doctor." The second purpose is that it personalizes the patient. A noncommunicating patient is often unable to communicate personality or interests to staff and, therefore, may have difficulty establishing a relationship with staff. A trusting relationship with staff is an important component of quality health care, hence a communication book that acts as a portfolio of the person's life can trigger conversations with staff and visitors. Finally, if family and staff are involved in the construction of the communication book, this increases their involvement in the care of the patient and increases understanding of the patient's particular problems. It is recommended that if a communication book is needed, it should contain personalized items, and staff and family should be involved in identifying what should go into the book and should provide some of the material. Suggestions for the content of a communication book are contained in Table 8–2.

STEP 3: PATIENT AND FAMILY EDUCATION AND COUNSELING

Patient education is integral to the successful management of chronic diseases. Informed patients are more empowered to actively participate in decisions about their care. Patient education can allay anxiety, enhance compliance and adjustment, and increase patient satisfaction with the quality of care (O'Mahoney, Rodgers, Thomson, Dobson, & James, 1997). Verbal education in conjunction with written information is the education process preferred by most patients and is the method considered most effective in enhancing patient recall (Ley, 1982). Written patient education materials ensure that the information provided to patients is consistent, and because patient education material can be referred to when required and under less stressful circumstances than a hospital environment, they aid patient recall and encourage self-paced learning (Bernier, 1993). It is, therefore, important not only to verbally explain the communication and swallowing disabilities to family and friends, but also important to provide appropriate written patient education materials as well.

The appropriateness and timeliness of the education material for the patient is a complex issue. Patients with aphasia need to have materials that have been modified because of the limitations of aphasia. There is a growing recognition that people with aphasia are particularly disadvantaged by their impairment, and this condition has ethical, as well as practical, implications. Application of aphasia-friendly principles can improve the readability of written stroke patient education materials. The six principles for written information are as follows:

1. Use average-length words and short sentences.
2. Keep to the main message only.
3. Use helpful icons as much as possible.
4. Keep plenty of white space.
5. Give the reader plenty of time.
6. Use multimodal support communication (i.e., read the information aloud with the patient) (www.shrs.uq.edu.au/cdaru/aphasiagroups).

Similar design principles apply when developing any patient education material. An attractive and appropriate format is important to motivate the reader to interact with the material and to enhance the readability and understanding of the information (Chapman &

TABLE 8–2

SUGGESTED TOPICS FOR A COMMUNICATION BOOK.

Topic	Description/Examples
Me (patient details)	Full name, date of birth, address (include photograph of home), place of birth (include photograph from home town or school), hobbies (include photographs or actual products), previous work, and so forth.
Family	A rough family tree is useful, particularly if the family is extensive and involved with the patient's care. Photographs are again useful for identifying family members.
People in the hospital	Again photographs of key staff are useful here. Writing their profession and contact details underneath is a way for patients and family to identify the myriad of staff involved in stroke care in a hospital. If the patient is severely aphasic, use a photograph of the staff member undertaking a usual role (e.g., the physical therapist walking with the patient up and down steps).
What I like to talk about	Some conversational topic triggers can be photographs, newspaper clippings, theater or event tickets, letters, awards, completed handcrafts, or just words and sentences.
I find it helpful if you . . .	List communication strategies for the patient, for example, slow down, write down the key words, give me time to respond, do not finish my sentences for me, do not pretend you understand me, be patient, do not look as though you are in a hurry, show that you know I am not stupid.
I need . . .	These may be generic key words or pictures (e.g., toilet, shave, toothbrush) or may be specific to the patient (e.g., glasses, hearing aid, dentures, cane, make up, warm clothes, robe, and so forth)
I want to talk about . . .	What happened, my stroke, my speech problem, my walking problem, the pain in my shoulder, the possibility of another stroke, when I can go home, how I feel.
Feelings	Glad to see you; not a good day; feeling down; am pleased with myself.
Aphasia	I have aphasia. I know what I want to say, but cannot find the words. I do not always understand what people say. I cannot read very well. I am having trouble writing. It is very frustrating. Everything is very confusing.

Langridge, 1997). Wellwood, Dennis, and Warlow (1994) found that only 12% of patients with stroke received patient education materials in the hospital. It is important that all patients with stroke are provided with patient education material about stroke.

It is well recognized that best practice in designing patient education materials begins with a clear understanding of the consumer's informational needs and abilities (Coulter, Entwistle, & Gilbert, 1999). In designing patient education materials for older people with communication disability, it is necessary to find out what the prospective readers want to know; write the text recognizing the literacy levels in this age group; and recognize the language, literacy, visual, and cognitive difficulties that may accompany stroke.

What information needs to be provided through patient education materials in the acute phase? If the person has had a stroke and it has resulted in aphasia, it is important that the speech-language pathologist does not assume other staff have adequately described what a stroke is to the patient in aphasia-friendly terms. It is also important to repeat the information as many times as the patient or the family need. There is a common misconception that a stroke is a heart attack. Explaining a stroke in terms of a brain attack can help patients and their families understand that it is the brain that is damaged, not the heart. The notion that it is an interruption of blood supply to the brain, either through a blood clot or bleeding, is an important concept to convey. The damage that stroke causes to the brain and the associated symptoms (e.g., hemiparesis, aphasia, facial weakness) is another difficult concept for nonmedical people. Finally, it is important to label and describe the communication and or swallowing impairments. Aphasia and dysarthria are not well-known disorders within the general community, and it is important that the patient and family members have a term to use to describe the language difficulties to others, to look up texts and search the Internet for information, and to attribute their difficulties to a specific language disorder rather than thinking that the stroke has affected the patient's mind.

Once terms such as *stroke* and *aphasia* have been explained, questions such as "Will it happen again?" "Will he get better?" "Will he always talk like this?" and "Will he be able to work/drive/play golf again?" need to be answered. Speech-language pathologists may not wish to cross professional boundaries by responding to medical or mobility-related questions; however, again it is important not to assume that other professionals will answer questions in a way that can be understood by people with communication disabilities. The speech-language pathologist may ask the physician or physical therapist to explain prognoses in these areas to the patient; then it may be useful to follow up with comprehension checks, asking the patient and the family about what was said. Further information or patient education material on the subject may be given to supplement the information provided by the other professionals.

Audiologists and speech-language pathologists are often required to act as advocates for people in the hospital who are communicatively disabled. The clinician's role can be one of an interpreter when other staff cannot understand the message of a patient who is communicatively disabled or cannot get a message across. Another role may be to facilitate communication with the patient, asking staff to respond to the patient's specific informational needs or to put forward the view of the patient who is unable to communicate it adequately. This role as communication facilitator or advocate is similar to that of interpreter or intermediator, and it is an important role in busy hospitals where communication about health care should be a primary concern.

STEP 4: IMPLEMENT IMPAIRMENT-BASED TREATMENT (OPTIONAL)

Once the patient's communication and swallowing status has been assessed, staff and family informed of the results, and everyday communication optimized, clinicians may choose to implement impairment-based therapy. There has been considerable discussion in the literature about the effectiveness of impairment-based language treatment in the early stages poststroke or in acute care (Fridriksson & Holland, 2001; Holland & Fridriksson, 2001; Marshall, 1997; Peach, 2001; Wertz, 1997). The major thrust of the argument put forward by Marshall (1997) and Holland and Fridriksson (2001) is that the focus in the acute phase should be support, counseling, and education rather than direct structured impairment-based language therapy. The acute phase was defined as before the beginning of a formal, daily rehabilitation program, usually 1 to 2 weeks poststroke, but maybe 3 to 4 weeks in severe cases. All authors conclude that evidence for and against early language treatment is not completely clear, hence further studies are needed in this area.

In the meantime, while the debate about the effectiveness of impairment-based treatments in the acute stage continues, it is evident that the role of the speech-language pathologist should always encompass education and counseling of patients who are communicatively disabled. There is also a role for speech-language pathologists in planning for discharge.

STEP 5: DISCHARGE PLANNING

Safe discharge must be a priority for all hospital-based health professionals. What are the specific issues for older people with communication disabilities? Older people may not have sufficient support in the community upon discharge, and older people with communication disability face special challenges as they attempt to reenter a communicating world.

The first step in the discharge process should be to find out what everyday communication is required for the patient to be discharged. One method is to interview the patient together with the spouse or family member to determine the key communication issues when the patient returns home. The Interview Schedule in the Functional Communication

Therapy Planner (Worrall, 1999; see Chapter 7) is a useful starting point. Safety issues are paramount, so asking about how the patient would contact someone in an emergency may be important if the family member intends to leave the patient home alone. Establishing effective communication between patient and family members is another important requirement before discharge. The FCTP interview also asks about household duties, managing finances, and transport issues as well as examining leisure activities. The importance of the patient returning to these activities after discharge is determined through the interview.

Before patients with moderate and severe communication disabilities are discharged home, speech-language pathologists should also be encouraged to visit the patient's home, if possible with the patient and the family present. This will depend on the hospital's policy on home assessments, but such assessments can be useful. Adaptations that facilitate communication may have already been made in the home. For example, a speech-language pathologist could spend time rehearsing the patient on skills required for telephoning in an emergency. The tasks may include dialing the number, providing a name and address, and indicating what emergency service is required. However, after visiting the patient's home, the speech-language pathologist may observe that the telephone has been preprogrammed for the emergency number so the patient need only push one button that has the emergency sign on it. Because the emergency operators trace the address of an incoming telephone call, providing a name and address is unnecessary. The only task left is to indicate the type of emergency service required. Hence, home visits provide information about the person's communicative needs in the home. The visit will also often demonstrate that the patient can perform better at home, surrounded by familiar people and a familiar environment.

ISSUES IN ACUTE CARE MANAGEMENT

Acute speech-language pathology care is a process. Although it has been described as a simple series of steps in this chapter, it is actually a complex process that demands a high level of skill by a speech-language pathologist. Johnson et al. stated that the key issues in acute speech-language pathology practice are

1. Appreciation of the importance of rapid access to information by all members of the health care team
2. Knowledge of appropriate observation and treatment methodologies for patients during periods of rapid change in health status
3. Communication with a broad audience of other professionals
4. Dealing with patients and families during times of crisis
5. Providing information that has immediate effect on patient care
6. Potential for significant clinical errors in judgment and/or practice
7. Observing immediate effects of illness, drugs, and surgical management on patient performance, function, and outcome

8. Dealing with issues related to patient advocacy and/or ethics

9. Understanding the role of the speech-language pathologist in assuring the best outcomes—both rehabilitative and medical. (1998, pp. 101–105)

The significant errors that can potentially be made by speech-language pathologists practising in acute care settings mentioned by Johnson et al. (1998) are reproduced in Figure 8–2.

Palmer and Hunter (1998) reminded speech-language pathologists about another significant issue for older inpatients in particular. Polypharmacy, when many older people are on numerous medications, each with side effects and interaction effects, is a major issue in acute care. Sometimes adverse effects are the reason for admission, whereas in other cases the older patient's usual medications interact with essential new medication prescribed on admission. This situation may have an effect on the patient's functioning in hospital.

There are also substantial ethical issues confronting the speech-language pathologist in the acute care setting. As Palmer and Hunter (1998) stated, autonomy or the individual's right to self-determination has become the prominent principle of modern medical ethics. This principle means that patients may choose not to have treatment. One of the first considerations, however, must be the patient's competence to make decisions. This consideration is usually a team decision, and the speech-language pathologist is often a key member of this decision-making team, especially in the case of a person with a severe speech or language impairment. The number of older people making advanced health care directives (i.e., living wills, enduring power of attorney for health care) is increasing (Tippett & Sugarman, 1996). Therefore, the team must be aware of any legally binding documents that direct the health care team in terms of the wishes of the patient regarding treatment. Although the ethical issues often revolve around dysphagia in the hospital setting, the principles remain the same for all health care.

Audiology Intervention

Many of the issues described previously for speech-language pathologists in the acute care setting apply to audiologists. There are instances when the audiologist is a key health care professional in the management of an older patient in acute care. This is not as common as for the speech-language pathologist, but will occur when the older person's primary reason for hospitalization is related to hearing (e.g., ear surgery, sudden onset of hearing loss) or when the older person has another primary condition (e.g., stroke, cancer) but a hearing problem is compromising the treatment process. The management steps in such cases and the role of the audiologist would be similar to those described previously for the speech-language pathologist. The audiologist will need to conduct screening assessment and diagnosis; assist the patient, family members, and staff to communicate effectively while

1. Failure to communicate results of high-risk or invasive procedures accurately or in a timely manner.
2. Failure to document detailed recommendations in the chart (especially diet changes or aspiration precautions).
3. Failure to respond to referrals or requests for information from families or physicians in a timely manner, especially when this delay causes interruption to other care or delays discharge from the acute care setting.
4. Performing any procedures without having demonstrated competency.
5. Failure to supervise noncertified personnel when they are completing procedures.
6. Failure to communicate results from language, speech, or swallowing testing that have diagnostic significance and could change the medical plan of care.
7. Failure to observe or report significant changes in patient behavior that may signal an alteration in the medical or psychological status.
8. Performing procedures outside the scope of practice.
9. Performing procedures that are experimental or of questionable benefit without appropriate informed consent.
10. Making diagnostic statements or drawing conclusions that are not substantiated by observation or test data.
11. Failure to make appropriate referrals when indicated.
12. Failure to follow up on recommendations previously made.
13. Failure to explain and document important information to the patient and/or the family.
14. Failure to assure patient confidentiality.
15. Providing services that would be viewed as incomplete or faulty by a group of your peers.
16. Failure to limit opinions and decisions to topics directly related to speech, language, swallowing, cognition disorders, and their sequelae.
17. Failure to follow basic procedures for infection control, universal precautions, and safety.

FIGURE 8–2. Potential significant errors in speech-language pathology practice in hospitals. Reproduced with permission from Johnson, A. F., Valachovic, A. M., & George, K. P. (1998), Speech-language pathology practice in the acute care setting: A consultative approach. In A. F. Johnson & B. H. Johnson (Eds.), *Medical speech-language pathology: A practitioner's guide* (pp. 96–130). New York: Thieme.

the patient is in the hospital; provide education and counseling to the patient and the family; and be involved in intervention and discharge planning.

In terms of a screening assessment, it may be necessary at times for the audiologist to conduct a test while the patient is in a hospital room because the patient is too ill or frail to be moved to the audiology clinic. On such occasions, the audiologist would assess the patient by asking a number of questions about his or her hearing history, by testing air conduction pure-tone thresholds using a screening audiometer with either circumaural headphones or insert earphones to decrease the effects of ambient noise, and by using a self-report assessment measure (see Chapter 5 for examples of suitable tools). This assessment does not complete the diagnosis, as further comprehensive assessment will be required in the audiology clinic when the patient is feeling better, but it provides useful preliminary information.

If the patient has a hearing impairment that is making communication difficult while in the hospital, then the audiologist can consider a number of options to help. First, there are those options that involve improving the hearing ability of the patient. This improvement can be achieved by providing the patient with a hearing aid or an assistive listening device (e.g., personal amplification system, telephone amplifier, earplugs for television; see Pichora-Fuller, 1997 for review). If the patient already has a hearing aid at home, it is important that the audiologist helps the patient to retrieve it. If the patient does not have a hearing aid, then the provision of a personal amplification assistive listening device would be most appropriate (see Chapter 9 Figure 9–3). The safety of such expensive equipment can be an issue in the hospital environment, and it is important that the audiologist assist the patient in this regard. Second, the audiologist could provide education to staff and family about the most effective means of communicating with the patient (see Chapter 9, Table 9-4). For example, it is important that the patient can see the speaker's face clearly, that speech is clear and at a slightly slower pace, that gesture is used as much as possible, and that the speaker always checks that the patient has understood. It may be necessary to write down messages in order for the patient to understand, and a notebook or small white board could be provided to assist with message writing. In addition, there are numerous educational materials on hearing impairment that could be provided to the patient, family, and staff. For example, the Self Help for Hard of Hearing (SHHH) organization in the United States has developed a program for hospitals that includes

- a guidebook on *People with Hearing Loss and Health Care Facilities*
- a staff training video called *I Only Hear You When I See Your Face*
- *Patient with Hearing Loss* brochures
- *Tips for Communication* cards

- *Tips for Staff* posters
- stickers of the International Symbol of Access for Hearing Loss

As described in the preceding section on speech-language pathology intervention, the audiologist may need to act as a communication facilitator in the hospital setting and as an advocate for the patient with hearing impairment. For discharge planning, there are times when the audiologist will also need to be involved in the home visit to determine the needs of the older person. There are numerous assistive listening devices for use around the home that could be recommended should the older person require them (see Pichora-Fuller, 1997).

Outpatient Services

The focus of rehabilitation for inpatients in a hospital is diagnosis, counseling, education, ensuring quality health care through effective communication, perhaps some initial impairment based treatment, and safe and appropriate discharge planning. Once the patient returns to the community, the emphasis changes. Patients with stroke are faced with the chronicity of the problem and are reminded every day of their activity limitations and participation restrictions. Frustration and depression may also become major problems. At this time, long-term treatment plans are made and rehabilitation begins in earnest.

The patient may seek ongoing treatment in an outpatient facility, day care center, rehabilitation unit, or clinic. Whatever the name of the facility, the rehabilitation model of service delivery (see Chapter 3) should be the primary approach used. In addition, because the final outcome is successful reintegration into the community, a more social model of practice may also be implemented. To illustrate the process of intervention for patients who are receiving treatment as an outpatient, the story of Doug and Beryl Worthington described earlier is now continued.

Audiology and Speech-Language Pathology Intervention

The case study shows how Doug and Beryl created a new life together. While initially the emphasis in the hospital was on medical matters such as Doug's dysphagia, the focus soon shifted to returning home and then, once he was safely at home, to reintegrating back into the community and restoring a sense of well-being. There was a progression in focus from the medical model to the rehabilitation model and then to the social model; however, these were only the primary approaches used at each stage. For example, there were aspects of the social model approach occurring within the hospital. It is important to keep the final goal of increased well-being in sight at all stages.

Case Study: Mr. Worthington (continued)

Finally, Doug was home. He was elated to be out of hospital and thought that he could now get on with his life. Beryl was fussing over him and never let him out of her sight. He was now able to walk with a cane although he was still a little shaky, and he was able to talk in short sentences, although he would often get the words mixed up.

In the first few weeks, many of Doug's old golfing buddies and friends from work came to see him. He could see the pity in their eyes as they struggled to talk with him, choosing instead to talk through Beryl. Each day became a struggle. Beryl was worried about him and would wake up every time he moved. He hated the thought of needing her help getting dressed. Doug was unable to help out much around the house. He felt useless, and he could see that Beryl was wearing herself out.

One day, during one of his visits to the hospital, his speech-language pathologist asked how things were at home and asked about Beryl. Doug could not stop crying. Although he was embarrassed, he agreed to see his physician. His physician prescribed anti-depressants and referred Doug and Beryl for counseling, which helped after a while. Things did not seem so bad. Beryl also spoke with the speech-language pathologist, and she started going out again with her friends, initially leaving Doug at home with another friend, and then by himself. Life was getting better. Doug was walking around the block now and was talking with some of the neighbors. He decided he would try a hearing aid again, and Beryl made an appointment for him with an audiologist whom the hospital audiologist had told them about.

Around this time, 2 months after his stroke, the speech-language pathologist introduced Doug to a group of people with aphasia. They met for a few hours each week at the hospital and did some speech therapy, but they also talked. They talked mainly about what it was like to have aphasia. What Doug liked about the group was that every person understood what he was going through. The speech-language pathologist was part of the group but, after a few months, she was not needed. The group listened while Doug spoke and he felt in the company of friends. When someone new came into the group, Doug was the first to welcome the person and take him or her under his wing. It was during this time that Doug met someone with aphasia who had been in the Polish prisoner of war camp around the same time as he had. They met for lunch, talked about old times, and developed a new friendship. Nine months after starting with the group, they both went to a conference about aphasia and spoke about their experiences. Doug became passionate about helping other people who had been through his experience of aphasia, so he became active in the aphasia association. Life was good again, and Beryl was having a hard time keeping up with him.

The process of care in outpatient facilities is largely similar to that described in community settings in Chapter 7. For audiologists providing outpatient services from a hospital or clinic, a number of group educational programs were described in Chapter 7. Programs that focused on hearing aids and programs, such as the *Active Communication Education* program that has an emphasis on the effects of hearing impairment on communication in everyday life, were discussed. A process of individual intervention based on the Client Oriented Scale of Improvement (Dillon, James, & Ginis, 1997) was also described.

For speech-language pathologists working in outpatient care or in a clinic that provides services for people with communication disability living in the community, both group and individual therapy were described in Chapter 7. The concept of centers exclusively for people with aphasia, and support organizations for people with hearing impairment, were introduced. If a local support organization or center is not available, the importance of establishing groups was emphasized. The steps involved in establishing a group for people with a communication disability in an outpatient or clinical setting were described. Individual therapy programs that have a predominantly rehabilitation or social model approach were described. The *Speaking Out* program (Worrall & Yiu, 2000) consists of 10 modules that address some everyday communication activities for people with aphasia, and the Functional Communication Therapy Planner (FCTP: Worrall, 1999) describes a step-by-step process for establishing, treating, and evaluating intervention goals with individuals who have aphasia.

In summary, there are a variety of options available for speech-language pathologists and audiologists who work in hospital settings. Within this context, it is easy to continue with the medical model approach. However, if the ultimate goal is to create a new life for older people who have been affected by a major illness such as stroke, then rehabilitation and social model approaches also need to be adopted in this setting. The patient should be referred to services that do provide these options if this is not feasible. One of the recurring themes in this text is that, in order to provide a relevant service to older individuals affected by communication disability, audiologists and speech-language pathologists need to listen to their patients. They need to know the issues for the patient at that point in time, they need to understand the patient's dreams and aspirations, and they need to know what annoys them. It is only through careful listening to patients that relevant services can be provided. Some patients may state that their speech is the main concern, whereas others may say they only wish they could hear their grandchildren on the telephone; others may describe the need to talk to people who understand their disorder. All of these can be linked to different levels of the WHO model (2001), and it is this eclectic approach of combining action at the levels of the body, the person, and society that clinicians can use to provide a valued service to older people with a communication disability.

🔑 KEY POINTS

- Older people constitute a large proportion of the caseload of hospital audiologists and speech-language pathologists.

- Although the medical model is the primary approach used, the rehabilitation and social models are also appropriate.

- The sources of communication difficulties in hospitals are the patients' communication impairments, the staff, and the environment.

- Older patients may have a range of preexisting hearing, speech, language, or voice impairments, but may also have been admitted due to a condition that is associated with a new communication disability.

- Patients who have been admitted to a hospital may be under emotional stress.

- There are many staff people in a hospital who communicate with older patients.

- Staff may not have the time or the skill to communicate with older patients.

- Staff may also hold agist stereotypical views of older people, which may lead to elderspeak.

- The physical barriers to a positive communication environment may include excessive noise, lack of privacy, or physical access to devices such as nurse call buttons.

- Hospital policies that improve communication accessibility for older patients are required.

- Creating a positive communication environment within the hospital is considered a social model approach.

- There is a common process for acute care that begins with the screening assessment and diagnosis, ensuring effective communication for patients while they are in the hospital, patient and family education and counseling, implementing impairment-based treatment (if appropriate), and discharge planning.

- Issues in acute care practice include the high level of skill required by clinicians who work in this setting, the potential errors that can occur, and the ethical dilemmas that may occur with older people in a hospital.

- When the primary reason for hospitalization is hearing related, the audiologist is a key health care professional.

- If hearing-related communication problems are occurring for older patients while in the hospital, the audiologist may provide important rehabilitation services (e.g., fitting a hearing aid or assistive listening device).

- Rehabilitation and social models of practice predominate over the medical model in the outpatient setting.

- Individual treatment and group therapy programs appropriate for outpatient settings are described in Chapter 7.

 ## CLASSROOM ACTIVITIES

1. Ask class members who have been patients in a hospital to reflect on what it was like. How easy was it to communicate with staff and family? What was the hospital environment like? Discuss what it would be like for older people with a communication disability, and then discuss ways in which speech-language pathologists and audiologists could help the older person while he or she is in the hospital.

2. Obtain some patient education materials about a topic such as stroke, aphasia, or hearing impairment. Ask the class to appraise the materials in terms of readability, content, and suitability for older people with a communication disability.

RECOMMENDED READING

Cornett, B. S. (1999). *Clinical practice management for speech-language pathologists.* Gaithersburg, MD: Aspen.

Johnson, A. F., & Jacobson, B. H. (1998). *Medical speech-language pathology. A practitioner's guide.* New York: Thieme.

McCooey, R., Toffolo, D., & Code, C. (2000). A socioenvironmental approach to functional communication in hospital inpatients. In L. E. Worrall & C. M. Frattali (Eds.), *Neurogenic communication disorders: A functional approach* (pp. 295–311). New York: Thieme.

 ## REFERENCES

Beech, J. R., Harding, L., & Hilton-Jones, D. (Eds.). (1993). *Assessment in speech and language therapy.* London: Routledge.

Bernier, M. J. (1993). Developing and evaluating printed education materials: A prescriptive model for quality. *Orthopaedic Nursing, 12*(6), 39–46.

Chapman, J., & Langridge, J. (1997). Physiotherapy health education literature. *Physiotherapy, 83*(8), 406–412.

Coulter, A., Entwistle, V., & Gilbert, D. (1999). Sharing decisions with patients: Is the information good enough? *British Medical Journal, 318,* 318–322.

Dabul, B.L. (1979). *Apraxia Battery for Adults.* Austin, TX: Pro-Ed.

Dillon, H., James, A., & Ginis, J. (1997). Client Oriented Scale of Improvement (COSI) and its relationship to several other measures of benefit and satisfaction provided by hearing aids. *Journal of the American Academy of Audiology, 8*(1), 27–43.

Elliot, E. (1984, August). My name is Mrs. Simon. *Ladies Home Journal,* 18, 21, & 150.

Enderby, P. M., Wood, V. A., & Wade, D. T. (1987). *The Frenchay Aphasia Screening Test.* London: NFER-Nelson.

Field, D. (1992) Communication with dying patients in coronary care units. *Intensive and Critical Care Nursing, 8,* 24–32.

Forster, S., Towers, E., & Buttner, A. (1999). *Access for people who are deaf and who have hearing impairments.* (Princess Alexandra Hospital Project Report.) Brisbane, Australia: Princess Alexandra Hospital.

Fridriksson, J. & Holland, A. (2001) Final thoughts on management of aphasia in the early phases of recovery following stroke. *American Journal of Speech-Language Pathology, 10*(1), 37–40.

Healthy Hearing. www.healthyhearing.com

Holland, A., & Fridriksson, J. (2001). Aphasia management during the early phases of recovery following stroke. *American Journal of Speech-Language Pathology, 10*(1), 19–28.

Jarrett, N., & Payne, S. (1995) A selective review of the literature on nurse-patient communication: Has the patient's contribution been neglected? *Journal of Advanced Nursing, 22,* 72–78.

Johnson, A. F., Valachovic, A. M., & George, K. P. (1998). Speech-language pathology practice in the acute care setting: a consultative approach. In A. F. Johnson & B. H. Jacobson (Eds.), *Medical speech-language pathology. A practitioner's guide* (pp. 96–130). New York: Thieme.

Kaplan, E. F., Goodglass, H., & Weintraub, S. (1983). *The Boston Naming Test* (2nd ed.). Philadelphia: Lea & Febiger.

Katz, R. C., Hallowell, B., Code, C., Armstrong, E., Roberts, P., Pound, C., & Katz, L. (2000). A multinational comparison of aphasia management practices. *International Journal of Communication Disorders, 35*(2), 303–314.

Keenan, J.S., & Brassell, E.G. (1975). *Aphasia language performance scales.* Murfreesboro, TN: Pinnacle.

Kersner, M. (1992). *Tests of voice, speech, and language.* London: Whurr Publishers.

Ley, P. (1982). Satisfaction, compliance and communication. *British Journal of Clinical Psychology, 21,* 241–254.

Llenore, E., & Ogle, K. R. (1999). Nurse-patient communication in the intensive care unit: A review of the literature. *Australian Critical Care, 12*(4), 142–145.

Logemann, J. A. (1998). Dysphagia: basic assessment and management issues. In A. F. Johnson & B. H. Jacobson (Eds.), *Medical speech-language pathology. A practitioner's guide* (pp. 17–37). New York: Thieme.

Lubinski, R. (1995). Environmental considerations for elderly residents. In R. Lubinski (Ed.), *Dementia and communication* (pp. 257–278). Clifton Park, NY: Delmar Learning.

Marshall, R. C. (1997). Aphasia treatment in the early postonset period: Managing our resources effectively. *American Journal of Speech-Language Pathology, 6*(1), 5–11.

McCooey, R. (2001). *Communication in the acute hospital setting.* Unpublished masters thesis, The University of Queensland, Brisbane, Australia.

McCooey, R., Toffolo, D., & Code, C. (2000). A socioenvironmental approach to functional communication in hospital inpatients. In L. E. Worrall & C. M. Frattali (Eds.), *Neurogenic communication disorders: A functional approach* (pp. 295–311). New York: Thieme.

Musson, N. D. (1998). An introduction to neurogenic swallowing disorders. In A. F. Johnson & B. H. Jacobson (Eds.), *Medical speech-language pathology. A practitioner's guide* (pp. 354–389). New York: Thieme.

National Center for Health Statistics. (1999). Retrieved 9 October 2001 from the World Wide Web: http://www.cdc.gov/nchswww/faq/avglsl.htm

O'Mahoney, P. G., Rodgers, H., Thomson, R. G., Dobson, R., & James, O. F. W. (1997). Satisfaction with information and advice received by stroke patient. *Clinical Rehabilitation, 11,* 68–72.

Palmer, T. R. & Hunter, M. N. (1998). Issues in geriatric medicine. In A. F. Johnson & B. H. Jacobson (Eds.), *Medical speech-language pathology. A practitioner's guide,* (pp. 131–149). New York: Thieme.

Peach, R. K. (2001). Further thoughts regarding management of acute aphasia following stroke. *American Journal of Speech-Language Pathology, 10*(1), 29–36.

Peterson, H. A., & Marquardt, T. P. (1994). *Appraisal and diagnosis of speech and language disorders* (3rd ed.). Englewood Cliffs, NJ: Prentice Hall.

Pichora-Fuller, M. K. (1997). Assistive listening devices for the elderly. In R. Lubinski & J. Higginbotham (Eds.), *Communication technology for the elderly: Vision, hearing, and speech* (pp. 161–201). Clifton Park, NY: Delmar Learning.

Poltl, S., & Hickson, L. (1990). Hearing status of elderly hospital inpatients. *Australian Journal of Audiology, 12* (2), 79–83.

Royal Brisbane Hospital Outcome Measure for Swallowing. (1998). Available from Speech Pathology Department, Royal Brisbane Hospital, Herston 4029, Queensland, Australia.

Self Help for Hard of Hearing. www.shhh.org.au

Shadden B. B., & Toner M. A. (Eds.). (1997). *Aging and communication: For clinicians by clinicians.* Austin, TX: Pro-Ed.

Sklar, M. (1983). *Sklar Aphasia Scale-Revised.* Los Angeles: Western Psychological Services.

Tippett, D. C., & Sugarman, J. (1996). Viewpoint. Discussing advance directives under the Patient Self-Determination Act: A unique opportunity for speech-language pathologists to help persons with aphasia. *American Journal of Speech Language Pathology, 5*(2), 31–34.

Wellwood, I., Dennis, M. S., & Warlow, C. P. (1994). Perceptions and knowledge of stroke among surviving patients with stroke and their carers. *Age and Aging, 23,* 293–298.

Wertz, R. T. (1997) Comments on "Aphasia treatment in the early postonset period: Managing our resources effectively." *American Journal of Speech Language Pathology, 6*(1), 12–18.

West, J. F. Sands, E., & Ross-Swain, D. (1998). *Bedside Evaluation Screening Test—Second Edition.* Austin, TX: Pro-Ed.

Whurr, R., (1996). *Aphasia Screening Test* (2nd ed.). London: Whurr Publishers.

World Health Organization. (2001). *International classification of functioning, disability and health.* Geneva: Author.

Worrall, L. E. (1999). *Functional Communication Therapy Planner.* Oxon, UK: Winslow Press.

Worrall, L. E., & Yiu, E. (2000). Effectiveness of functional communication therapy by volunteers for people with aphasia following stroke. *Aphasiology, 14,* 911–924.

Ylvisaker, M., Feeney, T., & Urbanczyk, B. (1993). A social-environmental approach to communication and behavior after traumatic brain injury. *Seminars in Speech and Language, 14,* 74–87.

Chapter 9

The Residential Care Environment for the Aged

Many speech-language pathologists and audiologists working in residential care facilities for the aged attempt to apply the medical or rehabilitation model of practice in that setting. In this chapter, it will be argued that a greater emphasis on the social model, focusing on participation, is more appropriate. The care facility is home for many older people and, therefore, the clinician needs to address issues about the environment as well as the individual. The chapter begins with a description of the important characteristics of residential care facilities for the aged from the perspective of speech-language pathology and audiology. The remainder of the chapter is devoted to intervention in residential care facilities: intervention for the individual resident, for the staff and visitors, and for the environment. A model of practice aimed at communication enhancement is presented.

The role of the speech-language pathologist or audiologist in residential care settings for the aged is particularly challenging. The majority of residents have some communication impairment, they are attempting to function in a difficult communication environment and, often, the clinician is only employed part time or as a consultant. This situation means that it may well be necessary to consider interventions that do the greatest good for the greatest number of residents, rather than providing an ideal intervention service for a small number of residents. Interventions that treat the environment will have an impact on all residents, not just those with known communication disability. This represents a paradigm shift away from traditional forms of treatment for the individual client with hearing, speech, or language problems. To understand why this shift is necessary, it is important to first understand the nature of the residential aged care environment for the aged.

Characteristics of Residential Care Facilities for the Aged

The nature of residential care facilities for the aged varies from country to country. In general, however, facilities can be described in terms of the number of residents, ownership (e.g., government, private), source of funds for services (e.g., government, health insurance, resident, or some combination of these), location (e.g., rural, suburban, or metropolitan), and level of care. In the United States, residential care facilities for the aged are called assisted living, intermediate, or long-term care facilities, depending on the level of care or assistance required by the residents. In Australia, residences for those who need less assistance with daily living are called low-care facilities or hostels, and places for those with greater long-term needs are called high-care facilities or nursing homes. In the United Kingdom, there are residential and retirement homes for those who need limited assistance and nursing homes for people who require full-time nursing care.

Clearly, the characteristics of the facility, and in particular the funding arrangements, have an impact on the way a facility functions (e.g., types of services offered, staffing levels). For example, recent changes to Medicare funding for services in residential care facilities for the aged in the United States have had the effect of limiting speech-language pathology services in long-term care environments (ASHA, 2000). Funding arrangements for residential care facilities for the aged are constantly changing and vary considerably from country to country, and it is important that audiologists and speech-language pathologists stay up-to-date with changes in their own regions. Issues of funding aside, the focus of this section is on the common features of residential care environments for the aged that are important from a communication perspective: the residents, staff members who are the residents' most frequent communication partners, and the communication environment within the facility. What communication happens? Who talks to whom and why? Is communication valued?

The Residents

In developed countries, such as the United States, the United Kingdom, and Australia, approximately 5 to 6% of people aged over 65 years (Australian Institute of Health & Welfare, 1997; Federal Interagency Forum on Aging-Related Statistics, 2000) live in care facilities. This increases to approximately 30% of the population for people aged over 85 years. Residents typically have a number of chronic illnesses necessitating the levels of assistance provided in a care facility. The major chronic conditions of residents in developed countries such as the United States, the United Kingdom, Australia, and Canada are (in decreasing order of prevalence) dementia, other mental disorders, cerebrovascular disease, chronic obstructive pulmonary disease, heart disease, and diabetes. Recent data from ASHA's National Outcomes Measurement System (ASHA, 1999) suggest that cerebrovascular disease, respiratory disease, and central nervous system diseases account for over 50% of the primary medical diagnoses for residents treated by speech-language pathologists in skilled nursing facilities in the United States.

Older people come to live in a residential care facility when they are unable to continue to live in the community. The move indicates a growing need for assistance with daily living and usually occurs because of the older person's increasing health problems, coupled with the decreasing ability of the community-based support services (i.e., family, friends, professional agencies) to provide adequate assistance. Moving from the community is less often a choice than a change that is thrust upon the older person, and it is important for clinicians to remember the magnitude of this event. The older person may have moved from a three-bedroom home of his or her own, with friends and family nearby, to a single room in a hospital-like environment, surrounded by strangers. Kaakinen (1995) pointed out the importance of this change from the speech-language pathology and audiology perspective. That is, effective communication is an essential component of coping with this transition and responding to it in a positive way.

Numerous research studies have documented the high prevalence of communication impairments in older people living in residential care facilities, a significantly higher prevalence than is found in the wider elderly community. One of the largest studies of this population was carried out in Australia by Worrall, Hickson, and Dodd (1993), who conducted screening tests of hearing, cognition, language, voice, speech, and pragmatics in 434 residents of care facilities for the aged. The percentage of residents who failed each test is shown in Figure 9–1. It can be seen from this figure that the most common communication impairment was hearing impairment, occurring in 81% of the population. Overall, 95% of the 434 participants had at least one communication impairment. There were originally 535 residents in the study, but only 434 were capable of completing the basic elements of the test battery (i.e., pure-tone audiometry). In most of these cases, the perceived reason for ineligibility was that the person was in the advanced stages of dementia. Thus, many of the 101 residents who could not be assessed had a cognitive communication impairment.

Another feature of the test results was the multiplicity of impairments in this population: combinations of hearing, speech, language, cognitive, voice, and pragmatic disorders.

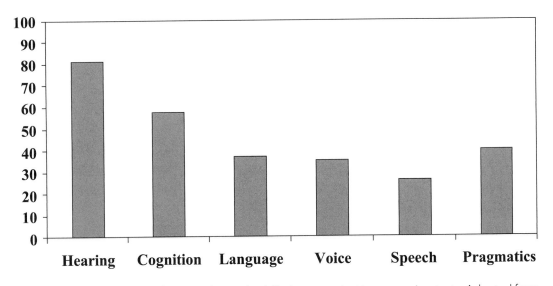

FIGURE 9–1. Percentage of 434 residents who failed communication screening tests. Adapted from Worrall, Hickson, & Dodd (1993).

In total, 70% of the residents who were assessed had more than one impairment, and the breakdown of the percentage of participants who failed two, three, or four tests, and so on, is shown in Figure 9–2. Twenty-one percent failed two screening tests, with the most common combination being hearing and cognitive disorders. Six percent of the sample failed all six screening tests.

Research data on the relationship between hearing impairment and dementia indicate that hearing impairment is a risk factor for cognitive decline in older people and that it may exacerbate the symptoms of dementia (Peters, Polter, & Scholer, 1988; Uhlmann, Larson, Thomas, Koepsell, & Duckert, 1989). Peters et al. conducted a longitudinal study of 38 older people with dementia and found that the decline in cognitive status was greater for participants with moderate hearing impairment than for those with normal or mild hearing loss. Uhlmann et al. compared 100 people with dementia of the Alzheimer's type to 100 people without dementia, matched for age, gender, and educational level. The mean hearing level of the group with dementia was significantly worse than the control group, and the prevalence of hearing impairment was significantly higher in the group with dementia (59% compared to 44% of the control group).

Hearing impairment is the most prevalent communication impairment in the residential population. Researchers have found that the prevalence of hearing loss ranges from 77 to 95% (Garahan, Waller, Houghton, Tisdale, & Runge, 1992; Gutnick, Zillmer, & Philput, 1989; Schow & Nerbonne, 1980; Worrall et al., 1993). Stumer, Hickson, and Worrall (1996)

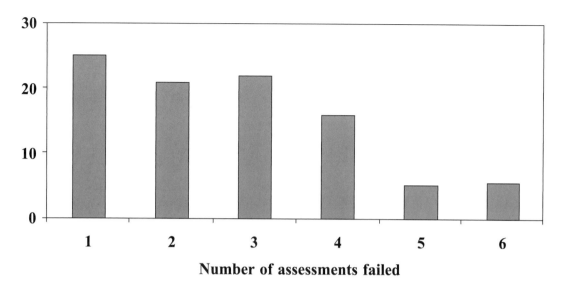

FIGURE 9–2. Percentage of 434 residents who failed different numbers of screening tests. Adapted from Worrall, Hickson, & Dodd (1993).

found that although 95% of 129 residents assessed in their study had a hearing impairment, only 27% reported any associated activity limitations and participation restrictions. This finding may be due to other health concerns taking priority for the residents and is no doubt related to the poor communication environment, which is discussed later in this section. Many residents not reporting any difficulties with hearing in everyday life in a facility suggests that conventional aural rehabilitation (i.e., hearing aid fitting) may not be acceptable to many residents. Older people make decisions about whether to wear hearing aids based on their communication needs: If a need is not recognized, then the hearing aid will not be worn.

Other impairments that were not assessed by Worrall et al. (1993) and may need to be considered by speech-language pathologists and audiologists working in residential care facilities for the aged are vision impairments and swallowing difficulties. Erber and Scherer (1999) reported that many residents have dual sensory loss (i.e., both hearing and vision impairments), and some of the possible consequences are breakdown in communication, loss of independence, social isolation, depression, and dementialike behaviors. Swallowing disorders are a common problem for residents seen by speech-language pathologists (ASHA, 2000). Sorin-Peters, Tse, and Kapelus (1989) reported that 13% of the residents in their study had swallowing difficulties. Swallowing problems have important nutritional implications, with reports of malnutrition in residents in care facilities in the United States ranging from 12 to 70% (Cooper & Cobb, 1988).

The Staff

Staff who work in residential care facilities for the aged are all potential communication partners for the residents. The major category of staff is nursing, consisting of nurses with various levels of training, and nursing assistants. Burgio and Scilley (1994) report that, in the United States, the majority of residents' care is provided by nursing assistants. In addition to nurses, most facilities also have personal care assistants, physicians, housekeepers, pastoral caregivers, and administrators. Depending on the funding to the facilities, some facilities may have (either on staff or on a consultancy basis) physical therapists, occupational therapists, speech-language pathologists, dietitians, social workers, activities officers, recreational therapists, and volunteers. The staff is predominantly female, and high staff turnover rates are reported.

What do these potential communication partners know about communication? What are their attitudes toward communication with residents? Evidence suggests that staff do not necessarily see the importance of communication for residents' quality of life and that communication is undervalued in preference to physical and medical care (Parker, 1987). Oliver and Redfern (1991) reported that nurse-resident interactions were typically of short duration, and most interaction (72%) was concerned with the physical aspects of nursing care.

This focus on physical care may well be related to time pressures in the work situation. In many facilities, nurses have to care for a number of residents who require a high level of assistance. The "if only there was more time" attitude is borne out by the results of a study by Kato, Hickson, and Worrall (1996). They interviewed 32 staff at one residential care facility for the aged and found generally positive attitudes about communication. Staff wanted more time to communicate with residents, and they were keen to have further training about communication. The authors concluded that "the problem appears to be one of resource allocation, rather than attitude" (p. 29).

Another issue that was evident in the Kato et al. (1996) study and in a number of other research reports was the lack of staff knowledge and awareness about the communication impairments of residents. Koury and Lubinski (1995) reported that nursing assistants had little knowledge of the nature of communication disability associated with dementia. Garahan et al. (1992) compared actual measured hearing impairment with file notes on hearing loss. In a sample of 121 residents, 77% had a hearing loss of some degree in the better ear; however, only 40% of this group had any documentation about the hearing loss in their files. Hopper, Bayles, Harris, and Holland (2001) also compared subjective reports with objective measures in 55 residents with dementia. All of the residents failed the hearing screening, yet only 15 (27%) were rated by nurses as having any hearing problems. Similarly, Burnip and Erber (1996) described how nursing staff frequently underestimate the effect of hearing loss on the communication of residents. In their Australian study on data collated for 44,012 residents, nursing staff identified 37.3% as having any hearing problems, a figure that is much lower than the actual prevalence for this population.

The Communication Environment

A number of research studies have shown that there tends to be little communication in residential care facilities and, when it does occur, it is poor quality communication (see Lubinski, 1995b for a review). To understand the communication problems faced by older people in residential care, speech-language pathologists and audiologists must understand the residents, their communication partners, and the environment in which interactions occur. Lubinski, Morrison, and Rigrodsky (1981) described the residential care facility for the aged as a communication-impaired environment. The environment is not just a passive backdrop for communication, but is an active contributor that affects how older people function. In this section, both the physical and social aspects of the environment that hinder effective communication are discussed.

THE PHYSICAL ENVIRONMENT

The physical residential care environment can be thought of at a macro and a micro level. The macro level consists of buildings, corridors, rooms, communal areas, gardens, and so forth. The micro level refers to more flexible components of the facility such as furniture, floor coverings, wall hangings, and chairs. Features of the environment that can adversely influence communication have been identified at both levels. At the macro level, facilities have been criticized for lack of space and privacy, few activity areas, and poor accessibility to communal rooms (Lubinski, 1995c). At the micro level, the major criticisms revolve around the poor sensory environment. From an acoustic point of view, hard floor and wall coverings typically used in residential facilities result in excessive noise and reverberation. Similarly, from a visual point of view, shiny reflective surfaces cause glare, and dimly lit corridors limit residents' ability to move about (Jones, Sloane, & Alexander, 1992). Another aspect of the micro physical environment that can be problematic for communication is the placement of furniture. For example, chairs lined up in rows against a wall are not a seating arrangement that is conducive to people sitting down to talk.

THE SOCIAL ENVIRONMENT

Investigation of the social world of residential care facilities for the aged has revealed still more barriers to communication. There are problems with resident-resident interactions and with resident-staff interactions. Resident-resident relationships, although not close, have nevertheless been found to be important for social support and for helping residents cope with the difficulties and stresses of life in a residential care facility (Guthiel, 1991). Unfortunately, resident-resident communication does not occur often (Bitzan & Kruzich,

1990). Kovach and Robinson (1996) studied communication between roommates in residential care and found that approximately half of the 50 residents surveyed never talked to their roommates. "Most of the reasons for this centered around physical barriers to communication such as hearing problems and speech impediments" (p. 627).

Lubinski (1995b) and Kaakinen (1995) provided summaries of the research on impoverished resident communication. Residents may not talk because they believe they have few meaningful contributions to make to conversation. They see that they have few people to communicate with, few topics for conversations, and few reasons to talk. Residents are also aware of restrictive unwritten rules that limit communication (Kaakinen, 1995, p. 39; Lubinski, 1995b, p. 7) such as

- not to talk to those with communication problems
- not to complain
- not to have private conversations when other people might be listening
- not to bother staff
- not to talk with the opposite sex
- not to talk about loneliness, dying, and illness, and
- not to talk too much.

As stated earlier in this chapter, resident-staff interactions have been found to be limited to mainly the physical aspects of care. Staff communication with residents has also been criticized in terms of the manner or style of the discourse. Some staff have been reported as frequently using elderspeak in residential care facilities for the aged. *Elderspeak* is a way of speaking based on agist stereotypes and is characterized by slow rate, increased loudness, greater repetitions, high pitch, exaggerated intonation, reduced complexity of syntactical structure, and simplified vocabulary (Coupland, Coupland, Giles, & Henwood, 1988). The effects of elderspeak are that the resident has fewer communication opportunities, there is less need for the older person to start a conversation, and there is a decrease in satisfaction with interactions (Ryan, 1991).

Baltes, Neumann, and Zank (1994) described the interactions between staff and residents as following a *dependency-support* script. This finding is important because of the link between autonomy and well-being, that is, the dependency pattern can lead to reduced quality of life for the resident. Dependency is a behavior that results in social contact and attention from staff, "a highly valued commodity in institutions" (p. 179). Some staff apply this script to all residents, expecting all to be dependent. The long-term consequences of this script are that the older person will do less for him- or herself and actual abilities will decline from lack of use. An example of *dependence-independence supportive* scripts, with dependent behavior beginning the interaction, is as follows. An older person is sitting in front of a tray of food staring at it. The staff member says "That's great, you're waiting for me to feed you" (*dependence-supportive*) or "Come on, you can do it by yourself" (*independence-supportive*). Another example, beginning with an independent behavior, is an older person putting on a shirt. The staff member takes the shirt and starts dressing the person (*dependence-supportive*) or makes the bed while the older person continues to dress (*independence-supportive*). Baltes et al. then go on to describe a training program aimed at reducing the dependency script.

In summary, the communication in residential care facilities is generally poor. This is because of complex interactions among the difficulties of the resident, the staff, and the physical and social environment in which they find themselves. What can audiologists and speech-language pathologists do to improve this situation? The following sections contain a model of practice for work in residential care facilities for the aged. In addition, numerous ideas for intervention are presented. The methods chosen will largely depend on the clinical time available and the funding arrangements for services.

Model of Practice for Speech-Language Pathologists and Audiologists

The current practice of speech-language pathologists in care facilities for the aged in the United States is described by data submitted to the ASHA National Outcome Measurement System (NOMS: ASHA, 1999). Sixty-six clinicians from 48 skilled nursing facilities submitted outcome data on 392 patients. An average of approximately 10 hours per patient was spent on speech-language pathology intervention. The majority of hours (8.8 hours) was spent in individual treatment, 3.3 hours were spent conducting group treatment, 1.6 hours were spent in training or consultation, and 1.4 hours were spent in evaluation or assessment. These data suggest that the focus of current practice in the United States is on conventional individual modes of intervention, applying either a medical or rehabilitation model of practice (see Chapter 3). Comparable figures for audiology practice or speech-language pathology practice in other countries are not available.

In terms of the models of practice presented in Chapter 3, it is argued here that work in residential care facilities lends itself to the social model of practice. In this model, the focus is on participation and the society in which the older person exists; in this case, the society is the residential care facility for the aged. This is not to say that the clinician should ignore the individual resident's communication impairments and activity limitations. The ideal service for an older person living in a residential care facility would include both individual intervention (e.g., hearing aid fitting, aphasia therapy) and intervention at the level of the society (e.g., training for staff, decreasing background noise in the environment). It is argued, however, that the most cost-effective benefit for the resident (and indeed all the residents in the facility) will come from societal level intervention. For example, staff education programs can be considered a societal level intervention, and if staff learn to value communication and become better communicators, it will positively affect their interactions with all residents.

Pye, Worrall, and Hickson (2000) also presented the argument that it is not appropriate to treat the individual in isolation when the environment clearly adversely affects their ability to communicate. In line with the WHO framework (2001), they advocate that intervention should be at the levels of body, activity, and participation. The authors identify three steps in the process of meeting the challenge of working in a residential care facility for the aged:

1. Acknowledge that the medical model of practice generally used in acute care hospital settings is not appropriate for work in residential care facilities for the aged. Although audiologists and speech-language pathologists still have to understand the individual's communication impairments, and comprehensive communication assessments may be necessary, the impairments should not necessarily be the focus of intervention.

2. Increase the range and quality of communication activities in the facility. Residents need opportunities to communicate, as well as the ability to do so.

3. Facilitate participation in this environment. By targeting participation restriction issues in a residential care facility, the speech-language pathologist or audiologist can have a significant impact on improving the quality of life of all residents, not just those clients with specific communication disabilities.

In the remainder of this section, interventions for the residents (individual and group programs), the staff, and the physical and social environment are presented. This division is for ease of presentation only and is not meant to imply that the clinician should choose one way or another. Holistic intervention incorporating a number of areas is preferable and, in the final section of the chapter, case studies are described to illustrate this approach.

Intervention for the Residents

INDIVIDUAL PROGRAMS

It is important for the communication impairments of residents to be assessed and documented on admission to the facility and at regular intervals (i.e., every 6 months) postadmission. The reasons why such assessments are important are that (a) funding is often linked to the impairments of residents (Pye et al., 2000), and (b) the clinician needs to be aware of the residents' difficulties so that he or she can develop appropriate interventions and begin the process of resident, family, and staff education. In terms of funding, if speech-language pathologists and audiologists do not document the high prevalence of impairment in the residential care facility, then there will be insufficient funds to employ speech-language pathologists and audiologists. As stated earlier in the chapter, Burnip and Erber (1996) investigated nursing staff awareness of communication impairments and found that nurses seriously underestimate the prevalence of communication impairments among residents. This has resource implications in Australia because financial allocations for residents are based on the amount of care they will require. The tool used currently to determine level of care is the Resident Classification Scale (RCS; Commonwealth Department of Health and Family Services, 1997). The RCS contains items about the speech, language, hearing, and swallowing impairments of residents. If these are not assessed appropriately and recorded, the facility will receive less funding per resident. This reduced funding will, in turn, adversely affect the availability of appropriate resources for residents.

Lubinski (1995b) described a similar instrument to the RCS called the Resident Assessment Instrument (RAI), which is used in the United States. Assessments are conducted at set intervals (e.g., quarterly, annually) or when a significant change in condition is observed. The RAI consists of two components that are used to quantify and describe the status of each resident: the Minimum Data Set (MDS) and the Resident Assessment Protocols (RAPs). The MDS consists of 74 items, which cover the resident's functional status in 16 domains, one of which is Communication/Hearing. Items are scored by nurses in consultation with residents, family, and staff. If a communication and/or hearing difficulty is identified on the MDS, then the RAPs are completed for that particular domain. These protocols are more descriptive and can include information about the cause of a problem, risk factors, resident's strengths and weakness, and any other information that can help guide further intervention (Hopper et al., 2001). Individual care plans are formulated based on MDS and RAPs results. The importance of such tools from the perspective of speech-language pathology and audiology is obvious: Communication impairments need to be recognized by nursing staff in order for specialist intervention to occur. This importance is highlighted by a recent study conducted by Hopper et al. (2001). Of 55 residents with cognitive communication and hearing impairments, less than half were rated on the MDS as having any communication or hearing problems, and, of these, none had been referred for further assessments by a speech-language pathologist or audiologist.

When the opportunity does arise for audiologists and speech-language pathologists to assess individual residents, an important point to remember is the multiplicity of impairments in this population. In particular, as stated earlier in the chapter, there is a high prevalence of dementia and hearing impairment, and these conditions might affect other assessment procedures. The effect of hearing impairment on assessment results is highlighted in a study by Weinstein and Amsel (1986). They showed that amplification improved the performance of residents with moderate to severe hearing impairment on a mental state examination,

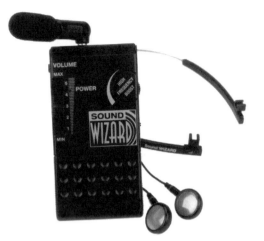

FIGURE 9–3. Example of a personal amplification assistive listening device. (Photograph used with permission from HITEC Group Int'l, Inc.)

suggesting the possibility that some of these residents would have been incorrectly assessed as having dementia if the amplification had not been provided. If a resident does not have a hearing aid, then a personal amplification assistive listening device could be used in this situation. These one-to-one, relatively inexpensive communication devices generally consist of a small body-worn case containing a microphone and amplifier (see Figure 9–3). The signal is presented to the listener via a standard set of headphones, thus customized ear molds are not required. Indeed, Rizzolo and Snow (1989) reported that the use of such devices was helpful in many circumstances in a residential care facility for the aged (e.g., for case history interviews, medical examinations, and interactions among staff and residents).

In the instance where an audiologist is assessing the hearing of a resident with dementia, it is essential that the clinician modify the assessment process to obtain accurate thresholds. Techniques for this process are outlined in Chapter 4. It is also important that the audiologist validate results by observing the resident in communication situations. For example, is the pure-tone audiometry finding of a severe hearing impairment in line with the resident's responses to sounds in the residential care facility? If this is not possible because the resident is assessed in an audiology clinic outside the care facility, then the audiologist could validate results by interviewing staff and/or significant others about the resident's communication.

To formulate a comprehensive intervention program for the individual resident, it is necessary for the clinician to assess the residents' communication activity limitations and participation restrictions, as well as their impairments. Few activity or participation level measures exist for older people living in residential care facilities. In audiology, the Nursing Home Hearing Handicap Index: Self Version for Resident and Staff Version (Schow & Nerbonne, 1977) may be used (see Chapter 5 Appendix D). This assessment can be useful, although experience suggests that the response scale needs to be modified to a 3-point, rather than a 5-point, scale for this population (Stumer et al., 1996). Currently, there is no speech-language pathology assessment designed specifically for this population. Pye et al.,

(2000) stated that the nature, duration, and quality of everyday communication in the facility need to be determined, and that, as no specific tools exist, this is best undertaken by observing the residents' communication, or by asking them and/or their significant others about communication. It is possible that some of the assessments of activity limitations and participation restrictions and quality of life previously described in Chapters 5 and 6 may also be used with residents; however, more research is necessary to determine their applicability to this population.

Pichora-Fuller and Robertson (1994) described another method of determining the everyday communication needs of residents. Although designed for residents with hearing impairment, the technique could be expanded for use with all residents. In this approach, residents were asked "When in your everyday life is it important to hear?" The 14 key situations identified by residents are shown in Figure 9–4. In terms of hours per month, the situations that residents were most commonly involved in were in the dining room and watching television. For speech-language pathology assessment, the question could be modified to "When in your everyday life is it important to be able to talk?" The situations when understanding, reading, and writing are important may also be elicited using this type of question. The communication needs identified can subsequently become the focus of intervention.

Once the individual resident's communication impairments, activity limitations, and participation restrictions have been assessed, then an individual intervention program can

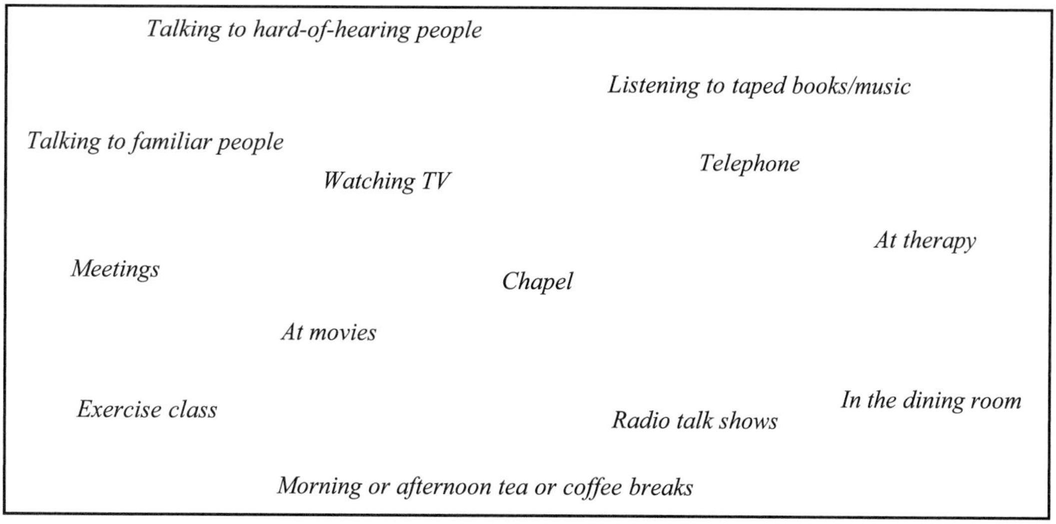

FIGURE 9–4. Situations and activities in which residents say it is important for them to hear. Adapted from Pichora-Fuller & Robertson, (1994).

be designed if necessary. The Functional Communication Therapy Planner (FCTP; Worrall, 1999), as discussed in Chapter 7, is a step-by-step process for establishing, treating, and evaluating intervention goals that can be used in this situation. Intervention goals aimed at improving communication can be set collaboratively by the resident, the clinician, staff, and significant others. Typically, the goals identified relate to everyday activities undertaken by the resident in the care facility. For example, the goal for a resident with hearing impairment may be to hear a roommate better. Intervention may take many forms: provision of an assistive listening device, education about hearing tactics, coaching the resident about what to do when communication breaks down, and so forth. In a speech-language pathology context, the goal for a client with dysarthria might be to converse at the dinner table. Intervention may include practicing strategies to improve intelligibility, rehearsing scripts for initiating and maintaining conversation, conversing at times when the room is quieter and no one is eating, and having conversational partners at the dinner table who are not hearing impaired.

Conventional individual intervention for residents with hearing impairment can be problematic. Hearing aids that might be suitable for older people living in the community can pose problems in the residential care facility. Pichora-Fuller (1997) provided a comprehensive description of the potential for assistive listening devices in this setting. Devices are available to enhance telephone and television listening, to improve listening in public rooms, to alert people with hearing impairment to an auditory signal by converting it to a visual or tactile signal (e.g., flashing light fire alarm), and to improve one-to-one communication. Assistive listening devices can be used in conjunction with hearing aids or on their own. Despite the wide range of available technology, however, the reported use of hearing aids and assistive listening devices by residents of care facilities has been very low. For example, Bradley and Molloy (1991) found that many hearing aids in nursing homes were not working or were in need of repair (32% of in-the-ear hearing aids, 63% of behind-the-ear hearing aids). In situations where audiologists are employed in a facility, the use of amplification is much better. For example, Lewsen and Cashman (1997) reported that 82% of residents used hearing aids regularly, and 88% used assistive listening devices regularly in their facility. An audiologist provided an on-site assessment and hearing aid dispensing service, and a hearing aid technician was available half-time to service and maintain amplification devices. This is not the norm, however, and, in the vast majority of cases, an audiologist works as a consultant only to a facility and visits the facility rarely. Lubinski, Stecker, Weinstein, and Volin (1993) surveyed audiologists and nursing home administrators in New York State to find out why audiological services were so limited when the demand was so high. The major reasons given were lack of funding, lack of onsite testing facilities, cost of transporting residents to offsite clinics, the physical health of residents, unfamiliarity of nursing staff with hearing loss and hearing aids, and the cognitive problems of residents.

So, what can be done at an individual level to assist residents with hearing impairment? First, the audiologist needs to work with the resident, staff, and significant others to choose the most appropriate form of amplification. A simple personal listening device, with body-worn amplifier and microphone, large controls, and walkman-style headphones (see Figure 9–3), may be more appropriate than a complicated, small, difficult-to-manage hearing aid. If a hearing aid is preferred, in-the-ear hearing aids have been found to be easier for older people to insert than behind-the-ear hearing aids (Upfold, May, & Battaglia, 1990). If television listening is the only activity of interest to the resident, then a dedicated assistive listening device might be best for that particular resident. Second, the research indicates that if hearing aid and/or assistive listening device fitting is to be successful, the residents need onsite support to manage these devices. If audiologists are not available, as is often the case, the support could be provided by staff (e.g., speech-language pathologists, nurses, personal care assistants), significant others, or volunteers. Whoever takes on this task has to have a commitment to the process, not just be allocated the task as another duty, and must have appropriate training provided by an audiologist. Dahl (1997) describes the successful use of trained volunteers in residential care facilities to provide support to residents with hearing impairment, staff, and significant others. Thirty-one volunteers with hearing impairment were recruited through the Canadian Hard of Hearing Association and attended an initial week-long training session and a follow-up session 3 months later. Volunteers were required to commit to visiting residents for one half day per week. A qualitative external evaluation of this project by Carson (1997) indicated that the benefits of this project were (a) the positive effect the role modeling by the volunteers had on residents and staff, (b) the acceptance of the volunteers by both residents and staff, (c) and the increased awareness by staff of hearing loss and its effects.

Palmer, Adams, Durrant, Bourgeois, and Rossi (1998) describe an individual intervention for a person with Alzheimer's disease and moderate dementia that exemplifies the benefits of appropriate amplification selection coupled with client support. The older person in this study was fitted with an in-the-ear hearing aid that had automatic signal processing and did not require a volume control, a feature that would have caused management difficulties. In terms of support, the older person's spouse was educated about hearing aid management and took on the role of caring for the hearing aid. Hours of hearing aid use were gradually increased. The fitting was deemed successful because the client eventually wore the hearing aid for approximately 15 hours per day without complaint. In addition, the spouse noted a reduction in problem behaviors such as pacing, negative statements, repeating, and searching. This result indicates the potential for successful intervention for people with hearing impairment and cognitive decline, if the traditional process of intervention is modified appropriately.

In summary, individual intervention for residents must begin with a comprehensive assessment of their communication impairments, activity limitations, and participation restrictions. The problems identified may then become areas for intervention, depending on the goals for intervention determined by the clinician in collaboration with the resident, the significant others, and the staff. It is important that staff provided with new technology in the form of hearing aids and assistive listening devices be given sufficient support to be able to make use of them.

GROUP COMMUNICATION PROGRAMS

Group communication programs have been recommended for residents, either as a supplement or as an alternative to conventional one-on-one treatment. These benefits may include generalization of strategies learned in individual therapy, conversational practice, opportunities to form friendships, as well as the psychological and emotional support that most members report from attending group programs. It is argued that such programs are extremely appropriate in the residential care environment, as they provide opportunities to communicate that older people otherwise do not have. However, not all residents will want to participate in groups, and not all will be suitable for group work. Group members are often chosen on the basis of the type of their communication disability (e.g., hearing impairment, aphasia, Parkinson's disease), but groups that have a common purpose (e.g., reading the daily newspaper, rehearsing intelligibility strategies, organizing a social event) may also be successful. The latter groups may include residents with a range of communication problems who are interested in the activity of the group. No matter how carefully the therapist chooses group participants, selection of the appropriate mix of group members does not always end in success. Group dynamics in communicatively disabled groups is the same as any other group or class. Balancing the number of talkers and nontalkers is considered a key to success.

It is important to establish goals for any group program, and the goals will vary depending on the participants. Goal setting could be accomplished collaboratively by group members, their significant others, and the clinician. There can be a mixture of goals for individuals within the group and for the group as a whole. For example, one member of the group may have the goal of initiating conversation more often, whereas another has the goal of using self-cueing strategies during word-finding difficulties. The group as a whole may have the goal of organizing the Christmas party or understanding aphasia. The conversation involved in both of these group activities is relevant to each member's individual goals.

Rustin and Kuhr (1999) have written an excellent book that contains numerous examples (113) of group activities for people with speech and language difficulties. Many of these would be appropriate for use with older people living in residential care facilities and, indeed, could be used for group programs in the community or in hospital settings. Each activity focuses on a different range of skills that the authors describe as foundation skills (e.g., eye-contact, listening, relaxation), interaction skills (e.g., greetings, answering questions, asking questions), affective skills (e.g., identification of feelings, trust, disclosures), and cognitive skills (e.g., social perception, problem solving, negotiating). For example, *persuasion* involves the following steps.

1. The group is divided into pairs. One member is chosen to sit down on a chair and his or her partner to stand up.
2. The person standing up is given two minutes to persuade the person sitting down to give up his or her chair. The person doing the persuading is instructed to use a range of strategies apart from physical violence. After two minutes, roles are reversed.
3. The group re-forms to discuss feelings evoked in the different roles. (Rustin & Kuhr, 1999, p. 220).

Jordan, Worrall, Hickson, and Dodd (1993) developed and evaluated an intervention program for groups of residents with specific communication disabilities relating to hearing impairment, Parkinson's disease, stroke, and dementia. The features of the program are listed in Figure 9–5. A trained volunteer facilitated the group sessions. Volunteers were recruited through a variety of sources including a local support group for people with hearing impairment and by advertising in a community newspaper. Volunteers attended two training sessions, each of 4 hours' duration, conducted by a speech-language pathologist. The content of the training sessions included information about

1. communication disability and older people;
2. specific disease processes related to the groups (i.e., hearing impairment, Parkinson's disease, etc.);
3. the content of the intervention program; and
4. the residential care facility.

The speech-language pathologist also provided support and guidance to the volunteers over the course of the program. The group intervention program was evaluated using three sources of information pre- and posttreatment: the clinician's evaluation of the resident's communicative competence, the caregiver's evaluation of the resident's communicative competence, and the resident's change in knowledge over the program period. A knowledge-based questionnaire was devised that asked the residents specific questions about the educational material covered in the group program. Of the 21 residents assessed, 13 participants (62%) showed improvement on at least one measure, 7 participants (33%) improved on two measures, and one participant (5%) improved on all three measures. For the group of 21 as a whole, significant improvements were found on the knowledge-based questionnaire only, and this improvement was most pronounced for the hearing-impaired resident group. Education is vital in chronic disease management. Information sharing enhances shared decision making between practitioner and resident, decreases anxiety, and

- Consists of four different programs for groups of residents with hearing impairment, Parkinson's disease, stroke, and dementia
- Developed by speech-language pathologists and audiologists
- Six weekly group sessions on different topics
- Each session is 2 hours
- Recommended group size is six to eight participants
- Potential participants are identified by the speech-language pathologist or audiologist in consultation with staff
- Groups are facilitated by a trained volunteer group leader
- A detailed manual is provided, with script and handout materials
- Each session is a mix of information giving, discussion, and practical components

Components of the hearing impairment program	■ The communication process: What is involved? What makes a good communicator? ■ Common misconceptions about hearing loss ■ Making your communication successful ■ Basic management of hearing aids ■ Basic assistive listening devices ■ Rules of conversation
Components of the dementia program	■ The communication process: What is involved? What makes a good communicator? ■ Making sure you get the message ■ Getting your message across ■ Strategies to overcome memory loss ■ Rules of conversation
Components of the Parkinson's program	■ What is Parkinson's disease? ■ The communication process: What is involved? What makes a good communicator? ■ How does Parkinson's disease affect your communication? ■ Making sure you get the message ■ Getting your message across ■ Strategies to overcome memory loss ■ Rules of conversation

continues

FIGURE 9–5. Outline of the *Communication and the Elderly* program. Adapted from Jordan et al. (1993).

Components of the stroke program	■ What is stroke? How may it affect you?
	■ The communication process: What is involved? What makes a good communicator?
	■ How does having a stroke affect your communication?
	■ Making sure you get the message
	■ Getting your message across
	■ Strategies to overcome memory loss
	■ Rules of conversation

FIGURE 9–5. Continued.

encourages realistic expectations and better coping strategies. It may also lead to the resident taking action that enhances communication, such as requesting a hearing assessment or joining an activity group. The results obtained in this study by Jordan et al. suggested that group intervention programs run by volunteers might be beneficial for residents with communication disability.

Jennings and Head (1997) conducted a resident education program focused on hearing impairment only. The goals of the program were (a) to increase residents' knowledge of hearing loss and the realistic benefits of hearing aids and (b) to improve communication interactions for residents with hearing impairment. Both individual and group sessions were included, and the authors commented on the advantage of the group setting over the individual. Information was provided on hearing aids, assistive listening devices, communication strategies, environmental coping, nonspeech information, and speechreading. Positive outcomes of the program were

1. increased resident attendance at activities in the facility,
2. more residents talking to those with hearing problems,
3. improvements in the residents' abilities to find solutions for everyday communication problems, and
4. increased knowledge of and ability to use assistive listening devices.

Intervention for the Residential Care Facility Environment

Speech-language pathologists and audiologists need to undertake activities in three major areas in order to enhance the communication environment of the residential care facility for the aged. First, staff education programs are necessary to increase awareness of the importance of communication and to provide staff with the skills to communicate more effectively with the residents. Second, modifications to the physical environment can mean that people are able to communicate more easily. Finally, changes to the social environment can facilitate communication and increase opportunities for interactions.

Lubinski (1995c) has developed a useful tool to use for evaluating the communication environment, a tool that will help the clinician know where to start. The Communication Environmental Assessment and Planning Guide contains a checklist of 44 questions about the physical environment (e.g., *Do caregivers control background noise during conversations and care?*) and 19 questions about the psychosocial environment (e.g., *Is communication an integral part of all interactions and activities?*). If problems are identified in any area, then an action plan is recorded on the guide.

PROGRAMS FOR STAFF

Lubinski (1995b) sees the in-depth in-service training of staff in residential care facilities for the aged as an expanding and nontraditional role for audiologists and speech-language pathologists. She points out that such training needs to be frequent because of the high staff turnover in many facilities. Training should not be totally didactic in nature and should include experiential components such as role play of communication scenarios. Staff programs can have both individual and group components, although the latter tends to occur most often, as group programs are more cost-effective. If possible, training should be provided to all members of the staff (e.g., nurses, activities officers, pastoral care workers), as they all form a part of the communication environment.

Areas that could be covered in a staff education program are

1. *The importance of communication to the quality of life of the residents.* The most effective way to get this message across to staff is to begin by encouraging them to consider their own lives and the elements that contribute to quality of life, that is, what is important to them. Responses typically revolve around relationships with family and friends. Communication is essential for the maintenance of such relationships. From that point, the staff members are asked to put themselves in the shoes of the residents and consider what is most important to them. Residents, too, value their relationships with family, friends, and staff.

2. *The importance of staff in the communication process.* The aim of this section of the program is for staff members to understand that they are major communication partners for residents and that they need to make the most of any communication opportunities that occur in the facility. Ask staff members to think about the communication opportunities that residents have in the facility. Who do residents get to talk to? When does conversation occur? Although the majority of staff may spend a great deal of time on physical aspects of care, it should be pointed out that many of these caregiving activities (e.g., showering, dressing, providing medication) can also be a chance to have a meaningful conversation with a resident.

3. *How staff can identify residents with communication problems.* The aim of this component of the program is to raise staff awareness about the communication problems of

residents. Insight into the communication difficulties of residents is the first step in the problem-solving process of effective communication with residents. Erber and Scherer (1999) provide a list of ideas to assist staff to identify residents with communication difficulty (see Figure 9–6).

4. *How staff can use problem-solving skills to facilitate effective communication with residents.* Table 9–1 contains a number of ideas for staff about how to improve communication with residents who have hearing impairment. Although it must be emphasized that these are potential strategies not to be used with all residents, they may help staff to accommodate to altered communication patterns of residents. It is important to emphasize that the main aim is to accommodate to each interactant's individual cues. This accommodation will avoid stereotypical communication behaviors such as elderspeak and the dependence-supportive scripts described earlier in this chapter. Although lists of strategies are useful as a basis for training, it is also important to include practice of these techniques. Such practice could be via role play during the education program and/or could be undertaken in real life. Koury and Lubinski (1995) pointed out that role plays are particularly useful because they encourage staff to actively participate and "Mistakes have no penalties; they occur in an informal, protected environment and serve to reinforce appropriate

---

Ask the resident and/or their significant others if he or she has hearing or vision or communication difficulties.

Check the resident's medical history for conditions associated with communication difficulties.

Check the resident's chart for specialist and speech-language pathology and audiology reports.

Observe the resident and note the following:

☐ Does the resident watch the speaker's lips intently?

☐ Does the resident rely on hearing aids or spectacles?

☐ Does the resident misunderstand what is said?

☐ Does the resident ask for repetition often?

☐ Does the resident have trouble understanding soft/high-pitched voices, rapid speech, or complex messages?

☐ Does the resident have trouble understanding at a distance, when he or she cannot see the speaker's face, or when there is any noise?

☐ Does the resident speak in an inappropriately loud voice and/or dominate conversation?

FIGURE 9–6. Tips to help staff identify residents with communication problems. Adapted with permission from Erber, N. P., & Scherer, S. C. (1999). Sensory loss and communication difficulties in the elderly. *Australasian Journal on Aging, 18*(1), 4–9.

TABLE 9–1

POTENTIAL STRATEGIES FOR STAFF TO COMMUNICATE EFFECTIVELY WITH RESIDENTS WITH HEARING IMPAIRMENT.

Gain the resident's attention	Make sure that the resident knows you are talking to him or her, for example, say the resident's name, tap the person on the shoulder, and establish eye contact.
Use topic cues	Cue the resident in to what you are going to talk about by identifying the topic first.
Simplify your language	Talk in short simple sentences. Avoid long and involved sentence constructions.
Comprehension checks	If you are not sure whether the resident has understood what you have said, ask him or her to repeat what you said.
Let the resident see your face	Residents can pick up a lot of information from your lips, face, and general body movements, so it is best to talk to them directly using a normal tone of voice.
Decrease glare	Many residents have vision as well as hearing problems and need to see your face as clearly as possible during conversation. Do not stand in front of a bright light or a window, as this will be distracting and will cast a shadow over your face.
Speak slowly	Speaking just a little more slowly than normal can help the resident to process what he or she hears.
Be patient	Try to avoid speaking for the resident by finishing his or her sentences, as this can be frustrating for the resident.
Decrease distance	Move closer to the resident when talking.
Decrease noise	Try to reduce the noise in the area where you are trying to talk or move the resident to a quiet location to talk.

Note: Adapted from Dodd, Worrall, & Hickson (1990) and Erber & Scherer (1999).

behavior" (p. 283). For real-life practice, the speech-language pathologist or audiologist could work with staff members and act as a coach (see Ylvisaker & Holland, 1985). If communication breaks down during a staff-resident interaction, the clinician could advise the staff member what to do and, if necessary, model an effective communication approach.

5. *How staff can assist residents with known communication disabilities who require specialized help.* Staff need to know how they can access audiology and speech-language pathology services for specific clients and what type of service will be provided (e.g., that advice will be placed in the personal care plans of clients). Residents with hearing impairment often need help with amplification devices. Although some general information can be provided in a group education program, there is such a wide range of hearing aids and assistive listening devices available that it is probably more appropriate in many cases to train a designated staff member (or volunteer) about the particular needs of individual residents. Training specific staff to assist those with specialized communication difficulties is an efficient and effective way to manage those clients.

Many staff education programs are designed by individual audiologists and speech-language pathologists for the particular facilities in which they are working, and Koury and Lubinski (1995) provide excellent, practical guidelines for how to proceed. There have been, however, some published staff training packages, namely, the FOCUSED program (Ripich, Wykle, & Niles, 1995), *Older Voices: An Inservice Training Program on the Communication Needs of Older Persons* (ASHA, 1991), and *Coping With Communication Disorders in Aging* (Shadden, Raiford, & Shadden, 1983). These programs and the methods described earlier could be used for training family members and volunteers, as well as staff.

ENHANCING THE PHYSICAL ENVIRONMENT

A number of ideas for enhancing communication by modifying the physical and social environments in residential care facilities are presented in Table 9–2. In terms of the physical environment, changes that result in less background noise and reverberation are particularly helpful for communication as the vast majority of residents have hearing impairment. The visual environment is also important because communication is typically auditory-visual, and residents need to be able to see the speaker's face clearly to pick up speechreading cues. Some of the physical changes are simple (e.g., rearranging chairs), whereas others are more complex (e.g., moving communal areas). Lubinski (1995c) pointed out that the speech-language pathologist or audiologist needs the support of decision makers within facilities to make changes to the environment. Discussion needs to take place so that these decision makers understand why communication is important and how changes to the environment can enhance communication.

ENHANCING THE SOCIAL ENVIRONMENT

It can be seen from Table 9–2 that ideas for improving the social environment involve all key participants in the environment: residents, staff, significant others, and volunteers. The aim is to increase the amount of communication that occurs between all stakeholders by increasing communication opportunities and decreasing barriers to participation. At the resident-resident communication level, one of the ideas is matching talkers with talkers as

TABLE 9–2

IDEAS FOR ENHANCING THE COMMUNICATION ENVIRONMENT IN RESIDENTIAL CARE FACILITIES FOR THE AGED.

Physical environment	Provide private places for people to converse.
	Arrange seating in face-to-face configurations.
	Personalize the resident's environment: Let the resident make decisions about room design, color, furniture, and so forth.
	Decrease noise from unattended televisions, radios, and stereos.
	Decrease noise and reverberation, particularly in communal areas such as dining rooms, for example, by use of carpeting and sound-absorbent walls and ceilings.
	Place communal areas away from major sound sources such as elevators, air conditioners, and ice machines.
	Provide assistive listening devices for residents with hearing impairments to use for communication, for example, loops, infrared devices, frequency modulated (FM) systems.
	Place notices and bulletin boards at eye level.
	Ensure that illumination can be increased or decreased as required, for example, with light dimmer switches, curtains.
	Improve visual contrasts, for example, use dark printing on a light background for signs.
	Remove shiny surfaces that reflect glare into residents' eyes.
	Use visual coding to help residents find their way to different parts of the facility.
Social environment	Establish a buddy system where a resident orients a new resident to the facility.
	Match talkers with talkers in room sharing, dining room seating, and so forth.
	Encourage residents to observe activities even if they do not want to participate.
	Include older people from the community as volunteers in the facility.
	Counsel and educate residents, family members, and staff about communication.
	Develop group activities that facilitate communication, for example, reminiscing and storytelling.
	Provide communication opportunities, for example, outings to other facilities, visits by volunteer organizations, social hours.
	Run problem-solving group sessions with staff, residents, and administrators to focus on the unwritten rules of the facility that might inhibit communication.

Note: Adapted from Erber (1994), Gravell (1988), Kaakinen (1995), Lubinski (1995a, 1995c), O'Connell & O'Connell (1980), and Pichora-Fuller (1997).

roommates. The importance of this idea is highlighted by a study of Kovach and Robinson (1996) who found that rapport was built between roommates who talked to each other and that roommate rapport was a predictor of life satisfaction. They recommend matching roommates who can communicate, rather than the situation that occurs at times where good communicators are matched with poor communicators in the hope that the good talker will help the roommate.

Other peer communication can occur between older volunteers and residents. Ozminkowski, Supiano, and Campbell (1991) evaluated the volunteer experience for 55 volunteers who ran group sessions in residential care settings for the aged. Activity sessions on writing and memory were aimed at facilitating residents' participation. Volunteers were also involved in life review sessions with individual residents. Volunteers were provided 4 hours of training. Satisfaction was evaluated after 1 year, and 95.5% of the volunteers reported they would recommend the experience to others. Most satisfied volunteers were those who had relatives in residential care facilities and those who had attended the training session and, therefore, knew what to expect.

Communication opportunities can be incorporated into the activities program of a facility. These programs are generally coordinated by an activities officer, a recreational therapist, a diversional therapist, or an occupational therapist. The audiologist or speech-language pathologist may be able to work with the coordinator to develop appropriate communication-centered activities. The clinician could discuss the communication needs of the residents with the activities officer and collaboratively develop appropriate communication-centered activities or activities that provide communicative opportunities. Budge (1998) reported that many residential care facilities have an activities program, but warns that these should not be a rigid list of daily activities with residents' names listed next to them. It is better if a more general program is devised and residents are allowed to choose what they would like to attend. Budge lists the features of a well-organized activities program, as follows:

- Activities should be flexible and varied and should reflect the interests and social histories of the residents.
- Residents, significant others, and staff should help with planning activities.
- Residents should not be forced to join in any activities; they have the right to say no.
- Residents should be encouraged to continue to attend activities and groups outside the facility.
- Visitors should be welcomed to join activities.

- A wide range of activities should be included so that the interests of all are catered for (e.g., cooking, poetry appreciation, discussion groups, gardening, aromatherapy sessions, happy hours, musical theme days, card games)

- Special event celebrations (e.g., birthdays, national holidays) should occur at least once a month.

Another communication opportunity occurs when a resident has visitors. It may be that significant others would benefit from counseling by the speech-language pathologist or audiologist about the specific communication difficulties experienced by the resident and how best to assist the person to communicate more effectively. In addition, the relatives and friends could be given advice about how to make the most of their visits from a communication perspective. Dannant (1998) described the concept of constructive visiting. The author suggests many activity ideas that could be useful for family and friends to include during a visit, for example, going for a walk, starting a hobby or craft together, playing games, discussing past interests, writing letters together, reading a newspaper or magazine together, working on a "This is your Life" book, and bringing in items for discussion (e.g., music, family photographs). A visit from family or friends can be a stimulating communication opportunity.

In this section, a number of ideas for enhancing the physical and social communication environment have been presented. The techniques chosen will depend on the facility in which the audiologist or speech-language pathologist is working.

Case Studies of Individual Intervention Programs in Residential Care Facilities

This section contains examples of two residents who received holistic intervention in a residential care facility for the aged. Along a continuum from the medical to the rehabilitation to the social model, the interventions suggested are more toward the social model end of the spectrum. In the first case, the intervention is provided by an audiologist for a resident with hearing impairment and, in the second case, the intervention is provided by a speech-language pathologist for a resident with dementia.

The residential care environment for the aged is an extremely complex communication environment and presents a major challenge for gerontological audiology and speech-language pathology. It is essential that intervention is multifaceted and addresses not only the individual resident and specific communication impairments, but also the broader issues of staff education and the physical and social environment of the facility. It is argued here that the social model of practice is most appropriate in the residential care setting. It is time for clinicians to think differently about the management of older people living in residential care facilities and to break away from their traditional one-to-one treatment role.

Case Study: Mrs. Mackenzie

Mrs. Mackenzie is 82 years old and has been admitted to a residential care facility following a fall that broke her hip. Prior to admission, she lived alone in her own home with support from her son and daughter-in-law who lived nearby. Mrs. Mackenzie's husband died 5 years ago. She began wearing an in-the-ear hearing aid in her left ear after her husband's death because of problems she had hearing the phone ring and hearing people at the door. She wore the hearing aid daily, had no problems managing it, and was happy with it.

Because Mrs. Mackenzie wears a hearing aid, the audiologist is called in to see her. Staff are not sure if the hearing aid is working, as they are still having a great deal of difficulty communicating with Mrs. Mackenzie. In the case history, Mrs. Mackenzie advises the audiologist that she cannot understand what is wrong with her hearing aid. It does not seem to be working as it once did and she cannot understand what people (staff and other residents) are saying to her. She copes better when talking to her family. The assessment reveals that Mrs. Mackenzie has a bilateral moderately severe sensorineural hearing loss. Her hearing aid is functioning well, but because her hearing has deteriorated since she received the aid 5 years ago, it is no longer providing enough amplification for her. The audiologist discusses the results with Mrs. Mackenzie, and they agree on an initial plan of action.

- The audiologist will take ear impressions for moulds for new behind-the-ear aids. Mrs. Mackenzie needs a stronger hearing aid, and a binaural fitting of this style of hearing aid is most suitable.

- The audiologist will contact Mrs. Mackenzie's family, discuss the arrangements with them, and ask if her son is prepared to attend the fitting appointment and assist with hearing aid management in the future.

- Mrs. Mackenzie will also discuss this with her family next time they visit.

- The audiologist will advise the staff of the difficulties that Mrs. Mackenzie is having at present and discuss appropriate communication strategies to use during conversations.

The audiologist subsequently fits Mrs. Mackenzie with her new hearing aids, enlists Mrs. Mackenzie's son as a support person, and returns to the facility 3 weeks later to check on her progress. Mrs. Mackenzie is using the hearing aids daily and is managing them well, with the exception of battery changing. Her son has been changing the batteries for her, and both Mrs. Mackenzie and her son are happy with this arrangement. She reports she is still having difficulty when communicating with staff when she is not wearing her hearing aids (i.e., when she is resting) and when trying to talk to other residents in the dining room. Following this session with Mrs. Mackenzie, the audiologist arranges a joint meeting with Mrs. Mackenzie, the head nurse for her ward, and Mrs. Mackenzie's son and daughter-in-law to discuss ways to deal with Mrs. Mackenzie's residual communication difficulties. The following plan of action is devised.

■ The head nurse will discuss Mrs. Mackenzie's difficulties with communication with the relevant staff members and document these on her personal care plan.

■ The audiologist will give a brief presentation on communication with people who have hearing impairment at a forthcoming staff meeting.

■ The audiologist will observe Mrs. Mackenzie in conversation in the dining room and make recommendations to improve the situation (e.g., modify seating arrangements, change communication partners).

■ The outcome of the plan will be evaluated in 3 months.

At the 3-month follow-up, Mrs. Mackenzie reports being much happier with her communication. She continues to wear her hearing aids daily and has made a good friend in the facility. She sits with her friend in the dining room, and they manage to converse adequately in that environment, although it is still difficult at times. Mrs. Mackenzie now accompanies her friend and attends some of the activities offered in the facility. She continues to have occasional problems with new members of the staff talking to her without her hearing aids on and, when that happens, she asks her son to intervene for her and talk to the head nurse about it. The audiologist considers that no further action is necessary at this time and advises Mrs. Mackenzie and her son to make contact if either believes further assistance is required.

Case Study: Mr. Creffield

Mr. Creffield has just been admitted to the facility. He has middle stage dementia of the Alzheimer's type (DAT) and has been admitted because his frail wife could not look after him any more. This situation has been very distressing for her and their two sons and two daughters. The speech-language pathologist assesses all residents on admission and develops a plan to enhance the resident's communicative well-being in the facility. The speech-language pathologist uses the Wellness-to-Opportunity framework (Lubinski & Orange, 2000) (Figure 9–7) as a blueprint for this plan. The framework aims to promote communicative wellness. Lubinski and Orange describe wellness approaches as those that target "healthy lifestyles and relationships through education, self-empowerment, and access to appropriate care" (p. 230). Communicative wellness applies this wellness approach and philosophy to communication issues. Therefore, the communication skills, effectiveness, and opportunity of the resident with dementia, the family, and staff are addressed within the context of a healthy lifestyle.

Assessment revealed that Mr. Creffield had many communicative strengths. His vision and hearing were only mildly impaired; he was physically fit and mobile; and he had retained good pragmatic skills with an open, friendly, and talkative style of communication. His discourse was not well organized, and he had many word-retrieval errors, but in general he was an easy person to converse with at a social level. His errors in naming family members were causing problems when the family came to visit, and he would occasionally become frustrated when he could not get his message across.

The main aim of the speech-language pathologist's plan for the next few months was to facilitate Mr. Creffield's integration into the facility and to help the family come to terms with the change. The plan involved

- Helping to select Mr. Creffield's roommate carefully, that is, someone who is also communicative and friendly.

- Helping to identify activities that Mr. Creffield might be interested in and that would therefore help maintain his communication skills.

- Developing a small personal portfolio of photographs and names of family members that he carries with him to prompt discussion and to facilitate retrieval of family names; this portfolio is noted in his chart so that staff are aware of its presence and purpose.

One month later, Mr. Creffield has settled in well, but his family remains distressed. The next month's plan is to spend more time with the family. Constructive visiting (Dannant, 1998) is described, and some conversational coaching in situ helps them to have a positive experience when visiting. One of the daughters offers to run an activity class (with her father) in woodworking, an activity they shared before. Her ongoing role as a volunteer has helped her father settle in well and has helped the family adjust. A son continues to take his father and mother to their favorite park and to other gardens they used to enjoy visiting. This plan has helped Mr. Creffield to maintain his communication skills and enhance his and his family's communicative effectiveness. It has enriched Mr. Creffield's communication opportunities and promoted wellness.

KEY POINTS

- The role of the speech-language pathologist and audiologist in residential care facilities for the aged is particularly challenging because the majority of residents have a communication impairment, they are attempting to communicate in a difficult communicative environment, and the clinician is generally not a full-time employee of the institution.

- Approximately 5–6% of the older population live in residential care facilities.

- Moving to a residential care facility may be a difficult transition for the older person and his or her family.

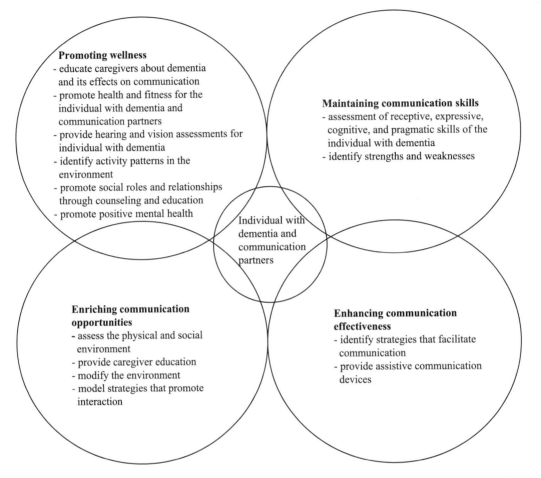

FIGURE 9–7. Modules in the Wellness-to-Opportunity framework for speech-language pathology intervention for people with dementia. Reprinted with permission from Lubinski, R., & Orange, J. B. (2000). A framework for the assessment and treatment of functional communication in dementia. In L. E. Worrall & C. M. Frattali (Eds.), *Neurogenic communication disorders: A Functional approach* (p. 229). New York: Thieme.

- Most residents who require speech-language pathology services have either had a stroke, have respiratory disease, or have a central nervous system disorder.

- Hearing impairment is the most common communication impairment, with 95% of residents having a hearing impairment.

- Multiplicity of communication impairments is common in the residential care facility population.

- There are many types and levels of staff who work in residential care facilities for the aged. Staff are predominantly female, and there is a high turnover rate.

- Staff-resident interactions are important but occur infrequently, are mostly associated with physical care, are often forms of elderspeak, and may create dependency.

- Many aspects of the physical environment of residential care facilities (hard floor coverings, lack of private areas, etc.) are not conducive to communication.

- Barriers to communication in the social environment include infrequent and poor resident-resident communication and unwritten restrictive rules of communication that residents believe exist.

- A social model of practice in residential care facilities for the aged is advocated because of the widespread impact it has on all residents.

- Communication impairments of residents need to be regularly assessed to inform staff and possibly those who fund residential care services of the communication impairments that exist.

- Individual intervention programs should be based on the assessment of residents' communication impairments, activity limitations, and participation restrictions. Specific goals for intervention should then be negotiated among the resident, the clinician, and other key stakeholders (e.g., staff, family) if necessary.

- Residents with hearing aids require onsite support with hearing aid use and management. Specific staff members or volunteers should be trained to provide support, if audiological support is not available.

- Several communication programs are available to use with groups of residents.

- Staff education programs are also mandatory aspects of providing a service to residential care facilities for the aged.

- Many strategies for enhancing the physical and social environments in the facility are presented.

CLASS ACTIVITIES

1. Ask which students in the class have been to a residential care facility for the aged. Ask those students to describe the physical environment of a resident's room: number of beds, seating arrangements, floor and wall coverings. Draw the descriptions on

the chalkboard and then ask the class to suggest changes to the environment that would improve communication for the resident.

■ Discuss the following scenarios with the class and ask them what they would do as the clinician working in the facility.

2. You observe that one of the nurses always talks to residents with hearing aids by shouting into the hearing aids.

3. You observe that a visiting spouse of a resident with aphasia always finishes his sentences for him and interrupts him while he is trying to speak.

4. After a group session with residents about the importance of communicative opportunities, a group of three residents comes to you and asks for a wider range of activities in the residential care facility.

5. A man with Parkinson's disease tells his volunteer that he is very concerned about his money, in particular, whether he has enough to pay for a few items that he would like to buy.

RECOMMENDED READING

Dahl, M. O. (1997). To hear again: A volunteer program in hearing health care for hard-of-hearing seniors. *Journal of Speech-Language Pathology and Audiology, 21*(3), 153–159.

Gravell, R. (1988). *Communication problems in elderly people: Practical approaches to management.* London: Croom Helm.

Jordan, F. M., Worrall, L. E., Hickson, L. M. H., & Dodd, B. J. (1993). The evaluation of intervention programs for communicatively impaired elderly people. *European Journal of Disorders of Communication, 28,* 63–85.

Kaakinen, J. (1995). Talking among elderly nursing home residents. *Topics in Language Disorders, 15,* 36–46.

Lubinski, R. (1995). State-of-the-art perspectives on communication in nursing homes. *Topics in Language Disorders, 15,* 1–19.

Pichora-Fuller, M. K. (1997). Assistive listening devices for the elderly. In R. Lubinski & J. Higginbotham (Eds.), *Communication technology for the elderly: Vision, hearing and speech* (pp. 161–200). Clifton Park, NY: Delmar Learning.

Pye, D., Worrall, L. E., & Hickson, L. (2000). The assessment and treatment of functional communication in an extended care facility. In L. E. Worrall & C. M. Frattali (Eds.), *Neurogenic communication disorders: A functional approach* (pp. 312–328). New York: Thieme.

Rustin, L., & Kuhr, A. (1999). *Social skills and the speech impaired* (2nd ed.). London: Whurr Publishers.

Worrall, L., Hickson, L., & Dodd, B. (1993). Screening for communication impairment in nursing homes and hostels. *Australian Journal of Human Communication Disorders, 21,* 53–64.

 ## REFERENCES

American Speech-Language-Hearing Association. (1991). *A trainer's manual.* Rockville, MD: Author.

American Speech-Language-Hearing Association. (1999). *National outcomes measurement system annual report—Skilled nursing.* Available from American Speech-Language-Hearing Association, 10801 Rockville Pike, Rockville, MD 20852-3279, USA.

American Speech-Language-Hearing Association. (2000). *Health care issues brief: Long term care.* Retrieved on 23 March, 2001 from the World Wide Web: http://professional.asha.org/slp/long_term.html

Australian Institute of Health and Welfare. (1997). *Aged and respite care in Australia: Extracts from recent publications.* Canberra: Australian Institute of Health and Welfare.

Baltes, M. M., Neumann, E-M., & Zank, S. (1994). Maintenance and rehabilitation of independence in old age: An intervention program for staff. *Psychology and Aging, 9*(2), 179–188.

Bitzan, J., & Kruzich, J. (1990). Interpersonal relationships in nursing home residents. *Gerontologist, 30,* 385–390.

Bradley, S., & Molloy, P. (1991). Hearing aid malfunctions pose problems for nursing homes. *The Hearing Journal, 44,* 24–26.

Budge, M. (1998). *Age matters: The art of keeping active and independent.* Sydney: MacLennan & Petty.

Burgio, L. D., & Scilley, K. (1994). Caregiver performance in the nursing home: The use of staff training and management procedures. *Seminars in Speech and Language, 15,* 313–321.

Burnip, L. G., & Erber, N. P. (1996). Staff perceptions of communication difficulty among nursing home residents. *Australian Journal on Aging, 15*(5), 127–131.

Carson, A. J. (1997). Evaluation of the To Hear Again project. *Journal of Speech Language Pathology and Audiology, 21*(3), 160–166.

Commonwealth Department of Health and Family Services. (1997). *The residential care manual.* Canberra: Australian Government Publishing Service.

Cooper, J. W., & Cobb, H. H. (1988). Patient nutritional correlates and changes in a geriatric nursing home. *Nutritional Support Services, 8,* 5–7.

Coupland, N., Coupland, J., Giles, H., & Henwood, K. (1988). Accommodating the elderly: Invoking and extending a theory. *Language and Society, 17,* 1–41.

Dahl, M. O. (1997). To Hear Again: A volunteer program in hearing health care for hard-of-hearing seniors. *Journal of Speech-Language Pathology and Audiology, 21*(3), 153–159.

Dannant, K. (1998). Constructive visiting. In M. Budge (Ed.), *Age matters: The art of keeping active and independent* (pp. 195–202). Sydney: MacLennan & Petty.

Dodd, B., Worrall, L., & Hickson, L. (1990). *Communication: A guide for residential care staff.* Canberra: Australian Government Publishing Service.

Erber, N. P. (1994). Conversation as therapy for older adults in residential care: The case for intervention. *European Journal of Disorders of Communication, 29,* 267–278.

Erber, N. P., & Scherer, S. C. (1999). Sensory loss and communication difficulties in the elderly. *Australasian Journal on Aging, 18*(1), 4–9.

Federal Interagency Forum on Aging-Related Statistics. (2000). *Older Americans 2000: Key indicators of well-being.* Retrieved on May 23, 2001 from the World Wide Web: http://www.agingstats.gov.

Garahan, M., Waller, J., Houghton, M., Tisdale, W., & Runge, C. (1992). Hearing loss prevalence and management in nursing home residents. *Journal of American Geriatrics Society, 40,* 130–134.

Gravell, R. (1988). *Communication problems in elderly people: Practical approaches to management.* London: Croom Helm.

Guthiel, I. A. (1991). Intimacy in nursing home friendships. *Journal of Gerontological Social Work, 17,* 59–73.

Gutnick, H. N., Zillmer, E. A., & Philput, C. B. (1989). Measurement and prediction of hearing loss in a nursing home. *Ear and Hearing, 10*(6), 361–367.

Hopper, T., Bayles, K. A., Harris, F. P., & Holland, A. (2001). The relation of minimum data set ratings to scores on measures of communication and hearing among nursing home residents with dementia. *American Journal of Speech-Language Pathology, 10,* 370–381.

Jennings, M. B., & Head, B. G. (1997). Resident and staff education within an ecological audiologic rehabilitation program in a home for the aged. *Journal of Speech-Language Pathology and Audiology, 21*(3), 167–173.

Jones, D., Sloane, J., & Alexander, L. (1992). Quality of life: A practical approach. In V. Minichiello, L. Alexander, & D. Jones. (Eds.), *Gerontology: A multidisciplinary approach* (pp. 224–265). Sydney: Prentice Hall.

Jordan, F. M., Worrall, L. E., Hickson, L. M. H., & Dodd, B. J. (1993). The evaluation of intervention programs for communicatively impaired elderly people. *European Journal of Disorders of Communication, 28,* 63–85.

Kaakinen, J. (1995). Talking among elderly nursing home residents. *Topics in Language Disorders, 15,* 36–46.

Kato, J., Hickson, L., & Worrall, L. (1996). Communication difficulties of nursing home residents. *Journal of Gerontological Nursing, 22,* 26–31.

Koury, L. N., & Lubinski, R. (1995). Effective in-service training for staff working with communication-impaired patients. In R. Lubinski (Ed.), *Dementia and communication* (pp. 279–291). Clifton Park, NY: Delmar Learning.

Kovach, S. S., & Robinson, J. D. (1996). The roommate relationship for the elderly nursing home resident. *Journal of Social and Personal Relationships, 13*(4), 627–634.

Lewsen, B. J., & Cashman, M. (1997). Hearing aids and assistive listening devices in long-term care. *Journal of Speech-Language Pathology and Audiology, 21*(3), 149–152.

Lubinski, R. (1995a). Environmental considerations for elderly patients. In R. Lubinski (Ed.), *Dementia and communication* (pp. 256–278). Philadelphia: Mosby Year Book.

Lubinski, R. (1995b). State-of-the-art perspectives on communication in nursing homes. *Topics in Language Disorders, 15,* 1–19.

Lubinski, R. (1995c). Environmental considerations for elderly residents. In R. Lubinski (Ed.), *Dementia and communication* (pp. 257–278). Clifton Park, NY: Delmar Learning.

Lubinski, R., Morrison, E. B., & Rigrodsky, S. (1981). Perception of spoken communication by elderly chronically ill patients in an institutional setting. *Journal of Speech and Hearing Disorders, 46*(4), 405–412.

Lubinski, R., & Orange, J. B. (2000). A framework for the assessment and treatment of functional communication in dementia. In L. E. Worrall & C. M. Frattali (Eds.), *Neurogenic communication disorders: A functional approach* (pp. 220–246). New York: Thieme.

Lubinski, R., Stecker, N., Weinstein, B., & Volin, R. (1993). Hearing health services in nursing homes: Perceptions of administrators and audiologists. *Journal of Long Term Care Administrators, 21,* 27–30.

O'Connell, P. F., & O'Connell, E. J. (1980). Speech-language pathology services in a skilled nursing facility: A retrospective study. *Journal of Communication Disorders, 13,* 93–103.

Oliver, S., & Redfern, S. (1991). Interpersonal communication between nurses and elderly patients: Refinement of an observational schedule. *Journal of Advanced Nursing, 16,* 30–38.

Ozminkowski, R. J., Supiano, K. P., & Campbell, R. (1991). Volunteers in nursing home enrichment: A survey to evaluate training and satisfaction. *Activities, Adaptation and Aging, 15*(3), 13–43.

Palmer, C. V., Adams, S. W., Durrant, J. D., Bourgeois, M., & Rossi, M. (1998). Managing hearing loss in a patient with Alzheimer disease. *Journal of the American Academy of Audiology, 9,* 275–284.

Parker, R. A. (1987). *The elderly and residential care: Australian lessons for Britain.* Aldershot, UK: Gower.

Peters, C. A., Polter, J. F., & Scholer, S. G. (1988). Hearing impairment as a predictor of cognitive decline in dementia. *Journal of the American Geriatrics Society, 36,* 981–986.

Pichora-Fuller, M. K. (1997). Assistive listening devices for the elderly. In R. Lubinski & J. Higginbotham (Eds.), *Communication technology for the elderly: Vision, hearing and speech* (pp. 161–200). Clifton Park, NY: Delmar Learning.

Pichora-Fuller, M. K., & Robertson, L. F. (1994). Hard-of-hearing residents in a home for the aged. *Journal of Speech-Language Pathology and Audiology, 18*(4), 278–288.

Pye, D., Worrall, L. E., & Hickson, L. (2000). The assessment and treatment of functional communication in an extended care facility. In L. E. Worrall & C. M. Frattali (Eds.), *Neurogenic communication disorders: A functional approach* (pp. 312–328). New York: Thieme.

Ripich, D. N., Wykle, M., & Niles, S. (1995). Alzheimer's disease caregivers: The focused program. A communication skills training program helps nursing assistants to give better care to patients with disease. *Geriatric-Nursing, 16*(1), 15–9.

Rizzolo, P., & Snow, T. (1989). Use of a hearing assistance device in nursing homes. *American Family Physician, 39,* 227–229.

Rustin, L., & Kuhr, A. (1999). *Social skills and the speech impaired* (2nd ed.). London: Whurr Publishers.

Ryan, E. B. (1991, July). *Attitudes and behaviors toward older adults in communication contexts.* Paper presented at the Fourth International Conference on Language and Social Psychology, Santa Barbara, CA.

Schow, R. L., & Nerbonne, M. A. (1977). Assessment of hearing handicaps by nursing home residents and staff. *Journal of the Academy of Rehabilitative Audiology, 10,* 2–12.

Schow, R. L., & Nerbonne, M. A. (1980). Hearing levels among elderly nursing home residents. *Journal of Speech and Hearing Disorders, 45,* 124–132.

Shadden, B., Raiford, C., & Shadden, H. (1983). *Coping with communication disorders in aging.* Tiggard, OR: CC Publications.

Sorin-Peters, R., Tse, S., & Kapelus, G. (1989). Communication screening program for a geriatric continuing care unit. *Journal of Speech-Language Pathology, 13,* 63–70.

Stumer, J., Hickson, L., & Worrall, L. (1996). Hearing impairment, disability and handicap in elderly people living in residential care and in the community. *Disability and Rehabilitation, 18*(2), 76–82.

Uhlmann, R. F., Larson, E. B., Thomas, S. R., Koepsell, T. D., & Duckert, L. G. (1989). Relationship of hearing impairment to dementia and cognitive dysfunction in older adults. *Journal of the American Medical Association, 261,* 2875–2878.

Upfold, L. J., May, A. E., & Battaglia, J. A. (1990). Hearing aid manipulation skills in an elderly population: A comparison of BTE and ITC aids. *British Journal of Audiology, 24*(5), 311–318.

Weinstein, B., & Amsel, L. (1986). Hearing loss and senile dementia in the institutionalized elderly. *Clinical Gerontologist, 4,* 3–15.

World Health Organization. (2001). *International classification of functioning, disability and health.* Geneva: Author.

Worrall, L. E. (1999). *Functional communication therapy planner.* Oxon, UK: Winslow Press.

Worrall, L., Hickson, L., & Dodd, B. (1993). Screening for communication impairment in nursing homes and hostels. *Australian Journal of Human Communication Disorders, 21,* 53–64.

Ylvisaker, M., & Holland, A. L. (1985). Coaching, self coaching and rehabilitation of head injury. In D. F. Johns (Ed.), *Clinical management of neurogenic communication disorders* (pp. 243–27). Boston: Little, Brown.

$\mathcal{C}hapter$ **10**

Implications for Theory, Practice, and Policy

This chapter summarizes the major themes from each of the three sections of the text: the Overview section, the Communication Changes With Age section, and the Practice in Different Gerontological Settings section. The implications that have emerged for theory, practice, and policy, including those for funding of services, are then discussed. Finally, some comments about the successful education of speech-language pathologists and audiologists in gerontology are provided.

Gerontological speech-language pathology and audiology are rapidly growing specialty areas of practice. Concerns have been raised, however, about whether the rapid increase in the proportion of older persons in the population will be matched by the capacity and willingness of service providers to deliver the necessary services for this client group (Paton, Sar, Barber, & Holland, 2001). The proportion of older people in the population will increase from approximately 12 to 20% in the next few years, and it must be of grave concern that research has shown that large numbers of students in the human and health professions have little or no interest in working with older persons (see Paton et al., 2001).

Barriers to student interest in gerontology include insufficient curriculum time and hence limited geriatric knowledge, the perceived lower status of work and financial compensation in gerontology, students' limited experience of healthy older people, students' perception of practicing clinicians' negative attitudes toward older people, and generally negative public attitudes toward older people (Paton et al., 2001). Many of these barriers are surmountable; however, there first needs to be recognition that gerontological practice is a specialist area of audiology and speech-language pathology that demands space in the curriculum. It is often assumed that practice with older people is the same as any form of adult practice. It is important to remember here the words of Palmer and Hunter (1998):

> Elderly people cannot be treated the same as if they were young adults who happen to be chronologically older. Because of physiological differences, a high frequency of functional and cognitive impairments, a lack of physiological reserve, a high frequency of multiple chronic illnesses, a greater number of sensory impairments, and an increased chance of being on multiple potentially interacting medications, the elderly must be approached in a specific age-appropriate manner. (p. 131)

Aged care and health care practices are rapidly changing to accommodate an aging society. New societal values are emerging that affect practice, and it is not appropriate for clinicians to maintain agist stereotypes and solely discipline-specific impairment-focused methods of intervention. It is time to move forward. The following summaries of the three sections of this text may help to encapsulate modern-day theories and practices in gerontological speech-language pathology and audiology.

Summary of Section I: Overview

Population aging is a major issue for speech-language pathology and audiology and indicates that gerontological practice needs to be considered a specialty area in the professions. Gerontology brings a broader perspective to case management than discipline-specific management. Four major theoretical frameworks in health and gerontology influence the practice of audiology and speech-language pathology with older people. First, the WHO's framework of Functioning, Disability, and Health (ICF; WHO, 2001) emphasizes the effects of communication changes with age in terms of the three levels of body structure and function, activity, and participation. The influence of environmental and personal factors is also considered. Second, the health-disease continuum is a concept that reminds professionals that the distinction between pathology and health is blurred, particularly in older people who have a multiplicity of age-related changes. Audiologists and speech-language pathologists have a role to play with all older people along this continuum, whether they have a recognizable communication disability or not. Third, healthy aging is a major policy trend in many countries, and it is argued that communication has a fundamental role in healthy aging. Therefore, clinicians must be increasingly involved in health promotion programs and prevention of communication disability in older people. Finally, the

Communication Accommodation Theory is an antiagist approach to conversational interactions that demands attention be paid to communication partners as well as to the older person with a communication disability. Under- or overaccommodation can lead to communication breakdown, lower self-esteem for the older person, and potentially increased dependency in the long term. Such communication behavior demonstrates a lack of respect for the older person.

There are potentially three models of practice that can be employed when working with older people. The medical model is characterized by a focus on impairment and a directive paternalistic style of clinical decision making. The rehabilitation model is characterized by a focus on the person with the impairment and the person's ability to function in everyday life. Typically, a process of informed decision making is used. In the social model, the focus is on the person in society, and the problems the person experiences are seen as being related not only to the client's own performance, but also to the disabling society in which the client lives. Shared decision making is generally applied. Different models of practice are necessary in different settings, with different clients. The clinician, therefore, needs to consider his or her own professional values, the organizational context, and the wishes of the client.

Summary of Section II: Communication Changes With Age

In this section, communication changes were discussed using the WHO model levels of impairment, activity limitations, and participation restrictions. In addition, the impact of communication changes on quality of life were described. Communication impairments that are of most concern to healthy older people are hearing loss, memory problems, and word-finding difficulties. Other changes have been found in comprehension, conversational discourse, speech, voice, and swallowing. Cognitive, vision, and hearing changes associated with healthy aging can complicate the differential diagnosis of pathological conditions such as dementia and aphasia. Although standard assessments can be applied with older people, it is necessary to take special care in conducting the assessment and in interpreting the results. It is argued, however, that for comprehensive rehabilitation, it is important to consider not just the impairments, but also the effects of those communication impairments on the individual's everyday life. The everyday effects are considered in terms of activity limitations and participation restrictions. Assessments of activity limitations take the form of direct observation or simulation of real-life tasks, or by asking the clients and/or their significant others about the clients' abilities in real life. There are a significant number of formal assessments of older people's activity limitations. It must be remembered, however, that the everyday activities of older people are different from the activities of younger people. In general, older people undertake more leisure activities, with a spouse or other older people, and spend a lot of time alone.

Participation is about an individual's involvement in life situations. It can be assessed through open-ended questions or through more direct questions about involvement in a range of social activities, for example, "What were you involved in two years ago?" and "What are you doing now?" There are few formal assessments of participation restrictions for older people with communication disabilities. Quality of life measures are becoming synonymous with participation. It is argued, however, that quality of life is a separate construct and is the unique perspective of each individual. Both health-related and nonhealth-related quality of life measures are described, some of which are generic for all populations, and some are specific to certain conditions. There are a number of difficulties in using quality of life measures for communicatively disabled populations. However, recommendations about the most appropriate measures are provided. Healthy older people rate their quality of life significantly higher than do younger people, but this does not apply to older people with communication disability who report a significantly poorer quality of life than do their peers. Older people consider social health, such as relationship with family, of paramount importance when they describe the quality of their lives. This choice has implications for the importance of speech-language pathology and audiology interventions that seek to enhance quality of life.

Summary of Section III: Practice in Different Gerontological Settings

Contrary to agist stereotypes, most older people live in the community. Speech-language pathologists and audiologists have both prevention and intervention roles with older people in the community. Health promotion programs that aim to maintain communication in healthy older people illustrate the preventative role. For people with a known communication disability living in the community, there are a number of group programs and individual interventions that are within the rehabilitation and social models of practice. It is argued that these models of practice are the most relevant for community settings.

In hospital settings, however, the medical model prevails. Older people are disproportionate consumers of health care, and it is important that speech-language pathologists and audiologists working in hospitals consider the specific needs of older patients. They should consider not just the older person and his or her impairments, but the older person's interactions in the hospital environment. This concept represents a shift from the traditional medical role in hospitals to encompass the broader rehabilitation and social models of practice.

The residential care facility is home for about 5% of older people. Again, although a medical model prevails in many facilities, it is particularly important in this context of a home environment to apply a rehabilitation and social model of practice. The role of the speech-language pathologist and audiologist in residential care facilities for the aged is particularly challenging because the vast majority of residents have a communication impairment, they are attempting to communicate in a difficult communicative environment, and the clinician is generally not a full-time employee of the institution. Much emphasis needs to be placed on improving staff-resident interactions because research shows they occur infrequently, are mostly associated with physical care, and are often forms of elderspeak that may create dependency. In addition, there are infrequent and poor resident-resident interactions, and unwritten restrictive rules limit communication opportunities for residents. Several communication programs are available for use with staff and groups of residents. The physical and social environments of residential care facilities for the aged also need direct intervention.

Implications for Theory

This section highlights the main questions in communication disability in aging for researchers and theorists. Students who want to or need to undertake research as part of their educational program or who are intending to pursue a research career, may find potential research questions in this section.

Healthy aging is an important concept in many societies. Governments and individuals see the benefit of preventing substantial decline and diseases in old age, but funding for healthy aging programs is not always available in mainstream health services. What role do audiologists and speech-language pathologists have in healthy aging? To answer this question, the role of communication in healthy aging and quality of life needs to be determined. There is a need for evidence about the relative strength of the relationship between communication and quality of life. The model described by Cruice, Worrall, and Hickson (2000), which links the three levels of the WHO model with quality of life, is an appropriate framework to test this relationship (see Figure 2–3, Chapter 2). As the professions move more toward evidence-based practice, statements such as "communication is important to quality of life" need to be substantiated by evidence.

Much of the discipline-specific knowledge in audiology and speech-language pathology is rooted in the impairment level. When examining activity, participation, and quality of life dimensions of older people with communication disabilities, multidisciplinary research efforts are often required. Hence, although the focus may be on older people with communication disabilities, the contributions of other disciplines such as social work, psychology, occupational therapy, and physical therapy are needed to appreciate the full perspective of the impact of a communication disability on activities, participation, and quality of life. A multidisciplinary model of practice applicable to older people with communication disability could be developed and evaluated.

In a discussion about the health-disease continuum in Chapter 2, it was suggested there is a subclinical population of older people with communication disabilities. These were described as older people with multiple and often mild communication-related impairments (e.g., a mild near and distance visual loss, a moderate hearing loss, and a mild cognitive loss) who exhibit communication activity limitations and participation restrictions. This population may be at risk for social isolation and may benefit from preventative services. Again, there is a need for evidence in this area. Do multiple and mild impairments create activity limitations and participation restrictions? Can preventative programs reduce social isolation?

The Communication Accommodation Theory has not been applied to interactions with people with communication disability. It has been used to study intergenerational interactions with healthy older people or with people from other cultures, but as yet, not with people who have a communication disability. Do underaccommodation and overaccommodation occur? Do they occur more frequently with older people with communicative disability? What are the speaker cues that allow accommodation? These questions may ultimately facilitate appropriate interactions among older people with communication disabilities and their conversational partners (e.g., family, staff).

Chapter 3 described three main models of practice: medical, rehabilitation, and social. Although the needs of the individual older person and the organization's preferred model of practice play a major role in the choice of model, Worrall (2000) argued that clinicians' own professional values influence the choice of approach used. Professional values are the beliefs that clinicians have internalized. Some clinicians may strongly believe that impairments can be cured and the clinician's role should be a curative one. Others may believe a curative approach is not appropriate for chronic conditions. It is probable that there is a relationship between clinician's professional values and their preferred model of practice.

There are many assessments of communication impairments; however, many are unsuitable for older people, particularly those frail aged in residential care facilities. There is also a growing number of measures of communication activity, but there are few measures of participation relevant to this population. This situation primarily stems from a lack of consensus about the concept of participation and how it should be measured. Multiple measures of quality of life are available, but few have a focus on communication or are appropriate for older people with communication disability. Refinement of the concepts of communication-related quality of life and participation is required, along with the development of measures appropriate for use with older people.

Finally, the issue of the appropriateness of elderspeak needs further research. Studies have shown that although it creates dependency, many older people in residential care facilities for the aged consider that it shows a caring attitude and, therefore, do not object to its use in their institution. There is a need to evaluate conversation that is caring (but not elderspeak) against the use of elderspeak alone. What are the features of caring communication that is not elderspeak? What do residents prefer?

Implications for Practice

This section highlights the main issues for the practice of gerontological speech-language pathology and audiology. These stem from the theoretical issues already described and may assist the clinician in providing a service soundly based in principles of gerontology.

Whichever setting the clinician works in, how can clinicians choose a model of practice that is appropriate for the context and the client and is not just based in their own professional values and their organization's perceived values? Certainly it is helpful to identify the predominant mode of practice in the organization. It is also helpful for clinicians to examine their own beliefs and make these explicit. A good example of an organization's beliefs being made explicit are those of the Connect (2001) network in the United Kingdom (www.ukconnect.org), an organization for people with aphasia. This organization has posted its values on its website (Figure 10–1) and makes these explicit to clients and visitors. Finally, but most important, it is essential to understand the goals and aspirations of the client. Asking the person about his or her needs is a vital step in determining the approach to use. Clinicians may choose to use different approaches for different clients, and this choice shows appropriate adaptability based on client's wishes.

The issues of multiskilling and the use of nonprofessional personnel are relevant to a discussion about interventions at the activity, participation, and quality of life levels particularly. For example, many residential care facilities for the aged have personnel who undertake activities with residents. Should these people be primarily responsible for carrying out activity-level group sessions for residents who are communicatively disabled? Volunteer stroke schemes are also prevalent in countries such as the United Kingdom. Volunteers visit people with

Respect

We value difference, diversity, and dialogue.

Communication

We believe in communication that is clear, open, and accessible to all.

Responsive

We listen actively to individuals and organizations and work together to build flexible, imaginative, yet realistic opportunities.

Participation

We believe that people have the right to participate fully in choices and decisions about therapy and life.

Equality

We are energetic in pursuing equal rights and new opportunities for people with communication disability.

Creative

We enjoy being open to and developing new ideas and practices.

Healthy

We care for and value people, communities, and environments.

Excellence

We offer long-term services that are high quality, effective, and efficient.

FIGURE 10–1. An example of explicitly stated values of an organization. Reprinted with permission from Connect—The Communication Disability Network www.ukconnect.org/about/index.html. See also Byng, S., Cains, D., & Duchan, J. (2002). "Values in Practice and Practicing Values." *Journal of Disorders of Communication 35*(2), 89–106.

aphasia in their own homes. Is this better than no services at all? Although Johnson and Jacobson (1998), among others, believe there is room for interdisciplinary collaboration, they express the fear that the discipline's expertise may be lost in the process. Although this fear may be true, a consultative approach, in which the qualified clinician supervises any intervention carried out by nonspeech-language pathologists or nonaudiologists, represents an innovative approach to service delivery for the older population.

How can speech-language pathologists and audiologists contribute to a healthy aging population? Apart from providing health promotion programs around communication issues for older people, there is also a need to examine the broader issue of maintaining older people in the community. There is a need to identify older people who are at risk of becoming socially isolated because of communication-related impairments. Therefore, it is important that audiologists and speech-language pathologists are included on teams that provide rehabilitation services for older people living in the community.

Practice within the residential care setting must be one of the most challenging for any clinician. There is a lack of evidence to help clinicians choose effective treatments and a lack of evidence about combinations of treatments that make up the entire package of service delivery. In this most challenging environment, the feasibility as well as the efficacy of interventions are important. In particular, there is a strong need for evidence-based interventions that are effective in training communication partners to accommodate appropriately with older people who have communication disabilities. The concept of treating the staff or the caregivers is not new, but clinicians need the tools to do it. This need also applies to assessing and providing intervention beyond the impairment level. Clinicians need the tools for the assessment of activity limitations, participation restrictions, and quality of life in the residential environment.

Implications for Policy

Policy is formulated at many levels. There are policies of departments, organizations, professions, governments, and nations. Policies can range from a simple mission statement on respect for older people, to health care policies that dictate funding of services, to complex laws that govern the legal rights of older people with cognitive impairment. Policies are in general a statement about how individuals should act; hence, there is a need for audiologists and speech-language pathologists not only to be knowledgeable about and abide by the policies of their governing agencies, but also to influence policy.

Probably the most significant effect of policy decisions is on the funding of services. Funding arrangements for health and aged care services vary markedly in different countries, and it is important that clinicians understand what is happening in their local environment. In the United States, there are two major government-run schemes that assist older people to meet health costs. Both schemes are administered by the Centers for Medicare and Medicaid Services (formerly the Health Care Financing Administration), a branch of the U. S. Department of Health and Human Services. The first is Medicare, which is a federal government program that pays for acute health care for people over the age of 65; the second is Medicaid, which is a state and federal program that supports health care for people who fall below the poverty line, many of whom are elderly. Almost all older Americans

(95%) are enrolled in Medicare, compared to 13% who are enrolled in Medicaid (Weinstein, 2000). Approximately 40% of all health care costs in the United States are funded by government through these schemes (Levit, Lazenby, Cowan, & Letsch, 1991). The remainder is paid for by private health insurance and/or directly by the consumer.

Medicare has two parts. Part A, which is funded from payroll deductions, is for approximately the first 100 days of hospital services and will only pay for those services that have been provided by or arranged by the hospital. Part B, for additional ancillary services after the first 100 hospital days have finished, includes home health and hospice care. Part B is a voluntary program funded by a combination of payroll deductions and contributions from subscribers. Medicare does not cover all costs related to medical expenses, and many older people take out insurance called Medigap to meet the shortfall. The system is complex and ever changing in response to government policy and financial issues. Clinicians should obtain up-to-date details from the ASHA website (www.asha.org) and/or from the Centers for Medicare and Medicaid Services site (www.cms.hhs.gov). Some particularly relevant features of Medicare, at the time of writing, are (Weinstein, 2000; White, 2001; www.asha.org)

- There is a Medicare Fee Schedule that assigns a relative value to each clinical procedure (e.g., individual speech-language treatment, swallowing evaluation, comprehensive hearing test) for speech-language pathology and audiology.

- A physician referral is necessary for Medicare payment of audiology and speech-language pathology services.

- After referral from a physician, audiologists may receive Medicare payments directly as independent practitioners.

- Medicare will pay for diagnostic audiological services when the diagnostic information is deemed to assist the physician to develop a treatment protocol or surgery.

- Medicare will not pay for audiological assessment related to hearing aid fitting only; that is, if a person has a hearing impairment but no other symptoms that warrant further investigation on medical grounds (e.g., unilateral impairment, vertigo), then the service is not funded.

- Aural rehabilitation services and cerumen management by audiologists are covered for hospital inpatients.

- Cochlear implant rehabilitation services and cerumen management by audiologists are covered if the audiologist is employed by a physician.

- Medicare does not fund hearing aid fitting.

- Speech-language pathologists cannot bill Medicare directly unless they establish a rehabilitation agency.

- Speech-language pathologists who bill through physicians' offices must be employees of that office.

Medicaid funds a range of aged care services for eligible older people. These include long-term care, home health care, adult day care, medical transportation, and respite care. Provisions for other services, such as hearing aids and dental care, vary from state to state. Medicaid is one of the major payers of long-term care in the United States. Weinstein (2000) points out "most people entering nursing homes do not qualify for Medicaid, however they become eligible once they have depleted the resources they had in paying for their own care prior to institutionalization" (p. 318). However, it is important for clinicians to remember that Medicaid may not be the only source of funding for services to an older person living in a care facility in the United States. The person may be able to pay for services with funds from Medicare, private health insurance, and/or personal own resources.

In contrast to the United States, most speech-language pathology and audiology services to older people in other English-speaking countries such as Australia, the United Kingdom, and Canada are funded through a publicly funded system that does not involve reimbursement issues. In Australia, for instance, there are two primary funding mechanisms. One is the usual health system (hospital and community health), which is administered at a state level. The other is a federal scheme for aging and hearing issues, and this scheme is the primary source of funding for services in residential care facilities as well as the primary source of funding for hearing services for older people. Indeed, the government department responsible for these areas is titled the Australian Department of Health and Aging (http://www.health.gov.au/). Health Canada (http://www.hc-sc.gc.ca/) is the primary source of funding for services in Canada; however, the provinces primarily administer the health system, so there is considerable variability between provincial services. The United Kingdom has an extensive publicly funded National Health Service (http://www.nhs.uk/). This service provides free speech and language therapy and audiology services to older people.

Funding policies and mechanisms are constantly changing in all countries, primarily driven by attempts to limit health-care costs. The most recent information is usually found on the websites of either government departments responsible for aging and/or health or from professional audiology and speech-language pathology organizations (see Worrall & Hickson, 2001).

Funding for speech-language pathology services may be limited in many settings such as hospitals and residential care facilities because communication is frequently undervalued by such institutions. Physical care is often the predominant focus of such organizations.

If audiologists and speech-language pathologists believe that communication is not valued within their organization, then there is a need to influence policy. Within large organizations this situation can seem like a mammoth task; however, strategies to make inroads into achieving this aim mostly revolve around linking communication to broader aspects of the organization. Many organizations have mission statements, strategic plans, quality improvement centers, accreditation procedures, outcome measures, and complaints procedures. Chapters 8 and 9 describe some strategies for creating a positive communication culture within hospitals and residential care facilities through influencing policies.

The Changing Role of Speech-Language Pathologists and Audiologists With the Aging Population

The increasing number of older people with communication difficulties has major implications for the role of speech-language pathologists and audiologists. It is currently estimated in the United States that 19% of the overall speech-language pathology caseload and 33% of the overall audiology caseload are older. By 2050, these caseloads are expected to increase to 39% and 59%, respectively (Shadden & Toner, 1997). It is, therefore, timely for the professions to carefully consider their roles with older people and to be proactive about how to meet the challenges of population aging. In this section, the traditional roles of speech-language pathologists and audiologists with older people are outlined, followed by a discussion of how these roles are expected to change in the future, and what needs to be done to prepare for these changing roles.

Traditional Roles

In 1988, ASHA published a landmark description of the roles of speech-language pathologists and audiologists working with older persons (ASHA, 1988). The description began with a list of general roles applicable to working with people of all ages and pointed out that the majority of these general roles are also appropriate for working with older clients. The list of roles for each profession included the identification of persons in need of speech-language pathology services, treatment planning, prevention or reduction of the handicapping effects of hearing loss, and serving as an advocate for persons who are hearing-impaired.

These traditional roles clearly represent the core business of the practice of audiology and speech-language pathology; however, it is important when working with the older population that practice is not limited to these roles. The ASHA (1988) document elaborated on a number of other service delivery roles that could be adopted by the professions (Figure 10–2). The key features of these roles were the need for flexibility in assessment and

- Reducing environmental, physical, and psychological barriers to communication

- Designing, managing, directing, and/or supervising communication enhancement programs

- Increasing emphasis on individual and family counseling

- Designing and implementing programs aimed at increasing communicative interactions among older people and significant others

- Using new technology to enhance older people's communication in social settings

- Increasing involvement in the evaluation and management of people with dementia

- Developing programs aimed at the maintenance of communication ability in older people

- Designing and implementing inservice programs for caregivers

- Facilitating support groups for older people with communication problems

- Providing advocacy for the communication needs of older people

- Promoting interdisciplinary case management for older people

FIGURE 10–2. New service delivery roles for speech-language pathologists and audiologists working with older people. Adapted from American Speech-Language-Hearing Association (1988).

management techniques and the focus on the functional communication of older people. The question in 1988 was, "How would these new roles become a reality?" Two major processes were identified as facilitating change: (a) greater involvement of practicing speech-language pathologists and audiologists at the policy level and (b) better professional preparation and education in gerontology.

It seems, however, that the professions have been slow to act in these areas. Over the past decade, there have been significant changes in health and aged care policies in many countries. The primary change in health systems of countries like the United States, Australia, Canada, and the United Kingdom has been the emphasis on increased accountability and cost reduction. Increased accountability has led to greater emphasis on reporting functional outcomes. In addition, with the expected rapid increase in the number of older people, many countries see the need to support health promotion and wellness programs for older people. These policy shifts have important implications for the roles of audiologists and speech-language pathologists with older people; however, there has been little response from the professions to date.

In terms of the education of speech-language pathologists and audiologists, it was reported as recently as 1998 that the professions are still poorly prepared for the increase in the aging population (Uffen, 1998). This situation is supported by evidence from a number of studies in the United States (Nerbonne, Schow, & Hutchinson, 1980) and Canada (Orange, MacNeill, & Stouffer, 1997). In 1980, Nerbonne et al. found that approximately one quarter of universities offering speech-language pathology courses either offered or planned to offer coursework in gerontology. By 1994, three quarters of the programs had some type of aging component, but this may not be enough because Orange et al. (1997) found that the majority of the clinicians they surveyed in Canada had gained their experience through on-the-job training or from continuing education courses, rather than their original professional preparation in the university program.

Hence, many university programs in speech-language pathology and audiology may not be adequately preparing future professionals for a role with older people. In addition, it appears from the literature that there is considerable diversity in the depth or extent of courses offered, with little recognition by university programs that specific gerontology courses are anything more than regular courses in adult communication disability. It is for this reason that this text was written. One goal of this text is to define some core knowledge for speech-language pathologists and audiologists as they enter the workforce. It is a means by which the reader can become prepared for population aging and reap the benefits of working with the elders of the world.

Future Roles

This text provides evidence that four major changes in emphasis may help meet the needs of older adults with communication disabilities.

1. Greater recognition needs to be given to the differences in work settings of speech-language pathologists and audiologists working with older people. There is a considerable difference between practice in an acute care hospital and practice in a residential care facility for the aged that provides long-term care. In addition, there are distinct differences between the roles of community-based speech-language pathologists and audiologists and those who work in a health care setting. Chapters 7, 8, and 9 describe the role of speech-language pathologists and audiologists in the three major work settings where the professions encounter older people (i.e., community, hospital, and residential care facility).

2. The role of the professions in community-based health promotion programs is relatively new, but has the potential to centralize the role of communication in older people's quality of life. There is a more detailed discussion of this concept in Chapters 3 and 7.

3. With the chronic nature of many communication difficulties in older people and the increased emphasis on accountability, there is a need to pay greater attention to the functional abilities of older people to meet their everyday communication needs. The medical or impairment-based model of traditional audiology and speech-language pathology intervention is being gradually broadened to include the functional approaches that emphasize everyday communicative activities and participation through communication. Chapters 5 and 6 describe the functional assessments applicable for older people with communication disabilities, whereas Chapters 7, 8, and 9 describe functional intervention approaches.

4. The theory and practice of the professions cannot be divorced from policy. Health and aged care policy changes have made a significant impact on speech-language pathology and audiology services in recent years. The professions need to not only respond to these changes and change the way services are delivered, but also provide input into policies at all levels.

Preparing for Change

Education is a key element for the development of speech-language pathologists and audiologists as specialists in aging. Figure 10–3 contains a list of the knowledge and skills that might be required. The material presented in this text assists audiology and speech-language

---

- Understanding of demographic and attitudinal issues in gerontology

- Skills in communicating appropriately with older people

- Understanding of government policies related to aging and the aged care industry

- Awareness of cultural and linguistic diversity in the aging population

- Skills to improve the communication environment for older people in various settings

- Skills and knowledge to provide high-quality education that targets the needs of staff and/or caregivers

- Skills in working collaboratively with other health professionals

- Skills to establish health promotion programs in the community or health care facility

- Skills to provide targeted rehabilitation to older people to improve functional abilities

- Skills in the use of technologies that may enhance the communication of older people

---

FIGURE 10–3. Knowledge and skills required by speech-language pathologists and audiologists specializing in aging.

pathology students to develop each of these attributes. To fully explore the area of communication disability in aging, it is not sufficient to know about communication disabilities that just happen to occur in people who are older. Gerontological specialists in both professions must develop a broader perspective of their roles and broader skills to work effectively with older people.

If an audiologist or speech-language pathologist finds gerontology interesting and exciting and chooses to seek employment working with older people, then he or she will probably be in high demand. It is likely there will not be sufficient numbers of trained professionals ready to meet the needs of the increasing numbers of older people. In particular, significant opportunities are available in the wellness and health promotion area of gerontological speech-language pathology and audiology.

This text has provided a broad view of gerontological speech-language pathology and audiology. It has emphasized to students that theory, practice, and policy all need to be integrated to be an effective clinician in this area. It has also highlighted the importance of viewing practice in these areas as a specialty within the professions. Such specialty needs to be recognized in the usual ways: Greater recognition of this growing area within the professions, increased input into professional preparation programs, and continued interdisciplinary research and practice.

It is hoped that this text has reflected our passion for gerontological speech-language pathology and audiology. Passion stems from positive personal experiences with older people with and without communication disabilities, observing the frequently suboptimal service for this population, experiencing the successes of innovative intervention programs, and the knowledge that one day, we too, will be old.

Creating passion in students leads to committed, dedicated, successful, and innovative clinicians. Ultimately, it is these dedicated clinicians who will change the system so that optimal services will be provided for older people with communication disabilities.

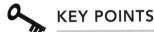

KEY POINTS

- Gerontological speech-language pathologists and audiologists need to be cognizant of the major theories in health and gerontology that influence practice with older people.

- Communication changes that occur in healthy aging and those associated with pathological conditions in older people can be described using the WHO dimensions of impairments, activity limitations, and participation restrictions; communication changes also affect quality of life.

- The three models of practice that can be employed in different gerontological settings are the medical, rehabilitation, and social models.

- For older people living in the community and for those in residential care facilities for the aged, rehabilitation and social models are most appropriate.

- In hospital settings, the medical model of practice is most common; however, there is scope to broaden this approach.

- A number of areas for further research in gerontological speech-language pathology and audiology practice are identified.

- Many aspects of practice requiring further development and evaluation are discussed.

- Funding of services for older people with communication disability is a major issue, and communication is not a priority issue for policy makers; therefore, there is a need for speech-language pathologists and audiologists to act as advocates in this regard.

- Traditional case-based and discipline-specific roles in speech-language pathology and audiology are slowly being broadened to encompass the rapid policy changes that have taken place in health and aged care.

- Education for speech-language pathologists and audiologists in the specialty area of gerontology is the key to the professions' response to population aging.

CLASS ACTIVITIES

1. Divide the class into small groups and ask each group to develop one of the research ideas presented in this chapter.

   - What is the research question that needs to be addressed?
   - How could such a question be tested?
   - What is an appropriate research plan to answer the question?
   - Who would the participants be?
   - What procedure could be used?
   - What measures could be taken?

2. Policy makers do not recognize communication as an important issue for older people. Ask the class to brainstorm ideas for increasing awareness about the importance of communication.

REFERENCES

American Speech-Language-Hearing Association. (1988, March). Position statement: The roles of speech-language pathologists and audiologists in working with older people. *ASHA*, pp. 80–84.

Bing, S., Cairns, D., & Duchan, J. (2002). Values in practice and practicing the values. *Journal of Communication Disorders, 35*(2), 89–106.

Connect. (2001). Retrieved from the World Wide Web on the 14th October, 2001, www.ukconnect.org/about/index.html

Cruice, M., Worrall, L., & Hickson, L. (2000). Measurement of quality-of-life in speech pathology and audiology. *Asia Pacific Journal of Speech, Language, and Hearing, 5*(1), 1–20.

Johnson, A. F., & Jacobson, B. H. (1998). Issues in medical speech-language pathology. In A. F. Johnson & B. H. Jacobson (Eds.), *Medical speech-language pathology. A practitioner's guide* (pp. 7–14). New York: Thieme.

Levit, K., Lazenby, H., Cowan, C., & Letsch, S. (1991). National health care expenditures, 1990. *Health Care Financing Review, 13*, 1–29.

Nerbonne, M. A., Schow, R. L., & Hutchinson, J. M. (1980). Gerontologic training in communication disorders. *ASHA, 22*, 404–408.

Orange, J. B., MacNeill, C. L., & Stouffer, J. L. (1997). Geriatric audiology curricula and clinical practice: A Canadian perspective. *Journal of Speech-Language Pathology and Audiology, 21*(2), 84–103.

Palmer, T. R., & Hunter, M. B. (1998). Issues in geriatric medicine. In A. F. Johnson & B. H. Jacobson (Eds.), *Medical speech-language pathology. A practitioner's guide* (pp. 131–149). New York: Thieme.

Paton, R. N. Sar, B. K. Barber, G., & Holland, B. E. (2001). Working with older persons: Student views and experiences. *Educational Gerontology, 27*, 169–183.

Shadden, B. B., & toner, M. A. (1997). *Aging and communication*. Austin, TX: Pro-Ed.

Uffen, E. (1998). Where the jobs are: Keeping an eye on the future. *ASHA, Winter*, 25–28.

Weinstein, B. E. (2000). *Geriatric audiology*. New York: Thieme.

White, S. C. (2001). Health care legislation, regulation, and financing. In R. Lubinski & C. Frattali (Eds.), *Professional issues in speech-language pathology and audiology* (2nd ed., pp. 213–228). Clifton Park, NY: Delmar Learning.

World Health Organization. (2001). *International classification of functioning, disability and health*. Geneva: Author.

Worrall, L. E. (2000). The influence of professional values on the functional communication approach in aphasia. In L. E. Worrall & C. M. Frattali (Eds.), *Neurogenic communication disorders: a functional approach* (pp. 191–205). New York: Thieme.

Worrall, L., & Hickson, L. (2001). International alliances. In R. Lubinski & C. Frattali (Eds.), *Professional issues in speech-language pathology and audiology* (2nd ed., pp. 77–94). Clifton Park, NY: Delmar Learning.

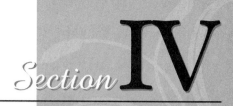

Section **IV**

Appendixes

List of Appendixes

Chapter 5 Appendixes

A Communicative Activities Checklist (COMACT)
B The Hearing Handicap Inventory for the Elderly (HHIE)
C Self-Assessment of Communication (SAC)
D Nursing Home Hearing Handicap Index (NHHI): Self Version for Resident
E The Denver Scale of Communication Function—Modified (DSCF-M)
F Client Oriented Scale of Improvement (COSI)

Chapter 6 Appendixes

A Social Activities Survey (SOCACT)
B Short Form-36v2™ Health Survey (SF-36)
C Rand Social Health Battery
D Medical Outcomes Study (MOS) Social Support Survey
E Ryff's Survey (Condensed) How I Feel About Myself

Chapter 7 Appendixes

A Keep on Talking Module: Communication and Well-Being
B Keep on Talking Module: What is Reading and Writing?
C Keep on Talking Module: Summary Action Plan
D Keep on Talking Module: Social/Communication Activities Table
E Keep on Talking Module: Social/Communication Activities Table
F Keep on Talking Module: Adult Aural Rehabilitation Group Outline
G Keep on Talking Module: Outline of the First Session of the *Active Communication Education* Program
H Keep on Talking Module: Outline of the Module on Conversation in Noise from the *Active Communication Education* Program
I Examples of communicative activities from the Functional Communication Therapy Planner (FCTP)

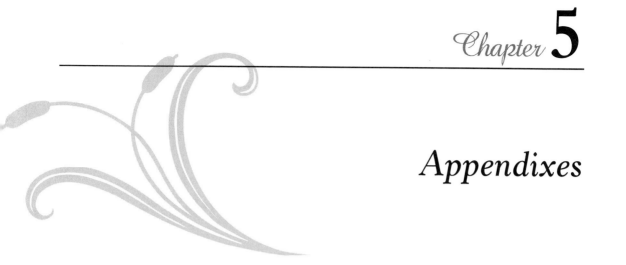

Chapter 5

Appendixes

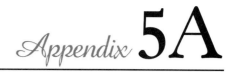

Appendix **5A**

Communicative Activities Checklist (COMACT)

How **OFTEN** do you do these activities? Please select (✓) **ONE** box only per line.

Activity	Daily	Weekly	Every 2 Weeks	Monthly	Rarely	Not at ALL	N/A
Talk to spouse							
Talk to family							
Talk to friends							
Talk to neighbors							
Talk to shopkeepers/tradespeople							
Talk to pets							
Talk on phone							
Talk in a small group of people							
Talk in a large group of people							
Give a speech at an informal group							

continues

Activity	Daily	Weekly	Every 2 Weeks	Monthly	Rarely	Not at all	N/A
Give a speech at a formal group							
Talk about photos							
Tell stories & jokes							
Place bets							
Order drinks							
Say prayers							
Listen to radio							
Listen to TV							
Listen to news							
Listen to sports programs							
Listen to a conversation							
Listen to a group of people talking							
Listen to a speech							
Read letters and cards							
Read mail catalogs							
Read pamphlets							
Read magazines							
Read newspapers							
Read novels/books							
Read the phone book							
Read forms & bills							

Activity	Daily	Weekly	Every 2 Weeks	Monthly	Rarely	Not at ALL	N/A
Read bank statements							
Read newsletters							
Do crosswords							
Read instructions & labels							
Read bus and train timetables							
Read map and directions							
Write letters and cards							
Write stories and newspaper articles							
Write shopping lists							
Write diary							
Write checks							
Fill in forms							
Write messages							
Do word puzzles & games							

Reprinted with permission from Cruice, M. (2001). *The effect of communication on quality of life in older adults with aphasia and healthy older adults*. Unpublished doctoral thesis.

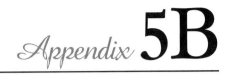

The Hearing Handicap Inventory for the Elderly

Instructions:

The purpose of this scale is to identify the problems your hearing loss may be causing you. Answer YES, SOMETIMES, or NO for each question. *Do not skip a question if you avoid a situation because of your hearing problem*. If you use a hearing aid, please answer the way you hear *without* the aid.

		Yes (4)	Sometimes (2)	No (0)
S–1.	Does a hearing problem cause you to use the phone less often than you would like?	____	____	____
E–2.	Does a hearing problem cause you to feel embarrassed when meeting new people?	____	____	____
S–3.	Does a hearing problem cause you to avoid groups of people?	____	____	____
E–4.	Does a hearing problem make you irritable?	____	____	____
E–5.	Does a hearing problem cause you to feel frustrated when talking to members of your family?	____	____	____
S–6.	Does a hearing problem cause you difficulty when attending a party?	____	____	____

		Yes (4)	Sometimes (2)	No (0)
E–7.	Does a hearing problem cause you to feel "stupid" or "dumb"?	____	____	____
S–8.	Do you have difficulty hearing when someone speaks in a whisper?	____	____	____
E–9.	Do you feel handicapped by a hearing problem?	____	____	____
S–10.	Does a hearing problem cause you difficulty when visiting friends, relatives, or neighbors?	____	____	____
S–11.	Does a hearing problem cause you to attend religious services less often than you would like?	____	____	____
E–12.	Does a hearing problem cause you to be nervous?	____	____	____
S–13.	Does a hearing problem cause you to visit friends, relatives, or neighbors less often than you would like?	____	____	____
E–14.	Does a hearing problem cause you to have arguments with family members?	____	____	____
S–15.	Does a hearing problem cause you difficulty when listening to TV or radio?	____	____	____
S–16.	Does a hearing problem cause you to go shopping less often than you would like?	____	____	____
E–17.	Does any problem or difficulty with your hearing upset you at all?	____	____	____
E–18.	Does a hearing problem cause you to want to be by yourself?	____	____	____
S–19.	Does a hearing problem cause you to talk to family members less often than you would like?	____	____	____
E–20.	Do you feel that any difficulty with your hearing limits or hampers your personal or social life?	____	____	____
S–21.	Does a hearing problem cause you difficulty when in a restaurant with relatives or friends?	____	____	____
E–22.	Does a hearing problem cause you to feel depressed?	____	____	____

continues

		Yes (4)	Sometimes (2)	No (0)
S–23.	Does a hearing problem cause you to listen to TV or radio less often than you would like?	_____	_____	_____
E–24.	Does a hearing problem cause you to feel uncomfortable when talking to friends?	_____	_____	_____
E–25.	Does a hearing problem cause you to feel left out when you are with a group of people?	_____	_____	_____

For Clinician's Use Only: Total Score: _____

Subtotal E: _____

Subtotal S: _____

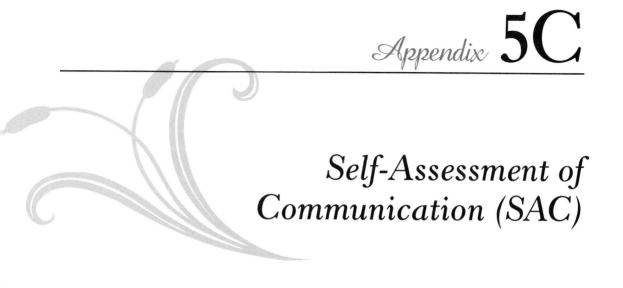

Self-Assessment of Communication (SAC)

Name _____

Date _____ Raw Score ___ × 2 = ___ − 20 ___ = × 1.25 = ___ %

Please select the appropriate number ranging from 1 to 5 for the following questions. Circle only one number for each question. If you have a hearing aid, please fill out the form according to how you communicate when the hearing aid <u>is not</u> in use.

Disability

VARIOUS COMMUNICATION SITUATIONS

1. Do you experience communication difficulties in situations when speaking with one other person? (for example, at home, at work, in a social situation, with a waitress, a store clerk, with a spouse, boss, etc.)

   1) almost never   2) occasionally   3) about half   4) frequently   5) practically
      (or never)   (about 1/4 of   of the time   (about 3/4   always
                        the time)   of the time)   (or always)

2. Do you experience communication difficulties in situations when conversing with a small group of several persons? (for example, with friends or family, co-workers, in meetings or casual conversations, over dinner or while playing cards, etc.)

   1) almost never   2) occasionally   3) about half   4) frequently   5) practically
      (or never)   (about 1/4 of   of the time   (about 3/4   always
                        the time)   of the time)   (or always)

3. Do you experience communication difficulties while listening to someone speak to a large group? (for example, at a church or in a civic meeting, in a fraternal or women's club, at an educational lecture, etc.)

   1) almost never   2) occasionally   3) about half   4) frequently   5) practically
      (or never)   (about 1/4 of   of the time   (about 3/4   always
                        the time)   of the time)   (or always)

continues

4. Do you experience communication difficulties while participating in various types of entertainment? (for example, movies, TV, radio, plays, night clubs, musical entertainment, etc.)

   1) almost never   2) occasionally   3) about half   4) frequently   5) practically
      (or never)   (about 1/4 of   of the time   (about 3/4   always
                         the time)   of the time)   (or always)

5. Do you experience communication difficulties when you are in an unfavorable listening environment? (for example, at a noisy party, where there is background music, when riding in an auto or bus, when someone whispers or talks from across the room, etc.)

   1) almost never   2) occasionally   3) about half   4) frequently   5) practically
      (or never)   (about 1/4 of   of the time   (about 3/4   always
                         the time)   of the time)   (or always)

6. Do you experience communication difficulties when using or listening to various communication devices? (for example, telephone, telephone ring, doorbell, public address system, warning signals, alarms, etc.)

   1) almost never   2) occasionally   3) about half   4) frequently   5) practically
      (or never)   (about 1/4 of   of the time   (about 3/4   always
                         the time)   of the time)   (or always)

Handicap

FEELINGS ABOUT COMMUNICATION

7. Do you feel that any difficulty with your hearing limits or hampers your personal or social life?

   1) almost never   2) occasionally   3) about half   4) frequently   5) practically
      (or never)   (about 1/4 of   of the time   (about 3/4   always
                         the time)   of the time)   (or always)

8. Does any problem or difficulty with your hearing upset you?

   1) almost never   2) occasionally   3) about half   4) frequently   5) practically
      (or never)   (about 1/4 of   of the time   (about 3/4   always
                         the time)   of the time)   (or always)

Handicap

OTHER PEOPLE

9. Do others suggest that you have a hearing problem?

   1) almost never   2) occasionally   3) about half   4) frequently   5) practically
      (or never)   (about 1/4 of   of the time   (about 3/4   always
                         the time)   of the time)   (or always)

10. Do others leave you out of conversations or become annoyed because of your hearing?

1) almost never (or never)	2) occasionally (about 1/4 of the time)	3) about half of the time	4) frequently (about 3/4 of the time)	5) practically always (or always)

Self-Assessment of Communication (SAC). Reproduced with permission from Schow, R. L., & Nerbonne, M. A. (1982). Communication Screening Profile: Use with elderly clients. Ear and Hearing, 3, 135–147.

Nursing Home Hearing Handicap Index (NHHI): Self Version for Resident

		Very Often				Almost Never
1.	When you are with other people do you wish you could hear better?	5	4	3	2	1
2.	Do other people feel you have a hearing problem (when they try to talk to you)?	5	4	3	2	1
3.	Do you have trouble hearing another person if there is a radio or TV playing (in the same room)?	5	4	3	2	1
4.	Do you have trouble hearing the radio or TV?	5	4	3	2	1
5.	(How often) do you feel life would be better if you could hear better?	5	4	3	2	1
6.	How often are you embarrassed because you don't hear well?	5	4	3	2	1
7.	When you are alone do you wish you could hear better?	5	4	3	2	1
8.	Do people (tend to) leave you out of conversations because you don't hear well?	5	4	3	2	1

9. (How often) do you withdraw from social   5   4   3   2   1
activities (in which you ought to
participate) because you don't hear well?

10. Do you say "what" or "pardon me" when   5   4   3   2   1
people first speak to you?

Total _____ × 2 = _____

−20

_____ × 1.25 = _____ %

Nursing Home Hearing Handicap Index (NHHI): Staff Version

	Very Often				Almost Never
1. When this person is with other people does he/she need to hear better?	5	4	3	2	1
2. Do members of the staff, family, and friends make negative comments about this person's hearing problems?	5	4	3	2	1
3. Does this person have trouble hearing another person if there is a radio or TV playing in the same room?	5	4	3	2	1
4. When this person is listening to radio or TV does he/she have trouble hearing?	5	4	3	2	1
5. How often do you feel life would be better for this person if he/she could hear better?	5	4	3	2	1
6. How often is this person embarrassed because he/she doesn't hear well?	5	4	3	2	1
7. When this person is alone does he/she need to hear the everyday sounds of life better?	5	4	3	2	1

continues

8. Do people tend to leave this person out of   5   4   3   2   1
    conversations because he/she doesn't hear
    well?

9. How often does this person withdraw   5   4   3   2   1
    from social activities in which he/she
    ought to participate because he/she
    doesn't hear well?

10. Does this person say "what" or "pardon   5   4   3   2   1
    me" when people first speak to him/her?

Total _____ × 2 = _____

$$-20$$

_____ × 1.25 = _____ %

Nursing Home Hearing Handicap Index (NHHHI): Self Version for Resident, and Nursing Home Hearing Handicap (NHHHI): Staff Version. Reproduced with permission from Schow, R. L., & Nerbonne, M. A. (1977). Assessment of hearing handicaps by nursing home residents and staff. *Journal of the Academy of Rehabilitative Audiology, 10,* 2–12.

The Denver Scale of Communication Function—Modified (DSCF-M)

PRE-THERAPY _____ POST-THERAPY _____

DATE _____

NAME _____ AGE _____ SEX _____

ADDRESS_____

_____

AUDIOGRAM (Examination Date)_____

Pure tone	250	500	1000	2000	4000	8000	Hz
RE	____	____	____	____	____	____	db (re:)
LE	____	____	____	____	____	____	(ANSI)

Speech _____ Discrimination Score (%)

SRT	Quiet	Noise (S/N =)
RE _____ dB	RE _____	_____
LE _____ dB	LE _____	_____

Hearing Aid Information:

Aided _____ For How Long _____ Aid Type _____

Ear _____ Satisfaction _____

Examiner _____

Instructions

I am going to say some statements relating to hearing loss. For each statement, I want you to tell me if you: (1) definitely agree, (2) slightly agree, (3) irrelevant, (4) slightly disagree or (5) definitely disagree. If you consider the statement to be irrelevant or unassociated to your communication problem, please tell me.

SCORING

(1) Definitely agree   (2) Slightly agree   (3) Irrelevant   (4) Slightly Disagree   (5) Definitely disagree

ATTITUDE TOWARD PEERS

1. The people I live with are annoyed by my loss of hearing. Comments:

   _____ 1. Definitely agree

   _____ 2. Slightly agree

   _____ 3. Irrelevant

   _____ 4. Slightly disagree

   _____ 5. Definitely disagree

2. The people I live with sometimes leave me out of conversations or discussions. Comments:

   _____ 1. Definitely agree

   _____ 2. Slightly agree

   _____ 3. Irrelevant

   _____ 4. Slightly disagree

   _____ 5. Definitely disagree

3. Sometimes people I live with make decisions for me because I have a hard time following discussions. Comments:

   _____ 1. Definitely agree

   _____ 2. Slightly agree

   _____ 3. Irrelevant

   _____ 4. Slightly disagree

   _____ 5. Definitely disagree

4. People I live with become annoyed when I ask them to repeat when was said because I did not hear them. Comments:

_____ 1. Definitely agree

_____ 2. Slightly agree

_____ 3. Irrelevant

_____ 4. Slightly disagree

_____ 5. Definitely disagree

5. Other people do not realize how frustrated I get when I cannot hear or understand. Comments:

_____ 1. Definitely agree

_____ 2. Slightly agree

_____ 3. Irrelevant

_____ 4. Slightly disagree

_____ 5. Definitely disagree

6. People sometimes avoid me because of my hearing loss. Comments:

_____ 1. Definitely agree

_____ 2. Slightly agree

_____ 3. Irrelevant

_____ 4. Slightly disagree

_____ 5. Definitely disagree

Socialization

7. I am not an "outgoing" person because I have a hearing loss. Comments:

_____ 1. Definitely agree

_____ 2. Slightly agree

_____ 3. Irrelevant

_____ 4. Slightly disagree

_____ 5. Definitely disagree

continues

8. I now take less of an interest in many things as compared to when I did not have a hearing problem. Comments:

_____ 1. Definitely agree

_____ 2. Slightly agree

_____ 3. Irrelevant

_____ 4. Slightly disagree

_____ 5. Definitely disagree

9. I am not a calm person because of my hearing loss. Comments:

_____ 1. Definitely agree

_____ 2. Slightly agree

_____ 3. Irrelevant

_____ 4. Slightly disagree

_____ 5. Definitely disagree

10. I tend to be negative about life in general because of my hearing loss. Comments:

_____ 1. Definitely agree

_____ 2. Slightly agree

_____ 3. Irrelevant

_____ 4. Slightly disagree

_____ 5. Definitely disagree

11. I do not socialize as much as I did before I began to lose my hearing. Comments:

_____ 1. Definitely agree

_____ 2. Slightly agree

_____ 3. Irrelevant

_____ 4. Slightly disagree

_____ 5. Definitely disagree

12. Since I have trouble hearing, I do not like to participate in activities. Comments:

_____ 1. Definitely agree

_____ 2. Slightly agree

_____ 3. Irrelevant

_____ 4. Slightly disagree

_____ 5. Definitely disagree

13. Since I have trouble hearing, I hesitate to meet new people. Comments:

_____ 1. Definitely agree

_____ 2. Slightly agree

_____ 3. Irrelevant

_____ 4. Slightly disagree

_____ 5. Definitely disagree

14. Other people do not understand what it is like to have a hearing loss. Comments:

_____ 1. Definitely agree

_____ 2. Slightly agree

_____ 3. Irrelevant

_____ 4. Slightly disagree

_____ 5. Definitely disagree

15. I do not feel relaxed or comfortable in a communicative situation. Comments:

_____ 1. Definitely agree

_____ 2. Slightly agree

_____ 3. Irrelevant

_____ 4. Slightly disagree

_____ 5. Definitely disagree

continues

Communication

16. Because I have difficulty understanding what is said to me, I sometimes answer questions wrong. Comments:

_____ 1. Definitely agree

_____ 2. Slightly agree

_____ 3. Irrelevant

_____ 4. Slightly disagree

_____ 5. Definitely disagree

17. Conversations in a noisy room prevent me from attempting to communicate with others. Comments:

_____ 1. Definitely agree

_____ 2. Slightly agree

_____ 3. Irrelevant

_____ 4. Slightly disagree

_____ 5. Definitely disagree

18. I am not comfortable having to communicate in a group situation. Comments:

_____ 1. Definitely agree

_____ 2. Slightly agree

_____ 3. Irrelevant

_____ 4. Slightly disagree

_____ 5. Definitely disagree

19. I seldom watch other peole's facial expressions when talking to them. Comments:

_____ 1. Definitely agree

_____ 2. Slightly agree

_____ 3. Irrelevant

_____ 4. Slightly disagree

_____ 5. Definitely disagree

20. Most people do not know how to talk to a hearing-impaired person. Comments:

_____ 1. Definitely agree

_____ 2. Slightly agree

_____ 3. Irrelevant

_____ 4. Slightly disagree

_____ 5. Definitely disagree

21. I hesitate to ask people to repeat if I do not understand them the first time they speak. Comments:

_____ 1. Definitely agree

_____ 2. Slightly agree

_____ 3. Irrelevant

_____ 4. Slightly disagree

_____ 5. Definitely disagree

22. Because I have difficulty understanding what is said to me, I sometimes make comments that do not fit the conversation. Comments:

_____ 1. Definitely agree

_____ 2. Slightly agree

_____ 3. Irrelevant

_____ 4. Slightly disagree

_____ 5. Definitely disagree

23. I do not like to admit that I have a hearing problem. Comments:

_____ 1. Definitely agree

_____ 2. Slightly agree

_____ 3. Irrelevant

_____ 4. Slightly disagree

_____ 5. Definitely disagree

continues

Specific Difficulty Listening Situations

24. I have trouble hearing the radio or the television unless I turn the volume on very loud. Comments:

_____ 1. Definitely agree

_____ 2. Slightly agree

_____ 3. Irrelevant

_____ 4. Slightly disagree

_____ 5. Definitely disagree

25. If someone calls me when my back is turned, I do not always hear him. Comments:

_____ 1. Definitely agree

_____ 2. Slightly agree

_____ 3. Irrelevant

_____ 4. Slightly disagree

_____ 5. Definitely disagree

26. If someone calls me from another room, I have much trouble hearing. Comments:

_____ 1. Definitely agree

_____ 2. Slightly agree

_____ 3. Irrelevant

_____ 4. Slightly disagree

_____ 5. Definitely disagree

27. When I sit talking with friends in a quiet room, I have a great deal of difficulty hearing. Comments:

_____ 1. Definitely agree

_____ 2. Slightly agree

_____ 3. Irrelevant

_____ 4. Slightly disagree

_____ 5. Definitely disagree

28. When I use the phone, I have much difficulty hearing. Comments:

_____ 1. Definitely agree

_____ 2. Slightly agree

_____ 3. Irrelevant

_____ 4. Slightly disagree

_____ 5. Definitely disagree

29. When I play cards, understanding my partner gives me much difficulty. Comments:

_____ 1. Definitely agree

_____ 2. Slightly agree

_____ 3. Irrelevant

_____ 4. Slightly disagree

_____ 5. Definitely disagree

30. At lectures or discussions I have much difficulty hearing the speaker. Comments:

_____ 1. Definitely agree

_____ 2. Slightly agree

_____ 3. Irrelevant

_____ 4. Slightly disagree

_____ 5. Definitely disagree

31. In church, when the minister gives the sermon, I have much difficulty hearing. Comments:

_____ 1. Definitely agree

_____ 2. Slightly agree

_____ 3. Irrelevant

_____ 4. Slightly disagree

_____ 5. Definitely disagree

continues

32. When a movie is shown, I have much difficulty hearing what is said. Comments:

_____ 1. Definitely agree

_____ 2. Slightly agree

_____ 3. Irrelevant

_____ 4. Slightly disagree

_____ 5. Definitely disagree

33. I have difficulty understanding announcements sent through the loudspeaker even when the speaker is in the same room. Comments:

_____ 1. Definitely agree

_____ 2. Slightly agree

_____ 3. Irrelevant

_____ 4. Slightly disagree

_____ 5. Definitely disagree

34. I have trouble understanding messages sent over the intercom. Comments:

_____ 1. Definitely agree

_____ 2. Slightly agree

_____ 3. Irrelevant

_____ 4. Slightly disagree

_____ 5. Definitely disagree

Denver Scale of Communication Function—Modified. Reproduced with permission from Kaplan, H., Feeley, J., & Brown, J. (1978). A modified Denver Scale: Test-retest reliability. *Journal of the Academy of Rehabilitative Audiology, 11*, 15–32.

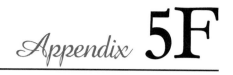

Client Oriented Scale of Improvement

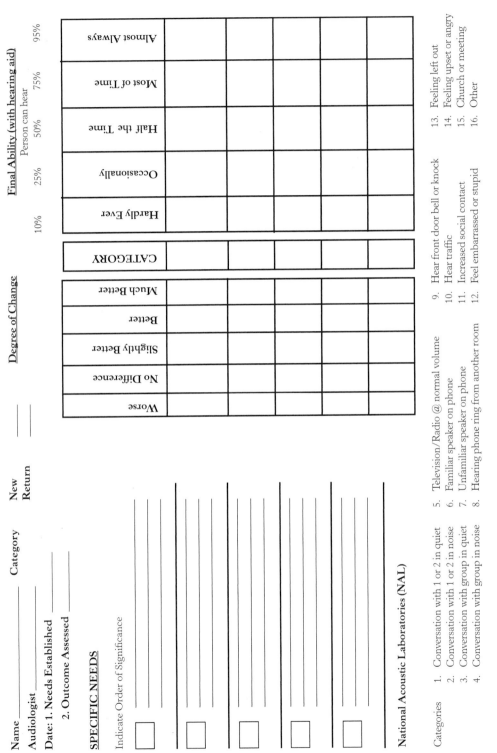

Name _____   Category _____   New ——
Audiologist _____   Return ——

Date: 1. Needs Established _____
2. Outcome Assessed _____

SPECIFIC NEEDS

Indicate Order of Significance

Degree of Change —— ——

Final Ability (with hearing aid)

Person can hear

	Worse	No Difference	Slightly Better	Better	Much Better	CATEGORY	Hardly Ever	Occasionally	Half the Time	Most of Time	Almost Always
							10%	25%	50%	75%	95%

National Acoustic Laboratories (NAL)

Categories

1. Conversation with 1 or 2 in quiet
2. Conversation with 1 or 2 in noise
3. Conversation with group in quiet
4. Conversation with group in noise

5. Television/Radio @ normal volume
6. Familiar speaker on phone
7. Unfamiliar speaker on phone
8. Hearing phone ring from another room

9. Hear front door bell or knock
10. Hear traffic
11. Increased social contact
12. Feel embarrassed or stupid

13. Feeling left out
14. Feeling upset or angry
15. Church or meeting
16. Other

Chapter 5 Appendix F. Client-Oriented Scale of Improvement. Reproduced with permission from Dillon, H., James, A., & Ginis, J. (1997). Client-Oriented Scale of Improvement (COSI) and its relationship to several other measures of benefit and satisfaction provided by hearing aids. *Journal of the American Academy of Audiology*, 8(1), 27–43.

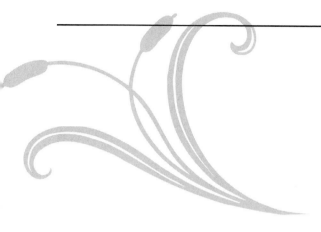

Appendixes

Social Activities Survey

How **OFFEN** do you do these activities? Please select (✔) **ONE** box only per line.

Activity	Weekly	Every 2 Weeks	Monthly	Rarely	Not at ALL	N/A
1. Visit exhibitions, museums, libraries						
2. Go to the movies, theatres, concerts, plays						
3. Go to restaurants						
4. Go shopping						
5. Watch television						
6. Read						
7. Exercise or play sports						
8. Take part in outdoor activities						
9. Travel or go on tours						
10. Play cards or other indoor games						
11. Work on hobbies						

continues

Activity	Weekly	Every 2 Weeks	Monthly	Rarely	Not at ALL	N/A
12. Play with or help children/ grandchildren						
13. Visit or help friends/relatives						
14. Go to family festivities or parties						
15. Go to church events or religious communities events						
16. Go to meetings of community voluntary organizations or charitable societies						
17. Go to professional events or union meetings						
18. Go to classes or lectures						
19. Go to clubs						
20. Go to political activities or occasions						

With **WHOM** do you **usually** do these activities? Please select (✓) **ONE** box only. Leave a blank for those that are not applicable (N/A).

Activity	By self	Spouse	Children	Relatives	Friends
1. visit exhibitions, museums, libraries					
2. Go to the movies, theaters, concerts, plays					
3. Go to restaurants					
4. Go shopping					
5. Watch television					
6. Read					
7. Exercise or play sports					
8. Take part in outdoor activities					
9. Travel or go on tours					
10. Play cards or other indoor games					
11. Work on hobbies					
12. Play with or help children/ grandchildren					
13. Visit or help friends/relatives					
14. Go to family festivities or parties					
15. Go to church events or religious communities events					

continues

Activity	By self	Spouse	Children	Relatives	Friends
16. go to meetings of community voluntary organizations or charitable societies					
17. go to professional events or union meetings					
18. go to classes or lectures					
19. go to clubs					
20. go to political activities or organizations					

Please select (✓) **ONE** only: I am satisfied with the activities I do   ❏

I would like to be doing more activities   ❏

I would like to be doing fewer activities   ❏

Is there anything that limits you in doing these social and recreational activities?

_____

THANK YOU for filling in this form

Social Activities Checklist (SOCACT). Reprinted with permission from Cruice, M. (2001). *The effect of communication on quality of life in older adults with aphasia and healthy older adults.* Unpublished doctoral thesis.

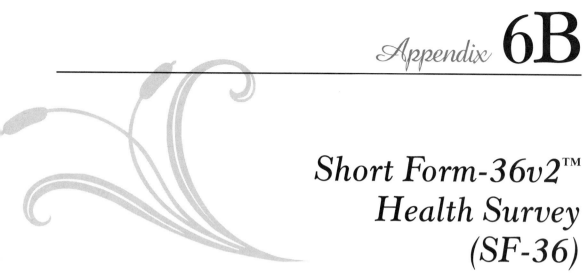

Short Form-36v2™ Health Survey (SF-36)

Instructions for Completing the Questionnaire

Please answer every question. Some questions may look like others, but each one is different. Please take the time to read and answer each question carefully by filling in the box that best represents your response.

EXAMPLE

This is for your review. Do not answer this question. The questionnaire begins with the section **Your Health in General** below.

For each question you will be asked to fill in a box in each line:

1. *How strongly do you agree or disagree with each of the following statements?*

	Strongly agree	Agree	Uncertain	Disagree	Strongly disagree
a) I enjoy listening to music.	❏	❏	❏	❏	❏
b) I enjoy readign magazines.	❏	❏	❏	❏	❏

Please begin answering the questions now.

Your Health in General

1. **In general, would you say your health is:**

Excellent	Very good	Good	Fair	Poor
❏	❏	❏	❏	❏

continues

2. <u>Compared to a year ago</u>, how would you rate your health in general <u>now</u>?

Much better now than one year ago	Somewhat better now than one year ago	About the same as one year ago	Somewhat worse now than one year ago	Much worse now than one year ago

3. The following questions are about activities you might do during a typical day. Does <u>your health now limit you</u> in these activities? If so, how much?

	Yes, limited a lot	Yes, limited a little	No, not limited at all
a) **Vigorous activities**, such as running, lifting heavy objects, participating in strenuous sports	❏	❏	❏
b) **Moderate activities**, such as moving a table, pushing a vacuum cleaner, bowling, or playing golf	❏	❏	❏
c) Lifting or carrying groceries	❏	❏	❏
d) Climbing **several** flights of stairs	❏	❏	❏
e) Climbing **one** flight of stairs	❏	❏	❏
f) Bending, kneeling, or stooping	❏	❏	❏
g) Walking **more than a mile**	❏	❏	❏
h) Walking **several hundred yards**	❏	❏	❏
i) Walking **one hundred yards**	❏	❏	❏
j) Bathing or dressing yourself	❏	❏	❏

4. During the <u>past 4 weeks</u>, how much of the time have you had any of the following problems with your work or other regular daily activities <u>as a result of your physical health</u>?

	All of the time	Most of the time	Some of the time	A little of the time	None of the time
a) Cut down on the **amount of time** you spent on work or other activities	❏	❏	❏	❏	❏
b) **Accomplished less** than you would like	❏	❏	❏	❏	❏

c) Were limited in the **kind** of work or other activities ☐ ☐ ☐ ☐ ☐

d) Had **difficulty** performing the work or other activities (for example, it took extra effort) ☐ ☐ ☐ ☐ ☐

5. During the <u>past 4 weeks</u>, how much of the time have you had any of the following problems with your work or other regular daily activities <u>as a result of any emotional problems</u> (such as feeling depressed or anxious)?

	All of the time	Most of the time	Some of the time	A little of the time	None of the time
a) Cut down on the **amount of time** you spent on work or other activities	☐	☐	☐	☐	☐
b) **Accomplished less** than you would like	☐	☐	☐	☐	☐
c) Did work or other activities **less** carefully than usual	☐	☐	☐	☐	☐

6. During the <u>past 4 weeks</u>, to what extent has your physical health or emotional problems interfered with your normal social activities with family, friends, neighbors, or groups?

Not at all	Slightly	Moderately	Quite a bit	Extremely
☐	☐	☐	☐	☐

7. How much <u>bodily</u> pain have you had during the <u>past 4 weeks</u>?

None	Very mild	Mild	Moderate	Severe	Very severe
☐	☐	☐	☐	☐	☐

8. During the past <u>4 weeks</u>, how much did <u>pain</u> interfere with your normal work (including both work outside the home and housework)?

Not at all	A little bit	Moderately	Quite a bit	Extremely
☐	☐	☐	☐	☐

continues

9. These questions are about how you feel and how things have been with you <u>during the past 4 weeks</u>. For each question, please give the one answer that comes closest to the way you have been feeling. How much of the time during the <u>past 4 weeks</u> . . .

	All of the time	Most of the time	Some of the time	A little of the time	None of the time
a) Did you feel full of life?	❑	❑	❑	❑	❑
b) Have you been very nervous?	❑	❑	❑	❑	❑
c) Have you felt so down in the dumps that nothing could cheer you up?	❑	❑	❑	❑	❑
d) Have you felt calm and peaceful?	❑	❑	❑	❑	❑
e) Did you have a lot of energy?	❑	❑	❑	❑	❑
f) Have you felt downhearted and depressed?	❑	❑	❑	❑	❑
g) Did you feel worn out?	❑	❑	❑	❑	❑
h) Have you been happy?	❑	❑	❑	❑	❑
i) Did you feel tired?	❑	❑	❑	❑	❑

10. During the <u>past 4 weeks</u>, how much of the time has your <u>physical health or emotional problems</u> interfered with your social activities (like visiting friends, relatives, etc.)?

All of the time	Most of the time	Some of the time	A little of the time	None of the time
❑	❑	❑	❑	❑

11. How TRUE or FALSE is <u>each</u> of the following statements for you?

	Definitely true	Mostly true	Don't know	Mostly false	Definitely false
a) I seem to get sick a little easier than other people	❏	❏	❏	❏	❏
b) I am as healthy as anybody I know	❏	❏	❏	❏	❏
c) I expect my health to get worse	❏	❏	❏	❏	❏
d) My health is excellent	❏	❏	❏	❏	❏

THANK YOU FOR COMPLETING THIS QUESTIONNAIRE!

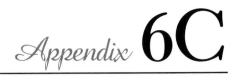

Rand Social Health Battery

Social Activities

1. About how many families in your neighborhood are you well enough aquainted with, that you visit each other in your homes?

   _____ families

2. About how many <u>close</u> friends do you have—people you feel at ease with and can talk with about what is on your mind? (You may include relatives.) (Enter number on line)

   _____ close friends

3. Over a year's time, about how often do you get together with friends or relatives, like going out together or visiting in each other's homes?   (Circle one)

Every day	1
Several days a week	2
About once a week	3
2 or 3 times a month	4
About once a month	5
5 to 10 times a year	6
Less than 5 times a year	7

4. During the <u>past month</u>, about how often have you had friends over to your home? (Do <u>not</u> count relatives.)   (Circle one)

Every day	1
Several days a week	2
About once a week	3
2 or 3 times in past month	4
Once in past month	5
Not at all in past month	6

5. About how often have you visited with friends at their homes during the past month? (Do not count relatives.)   (Circle one)

Every day	1
Several days a week	2
About once a week	3
2 or 3 times in past month	4
Once in past month	5
Not at all in past month	6

6. About how often were you on the telephone with close friends or relatives during the past month?   (Circle one)

Every day	1
Several times a week	2
About once a week	3
2 or 3 times	4
Once	5
Not at all	6

7. About how often did you write a letter to a friend or relative during the past month?   (Circle one)

Every day	1
Several times a week	2
About once a week	3
2 or 3 times in past month	4
Once in past month	5
Not at all in past month	6

8. In general, how well are you getting along with other people these days—would you say better than usual, about the same, or not as well as usual?   (Circle one)

Better than usual	1
About the same	2
Not as well as usual	3

9. How often have you attended a religious service during the past month?   (Circle one)

Every day	1
More than once a week	2
Once a week	3
2 or 3 times in past month	4
Once in past month	5
Not at all in past month	6

continues

10. About how many voluntary groups or organizations do you belong to—like church groups, clubs or lodges, parent groups, etc. ("Voluntary" means because you want to.)

_____ groups or organizations (Write in number. If none, enter "0")

11. How active are you in the affairs of these groups or clubs you belong to? (If you belong to a great many, just count those you feel closest to. If you don't belong to any, circle 4.)   (Circle one)

Very active, attend most meetings	1
Fairly active, attend fairly often	2
Not active, belong but hardly ever go	3
Do not belong to any groups or organizations	4

Rand Social Health Battery. Reprinted with permission from Donald, C. A., & Ware, J. E. (1982). The quantification of social contacts and resources. Santa Monica, CA: Rand Corporation.

Medical Outcomes Study (MOS) Social Support Survey

This brief, self-administered social support survey was developed for patients in the Medical Outcomes Study, a two-year study of patients with chronic conditions. It is easy to administer to chronically ill patients, and the items are short, simple, and easy to understand. It may also be appropriate for use with other populations.

How to score the survey

The survey consists of four separate social support subscales and an overall functional social support index. A higher score for an individual scale or for the overall support index indicates more support.

- To obtain a score for each subscale, calculate the average of the scores for each item in the subscale.

- To obtain an overall support index, calculate the average of (1) the scores for all 18 items included in the four subscales, and (2) the score for the one additional item (see last item in the survey).

- To compare to published means in the article referenced below, scale scores can be transformed to a 0–100 scale using the following formula:

$$100 \times \frac{(\text{observed score} - \text{minimum possible score})}{(\text{maximum possible score} - \text{minimum possible score})}$$

MOS Social Support Survey

People sometimes look to others for companionship, assistance, or other types of support. How often is each of the following kinds of support available to you if you need it? Circle one number on each line.

	None of the time	A little of the time	Some of the time	Most of the time	All of the time
Emotional/informational support					
Someone you can count on to listen to you when you need to talk	1	2	3	4	5
Someone to give you information to help you understand a situation	1	2	3	4	5
Someone to give you good advice about a crisis	1	2	3	4	5
Someone to confide in or talk to about yourself or your problems	1	2	3	4	5
Someone whose advice you really want	1	2	3	4	5
Someone to share your most private worries and fears with	1	2	3	4	5
Someone to turn to for suggestions about how to deal with a personal problem	1	2	3	4	5
Someone who understands your problems	1	2	3	4	5
Tangible support					
Someone to help you if you were confined to bed	1	2	3	4	5
Someone to take you to the doctor if you needed it	1	2	3	4	5

	None of the time	A little of the time	Some of the time	Most of the time	All of the time
Someone to prepare your meals if you were unable to do it yourself	1	2	3	4	5
Someone to help with daily chores if you were sick	1	2	3	4	5

Affectionate support

	None of the time	A little of the time	Some of the time	Most of the time	All of the time
Someone who shows you love and affection	1	2	3	4	5
Someone to love you and make you feel wanted	1	2	3	4	5
Someone who hugs you	1	2	3	4	5

Positive social interaction

	None of the time	A little of the time	Some of the time	Most of the time	All of the time
Someone to have a good time with	1	2	3	4	5
Someone to get together with for relaxation	1	2	3	4	5
Someone to do something enjoyable with	1	2	3	4	5

Additional item

	None of the time	A little of the time	Some of the time	Most of the time	All of the time
Someone to do things with to help you get your mind off things	1	2	3	4	5

Medical Outcomes Study Social Support Survey. Reprinted with permission from Sherbourne, C. D., & Stewart, A. L. (1991). The MOS Social Support Survey. Social Science and Medicine, 32, 705–714. This article is also available as *RAND Reprint 218*.

Ryff's Survey (Condensed) How I Feel About Myself

MY NAME _____ DATE _____

SPOUSE/FAMILY MEMBER NAME _____

This survey is about how you think and feel about your life. Please circle the number that shows how much you agree or disagree.

Circle **ONE** number for each statement.

There are no right or wrong answers.

Example a.   **I feel sad most of the time.**

Strongly disagree   1   2   3   4   5   6   Strongly agree

If you circled # 1, that means you strongly disagree—you are <u>not</u> sad most of the time.

Example b.   **I go out every day.**

Strongly disagree   1   2   3   4   5   6   Strongly agree

If you circled # 3, that means you agree some—you sometimes go out.

---

1. I have confidence in my own opinions, even if they are contrary to the general consensus.

Strongly disagree   1   2   3   4   5   6   Strongly agree

2. The demands of everyday life often get me down.

Strongly disagree   1   2   3   4   5   6   Strongly agree

3. In general, I feel that I continue to learn more about myself as time goes by.

Strongly disagree   1   2   3   4   5   6   Strongly agree

4. Most people see me as loving and affectionate.

Strongly disagree   1   2   3   4   5   6   Strongly agree

5. I have a sense of direction and purpose in life.

Strongly disagree   1   2   3   4   5   6   Strongly agree

6. In general, I feel confident and positive about myself.

Strongly disagree   1   2   3   4   5   6   Strongly agree

7. I tend to worry about what other people think of me.

Strongly disagree   1   2   3   4   5   6   Strongly agree

8. I am quite good at managing the many responsibilities of my daily life.

Strongly disagree   1   2   3   4   5   6   Strongly agree

9. I am the kind of person who likes to give new things a try.

Strongly disagree   1   2   3   4   5   6   Strongly agree

10. Maintaining close relationships has been difficult and frustrating for me.

Strongly disagree   1   2   3   4   5   6   Strongly agree

11. My daily activities often seem trivial and unimportant to me.

Strongly disagree   1   2   3   4   5   6   Strongly agree

12. I like most aspects of my personality.

Strongly disagree   1   2   3   4   5   6   Strongly agree

13. Being happy with myself is more important to me than having others approve of me.

Strongly disagree   1   2   3   4   5   6   Strongly agree

14. I often feel overwhelmed by my responsibilities.

Strongly disagree   1   2   3   4   5   6   Strongly agree

15. I don't want to try new ways of doing things—my life is fine the way it is.

Strongly disagree   1   2   3   4   5   6   Strongly agree

continues

16. I don't have many people who want to listen when I need to talk.

Strongly disagree   1   2   3   4   5   6   Strongly agree

17. I sometimes feel as if I've done all there is to do in life.

Strongly disagree   1   2   3   4   5   6   Strongly agree

18. Given the opportunity, there are many things about myself that I would change.

Strongly disagree   1   2   3   4   5   6   Strongly agree

19. I tend to be influenced by people with strong opinions.

Strongly disagree   1   2   3   4   5   6   Strongly agree

20. In general, I feel I am in charge of the situation in which I live.

Strongly disagree   1   2   3   4   5   6   Strongly agree

21. I gave up trying to make big improvements or changes in my life a long time ago.

Strongly disagree   1   2   3   4   5   6   Strongly agree

22. I feel like I get a lot out of my friendships.

Strongly disagree   1   2   3   4   5   6   Strongly agree

23. I find it satisfying to think about what I have accomplished in life.

Strongly disagree   1   2   3   4   5   6   Strongly agree

24. Everyone has their weaknesses, but I seem to have more than my share.

Strongly disagree   1   2   3   4   5   6   Strongly agree

Ryff's Survey (Condensed) "How I Feel About Myself." Thelander, M., Hoen, B., & Worsley, J. (1994). *York-Durham Aphasia Centre: Report on the evaluation of effectiveness of a community program for aphasic adults.* York-Durham Aphasia Center. Adapted from Ryff, C. D. (1989). Happiness is everything, or is it? Explorations on the meaning of psychological well-being. *Journal of Personality and Social Psychology, 57*(6), 1072.

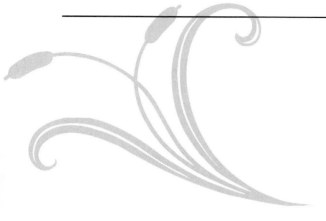

Chapter 7

Appendixes

Keep on Talking Module: Communication and Well-Being

Why is Communication Important?

It is important to communicate so that you can present your point of view, exchange ideas, learn new things, enjoy a joke, etc. Communication is a basic human function and is essential to well being. Perhaps it is easier to understand this if we consider the possible consequences of *NOT* being able to communicate effectively:

- frustration and anger at not being understood
- social isolation
- inability to exercise your rights

Question

Please write down below how you would feel or what you would do if those around you could not understand what you were saying.

_____

_____

_____

_____

An example of a reflective activity from the *Keep on Talking* program. Reproduced with permission from the author.

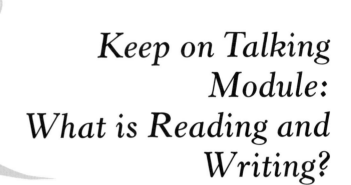

Keep on Talking Module: What is Reading and Writing?

Reading can be divided roughly Into 2 types:

1. **Recreational reading**

   Recreational reading is to do with leisure e.g., reading novels, magazines, newspapers, letters and cards. Reading can be a source of great enjoyment and learning. This can provide ideas for conversation.

2. **Essential reading**

   Essential reading allows us to find out important informtion, e.g., reading forms and bills, product instructions, medicine labels, bus timetables, telephone books, sales material, voting, bargains on "junk" mail.

Therefore reading is part of our everyday life and vital for communication with other people and with organizations. It keeps us in touch with our family, our friends, and our community.

Writing

In the same way, we write for RECREATIONAL reasons: letters, cards, newsletter articles, calligraphy, short stories. And for ESSENTIAL reasons: signing checks, filling out forms, voting, writing a shopping list, taking messages.

Writing, like reading, makes sure that we are active members of our community.

An example of an information handout from the *Keep on Talking* program. Reproduced with permission from the authors.

Keep on Talking Module: Summary Action Plan

How to "Keep on Talking" & Maintain Effective Communication

Please complete these statements so that you can refer to them in the future.

1. If I have problems with my hearing,

I will _____

I will _____

2. If I have problems with reading,

I will _____

I will _____

3. I have problems with writing,

I will _____

I will _____

4. If I have problems with my memory,

I will _____

I will _____

Keep on Talking Module: Social/Communication Activities Table

20 ___

What was I doing this time last year?	What am I doing now?	If there has been a change, why?	What can I do about this?
Social, Communication Activities:			
Reading, Writing Activities:			

Social/Communication activities table from the *Keep on Talking* program. Reproduced with permission of the authors.

Keep on Talking Module: Social/Communication Activities Table

Example

What was I doing this time last year?	What am I doing now?	If there has been a change, why?	What can I do about this?
Social, Communication Activities:			
■ attending Senior Citizens Club	■ staying home	■ poor health	■ finding a friend to go with
■ bowling	■ staying home	■ broken hip	■ join elderly fitness group
■ going to the movies	■ staying home	■ problems with hearing	■ go to Better Hearing Center
Reading Writing Activities:			
■ writing letters to relatives every 2 weeks	■ only writing Christmas cards	■ difficulty holding the pen	■ go to the Independent Living Center
■ reading novels and newspapers	■ only reading newspaper headlines	■ difficulty with glasses	■ have vision tested

Example of a completed Social/Communication activities table from the *Keep on Talking* program. Reproduced with permission of the authors.

Adult Aural Rehabilitation Group Outline

Outline handed to members of adult aural rehabilitation group. This group meets for 2 hours each week for 6 weeks.

SESSION ONE

1. INTRODUCTIONS, ORIENTATION
2. Discussion of what to expect from the group, what situations are difficult: development of list of individual problem areas
3. Presentation of information on hearing and causes of hearing loss

HANDOUTS: Note books, diagrams of the ear, list of purposes of the group
OUTSIDE WORK: Begin list of difficult situations

SESSION TWO

1. Discussion of difficult situations, introduction of Communication Profile for the Hearing Impaired (CPHI)
2. Presentation of information on the audiogram
3. Performance of brief speechreading test, discussion of speechreading

OUTSIDE WORK: Start on CPHI, speechreading assignment

SESSION THREE

1. Discussion of CPHI, discussion of speechreading assignment
2. Demonstration, pep talk on maximizing the chances for speechreading
3. Presentation of information on hearing aids

OUTSIDE WORK: Assertive speechreading assignment

SESSION FOUR

1. CPHI inventory due
2. Discussion of speechreading assignment, situation analysis

3. Videotape demonstration

4. More information on hearing aids

OUTSIDE WORK: Analyze two situations that you encounter in everyday living

SESSION FIVE

1. Conversation repair, demonstration, and practice

2. Discussion of CPHI inventory results, individual counseling

3. Presentation of information and demonstration of assistive listening devices

HANDOUT: List of assistive listening devices and addresses of suppliers

SUGGESTION: Attend a concert at the Koger Center; use their excellent infrared listening system

SESSION SIX

1. Review of specific strategies for difficult listening situations

2. Speechreading practice, situation management

3. Course evaluation: "Y'all tell us what you think"

4. Wrap-up

Reproduced with permission from the publisher. Montgomery, A., and Houston, K. T. (2000). The hearing-impaired adult: Management of communication deficits and tinnitus. In Alpiner, J. G., & McCarthy, P. A. (Eds.), (2000). Rehabilitative audiology: Children and adults (3rd Ed., p. 397). Baltimore: Lippincott, Williams and Wilkins.

Outline of the First Session of the Active Communication Education *Program*

The objectives of the session:

- ■ To welcome group members and enable them to get acquainted with the other people in the group.

- ■ To obtain personal details and preprogram measures of hearing activity limitations and participation restrictions, quality of life, and communicative function.

- ■ To explore the communication difficulties that the participants experience in everyday life.

- ■ To identify and prioritize their communication needs so that these can be the focus of the remaining sessions.

- ■ For participants to understand the aims of the program.

Materials: Folders for members to carry handouts; Handouts—chronicle homework sheet; whiteboard or butcher paper; whiteboard marker pen; pencils or pens; post-it stickers; name tag labels; tea and coffee

Introduction and Welcome to the Group (15 minutes)

Facilitators introduce themselves and describe the program, its aims, and how it will run. Each participant is invited to say who he or she is, what he or she has done in the past about hearing problems, why he or she has come along.

Communication Needs Analysis (20 minutes)

Ask the group to brainstorm about the questions:

What communication difficulties do you have in everyday life?

What activities do you have difficulty participating in because of your hearing loss?

Go around the group asking the participants to give **one difficulty at a time** until all possibilities are exhausted. It is important to keep this activity moving and not allow participants to discuss difficulties in depth at this stage.

List all difficulties on the whiteboard and link any that are similar.

Nominal Group Technique (15 minutes)

To prioritize the most important communication difficulties. Each participant is given 3 post-it stickers labeled 1, 2, and 3, and he or she is to come to the board and put a sticker next to the most important (label 1) and next to the least important (label 3).

Tea or coffee break (15 minutes)

Problem-Solving Process (40 minutes)

Take the top priority item and introduce the problem-solving process that will be applied. Steps in the process are:

- What is involved in the communication activity? Who, what, when, where, why?
- What are the sources of difficulty in the activity?
- What are some possible solutions?
- What information is necessary to apply the solutions?
- What practical skills are necessary to apply the solutions?
- How can you test the solutions?

Conclusion (15 minutes)

Discuss the modules that will be covered in the following sessions and give the participants the chronicle homework sheet.

Homework Activity: A Personal Chronicle of Hearing Loss

The aim of this task is for you to document how hearing loss has affected you and how you have coped with it. The chronicle can be either a page or a book! We suggest that you write your chronicle under the following headings:

■ When did you first start noticing your hearing loss? What impact has it had on you over the years? What does your family say about your hearing loss? How do you feel about your hearing loss?

■ How well do you think you have coped with the changes associated with hearing loss? How have you adapted to your hearing loss? Have you developed any strategies over the years? What strategies have worked? Have any not worked?

■ Describe an incident when you used a strategy that worked, then describe an incident that did not work.

■ If you had some advice to give to someone who also has a hearing loss, what would it be?

■ How do you describe yourself now? How do other people describe you? Have you changed over the years?

Outline of the Module on Conversation in Noise from the Active Communication Education Program

The objectives of the session:

- To work through the problem-solving process as applied to an example situation of conversation in noise.

- To identify component skills necessary for better communication in noise.

- To practice the component skills of requesting clarification

- To work through the problem-solving process as applied to a situation unique to each participant.

- **Materials:** Handouts: pages 106 to 117, Erber (1996); copies of the Wilson, Hickson, and Worrall (1998) article; whiteboard or butcher paper; whiteboard marker pen; pencils or pens; blank sheets of paper, name tag labels, tea and coffee

Introduction (15 minutes)

Ask the clients to complete a feedback form for the last session.

Discuss homework activities.

Write agenda for this session on the whiteboard.

Example of a Noisy Situation (30 minutes)

Ask each individual to look at the conversation in noise activity sheet and suggest ways to improve his or her ability to communicate in that setting.

continues

List on the board all the ideas participants have to improve the listening environment and optimize their chances of communicating well in that situation.

Present the key points in the Erber (1996) handout.

Identify necessary component skills (15 minutes)

After making the modifications to the environment to optimize their chances of communicating well in that situation, breakdowns in communication still occur. Ask the group to think of ways to repair these communication breakdowns.

Discuss the need to practice these repair strategies, as research has shown that there is a difference between what people say they will do and what they actually do.

Present the key points in the Wilson, Hickson, and Worrall (1998) handout.

Tea or coffee break (15 minutes)

Practice clarification skills (20 minutes)

Divide the group into two and use sentences from Exercise 9, page 84 (Kaplan, Bally, & Garretson, 1995). Ask participants what they would do in each of the situations. For example, the receptionist at your hearing aid dealer tells you, "Your appointment will be next Thursday at ? in the afternoon." You do not hear the time. What would you do?

Discussion of Individual Noisy Situations (15 minutes)

Have each group member draw a noisy situation that regularly presents him or her with difficulties in communication.

Work through the problem-solving process from Session 1 and ask group members to consider ways to repair likely breakdowns in communication.

Conclusion of Session and Discussion of the Next Module (10 minutes)

Examples of communicative activities from the Fuctional Communication Therapy Planner (FCTP)

Client: _____

Interviewer: _____

Date of interview _____

Others present at interview _____

Social interaction	Importance
Uses greetings	
Introduces others	
Maintains topic	
Requests actions or objects	
Answers questions	
Indicates emotions	
Relates stories or jokes	
Provides instructions	
Gives messages	
Initiates conversation	
Asks questions	
Seeks clarification	
Expresses opinion	
Responds to others' nonverbal behavior	

Managing finances	Importance
Checking and paying bills	
Writing checks	
Reading bank statements	
Paying rent/mortgage	
Reading financial literature	
Filling in forms	
Using cash	
Using a credit card	
Using an automatic teller machine/cash point	

Using the telephone	Importance
Looking up numbers in the telephone directory	
Dialing an emergency number	
Taking telephone messages	
Making appointments	
Making business calls	
Making social calls	

Preparing food	Importance
Reading labels on food packets	
Selecting and measuring ingredients	
Reading sell by/use by dates and calculating freshness	
Following recipes	
Using the microwave and oven	

Examples of communicative activities from the Functional Communication Therapy Planner (Worrall, 1999). Reproduced with permission from Worrall, L. (1999). *Functional Communication Therapy Planner*. Oxon, UK: Winslow Press, B2–B3.

Index

Note: Boldface numbers indicate illustrations.